Neurofibromatosis

Neurofibromatosis

Guest Editors

Rianne Oostenbrink
Ignacio Blanco
Enrico Opocher

MDPI

Basel • Beijing • Wuhan • Barcelona • Belgrade • Novi Sad • Cluj • Manchester

Guest Editors
Rianne Oostenbrink
Department of General Pediatrics
Erasmus MC
Rotterdam
The Netherlands

Ignacio Blanco
Metropolitana Nord Laboratory
Germans Trias i Pujol University Hospital
Badalona
Spain

Enrico Opocher
Pediatric Hematology, Oncology and Stem Cell Transplant Division
Padua University Hospital
Padua
Italy

Editorial Office
MDPI AG
Grosspeteranlage 5
4052 Basel, Switzerland

This is a reprint of the Special Issue, published open access by the journal *Cancers* (ISSN 2072-6694), freely accessible at: https://www.mdpi.com/journal/cancers/special_issues/NW96RVS221.

For citation purposes, cite each article independently as indicated on the article page online and as indicated below:

Lastname, A.A.; Lastname, B.B. Article Title. *Journal Name* **Year**, *Volume Number*, Page Range.

ISBN 978-3-7258-7198-8 (Hbk)
ISBN 978-3-7258-7199-5 (PDF)
https://doi.org/10.3390/books978-3-7258-7199-5

Cover image courtesy of Ignacio Blanco

Contents

About the Editors

Rianne Oostenbrink

Rianne Oostenbrink, MD, PhD, is Associate Professor at the Department of General Pediatrics, ErasmusMC—University Hospital, Rotterdam, The Netherlands. She is coordinating the national expertise center for Neurofibromatosis Type 1 at the Erasmus MC, which is embedded in the ENCORE (ErasmusMC Neurocognitive Research) Group. She is leading the national NF1 clinical network in the Netherlands. Further, she works as general pediatrician at the Department of General Pediatrics, ErasmusMC—Sophia Children's Hospital. As a clinical epidemiologist and clinical scientist, her research areas of interest are quality of life and neurocognitive problems in children with NF1, trial development in NF1, patient-shared decision making, and the development of prediction tools for both clinicians and parents. She has contributed to the EU-PEARL project as WP leader to develop platform trials in NF (EU patient-centric clinical trial platforms, IMI2-RIA project). She has performed international collaboration through the European Reference Network GENTURIS, European Neurofibromatosis Group (ENFG), CCAB of CTF-Europe.

Ignacio Blanco

Ignacio Blanco, MD, PhD, earned his medical degree and doctorate from the Autonomous University of Barcelona. He is a specialist in General and Digestive Surgery and is accredited in Human Genetics by the Spanish Association of Human Genetics. He is Clinical Director of the Clinical Laboratory Metropolitana Norte and Head of the Genetics Service at Hospital Germans Trias i Pujol. He coordinates the National Reference Centre (CSUR) for adult patients with phacomatoses and serves as the national lead for the European Reference Network GENTURIS on tumur predisposition. He is a member of the Advisory Committee for the Common Portfolio of Services in Genetics at the Spanish Ministry of Health and of the Advisory Commission on Rare Diseases of the Catalan Department of Health. His clinical work focuses on the diagnosis and follow up of individuals and families with genetic disorders, with special emphasis on neurofibromatoses and schwannomatosis. He leads competitive national and international research projects. He is an Associate Professor at the Autonomous University of Barcelona and the School of Health Sciences, TecnoCampus.

Enrico Opocher

Enrico Opocher is a Pediatric Oncologist from Italy, with a special interest in treating infants, children and young adults with solid and central nervous system neoplasms, including NF-1-associated LGG and plexiform neurofibroma. He has been trained between Padova, France and UK and now member of the ENFG group and within the scientific board of NF-1 lay groups and scientific societies such as SIOP Europe and SIOP—Brain Tumor Group. He has been collaborating with experts from many countries in establishing a more robust and standardized functional assessment and outcomes in children with NF1-optic pathway glioma, aiming at identifying sight-saving treatments to implement in prospective clinical trials.

Preface

In this Special Issue Reprint in *Cancers*, we have collected original research articles and comprehensive review articles focusing on the disease course, disease modifiers, and treatments of tumors in patients with neurofibromatosis type 1, NF2-related schwannomatosis, and non-NF2-related schwannomatosis.

Neurofibromatosis type 1 (NF1), NF2-related schwannomatosis (NF2), and non-NF2-related schwannomatosis (SWN) are rare genetic disorders predisposing to the development of various tumors of the central and peripheral nervous systems. Although often benign, these neoplasms can still cause significant morbidity due to their size and/or location and are rarely amenable to surgical resection.

It is therefore essential to translate pre-clinical advances into more effective treatment options for many of these tumors, as can be found in the paper of Pei-Yu Hung et al. In the discussion on how to position these treatments, Santelangelo et al contribute to understanding the natural course. Disease modifiers are discussed by Douwes et al, and biomarkers are discussed by Busciglio et al. and Iasella et al present the potential effects of monitoring patients, although different perspectives remain in Europe, as discussed by Taal et al. The papers of Curlee et al., Tops et al., Douwes et al. and Mladenov et al. discuss the challenges of treatment for NF1- and NF2-related Schwannomatosis, and their efficacy and toxicity.

As Editors, we hope that this Special Issue Reprint provides readers with an insight into the significant advancements made in the challenging, yet fascinating, field of neurofibromatosis.

Rianne Oostenbrink, Ignacio Blanco, and Enrico Opocher
Guest Editors

cancers

MDPI

Review

The Pathogenesis of the Neurofibroma-to-Sarcoma Transition in Neurofibromatosis Type I: From Molecular Profiles to Diagnostic Applications

Sabrina Busciglio [1,†], Ilenia Rita Cannizzaro [1,†], Anita Luberto [1], Antonietta Taiani [1], Barbara Moschella [1], Enrico Ambrosini [2], Sofia Cesarini [1], Mirko Treccani [3], Cinzia Azzoni [4], Lorena Bottarelli [4], Domenico Corradi [4], Vera Uliana [2], Davide Martorana [2], Valeria Barili [1,*] and Antonio Percesepe [1,2]

1 Medical Genetics, Department of Medicine and Surgery, University of Parma, 43126 Parma, Italy
2 Medical Genetics, University Hospital of Parma, 43126 Parma, Italy
3 Department of Food and Drug, University of Parma, 43126 Parma, Italy
4 Pathology Unit, Department of Medicine and Surgery, University of Parma, 43126 Parma, Italy
* Correspondence: valeria.barili@unipr.it
† These authors contributed equally to this work.

Simple Summary

Patients with Neurofibromatosis type 1 can develop different types of nerve sheath tumors, though only a small fraction become malignant. Distinguishing benign plexiform neurofibromas from early signs of malignant transformation remains challenging using imaging or clinical symptoms alone. This review examines the molecular evolution of these tumors, describing the key genetic and epigenetic changes that drive the transition from benign lesions to malignant peripheral nerve sheath tumors (MPNST). By integrating evidence from multiple "omics" studies, we highlight the biological hallmarks of each stage of progression and explore emerging biomarkers that may help to identify patients at higher risk. We also discuss new liquid biopsy approaches, which analyze tumor-derived DNA fragments circulating in the blood and may allow earlier detection of malignant transformation. Understanding these mechanisms can improve surveillance strategies and support more personalized care for patientswith NF1.

Abstract

Neurofibromatosis type 1 (NF1) predisposes to a spectrum of peripheral nerve sheath tumors, ranging from benign plexiform neurofibromas (PN) to atypical neurofibromatous neoplasms of uncertain biological potential (ANNUBP) and malignant peripheral nerve sheath tumors (MPNST). Tumorigenesis follows a multistep molecular cascade initiated by biallelic *NF1* inactivation, followed by *CDKN2A* loss and disruption of the Polycomb Repressive Complex 2 (PRC2). These events guide chromatin remodeling, widespread epigenetic dysregulation, and activation of oncogenic pathways such as RAS/MAPK and PI3K/AKT. Here, we integrate genomic, transcriptomic, and epigenomic studies to delineate the molecular trajectories underlying tumor progression and to define promising biomarkers for the early detection of malignant transformation. Emerging liquid biopsy approaches, based on circulating tumor DNA (ctDNA) analyses, reveal distinctive copy number variations (CNVs) and methylation patterns that mirror tissue-derived profiles, enabling the detection of malignant transformation. Together, these findings support a model in which cumulative genetic and epigenetic alterations drive the PN–ANNUBP–MPNST continuum. They also underscore the value of multi-omics and liquid biopsy-based strategies to improve early diagnosis, patient risk stratification, and personalized management of NF1-associated tumors, thereby advancing precision medicine in this complex disease spectrum.

Keywords: Neurofibromatosis type 1; malignant peripheral nerve sheath tumors; liquid biopsy; genomic profiling; epigenetic dysregulation; omics analysis

1. Introduction

Neurofibromatosis type 1 (NF1) is a common autosomal dominant genetic disorder, affecting approximately 1 in 2500–3000 individuals worldwide. It is caused by pathogenic variants in the *NF1* gene located on chromosome 17q11.2 [1,2].

Diagnostic hallmarks include benign neurofibromas, which can be cutaneous, subcutaneous, or plexiform (PN), carrying a significant risk of malignant transformation [3]. Among the most life-threatening complications is the development of malignant peripheral nerve sheath tumors (MPNSTs), which occur in approximately 8–13% of individuals with NF1 and represent a major cause of NF1-related mortality [4].

The tumor progression of PN leads to the MPNST development, which is a soft-tissue sarcoma characterized by high recurrence (30–70%) after resection and resistance to chemotherapy [5]. Beyond neural manifestations, NF1 is a multisystem disorder involving skeletal, cardiovascular, and endocrine systems and is associated with an increased risk of other malignancies [6]. Thus, the NF1 clinical spectrum encompasses benign, intermediate, and malignant lesions, reflecting a multistep neoplastic process driven by sequential genetic and epigenetic events.

2. Molecular Pathogenesis and Genetic Drivers of NF1-Related Tumors

2.1. NF1 Loss and the Initiation of Plexiform Neurofibroma (PN)

Approximately half of individuals with NF1 develop PNs, which are benign, often congenital nerve sheath tumors. These tumors arise from multiple deep nerve fascicles and their branches and are characterized by a tortuous, infiltrative growth pattern that extends along the length of a nerve and into surrounding tissues. Histologically, PNs display distinctive features, such as coarse collagen bundles interspersed with loosely arranged, haphazard spindle cells with ill-defined cytoplasmic borders and an absence of degeneration or necrosis, that clearly differentiate them from MPNST. Mitotic figures are rare, usually fewer than 1 per 50 high-power fields (HPF which corresponds to 0.2 mm^2). The tumor is composed predominantly of wavy Schwann cells (S100-positive), interlaced with a lattice-like network of fibroblasts (CD34-positive) and scattered degranulated mast cells. The nuclei of neurofibroma cells are characteristically comma-shaped, and only a small fraction (<2–5%) of cells show Ki-67 immunoreactivity, reflecting the low proliferative index of these lesions [7].

Bi-allelic inactivation in the *NF1* gene is the initiating event in neurofibroma formation [8–10] and a crucial precursor to malignancy, especially in NF1-associated MPNSTs [11,12]. The *NF1* gene encodes neurofibromin, a protein that acts as a negative regulator of RAS (Rat sarcoma virus) signaling. Neurofibromin contains a GTPase-activating protein (GAP)-related domain of approximately 300 amino acids, which stimulates the intrinsic GTPase activity of RAS, accelerating the conversion of active RAS-GTP to its inactive RAS-GDP state. Given the central role of RAS in cell cycle regulation and tissue growth, most studies have focused on its RAS-GAP function. Through this mechanism, neurofibromin negatively impacts several downstream proteins, including RAS–MEK–ERK (MAPK), RAS–AKT–mTOR, and RAS–Rac1 pathways [13].

Although individuals with NF1 inherit a germline variant in one *NF1* allele, a single mutated copy is insufficient for tumor formation. Rather, loss-of-function (LOF) mutations and complete absence of neurofibromin expression are necessary for the development of benign and malignant tumors [13]. This leads to continuous RAS signaling, which promotes cell proliferation via the MAPK cascade, and enhances cell survival by inhibiting apoptosis through the PI3K/AKT/mTOR pathway. Somatic loss of heterozygosity (LOH), for instance, represents a common mechanism of LOF of the remaining wild type allele in somatic cells such as Schwann cells, which give rise to neurofibromas [14,15]. LOH may arise in somatic cells through a number of mechanisms, including deletions, whole chromosome loss due to nondisjunction with or without re-duplication. However, mitotic recombination has been shown to be the most frequent common event accounting for LOH in NF1-associated tumors [15].

The constitutive RAS hyperactivation associated with biallelic *NF1* inactivation has been documented in both human and murine NF1-associated tumors [13]. The best-characterized downstream effector is the MAPK pathway: increased RAS-GTP activates RAF kinase, which sequentially phosphorylates MEK and ERK1/2 kinases, resulting in transcriptional activation of genes that promote cell proliferation and differentiation [16]. Dysregulation of this pathway is observed in the majority of MPNSTs, and BRAF mutations or amplifications, which can also activate ERK signaling, are particularly common in sporadic MPNST [17].

Another major RAS effector branch is the PI3K/AKT/mTOR pathway. Neurofibromin loss enhances PI3K and AKT activity, leading to phosphorylation and inactivation of the tuberin (TSC2) protein and consequent constitutive mTOR activation [16]. This axis supports cell survival, growth, and metabolism. Both mTORC1 and mTORC2 contribute to NF1 tumorigenesis, and pathway hyperactivation is consistently detected in NF1-deficient cells and tumors.

Together, these findings define *NF1* loss as the initiating molecular event that drives RAS pathway hyperactivation, laying the basis for benign PN formation and subsequent progression toward malignant transformation in NF1-associated tumors.

2.2. Key Cooperating Alterations in Progression to ANNUBP and Malignancy to MPNST

Patients with NF1-associated MPNST have lower survival rates and greater resistance to therapy compared to those with sporadic MPNST. However, complete resection of premalignant lesions can significantly reduce mortality and recurrence, highlighting the importance of early diagnosis and surgical excision of precursor lesions before tumors progress to high-grade or metastatic disease. There are dramatic histological alterations that distinguish PN from MPNST. Indeed, MPNSTs exhibit striking cytologic atypia, with cells showing nuclear enlargement, pleomorphism, and loss of characteristic neurofibromatous architecture. Instead, they form intersecting fascicles arranged in herringbone or storiform patterns. Mitotic activity is markedly increased (>10 mitoses per 10 HPF). While some regions may show more uniform, spindle-shaped cells, areas of perivascular hypercellularity and focal necrosis are common [18].

Interestingly, an intermediate stage between PN and MPNST, now classified as an atypical neurofibromatous neoplasm of uncertain biological potential (ANNUBP), may represent a pre-malignant step in the pathological continuum of malignant transformation [19]. ANNUBPs feature hyperchromatic nuclei, increased cellularity, and disruption of the typical neurofibroma architecture, sometimes with herringbone or storiform fascicular growth pattern, but lack necrosis. The ANNUBPs are histologically intermediate lesions that display increased cellularity, nuclear atypia, and low mitotic activity (>1 per 50 HPF but <3 per 10 HPF), without infiltrative growth. They often arise within pre-existing PNs and may show heterogeneous or reduced expression of Schwann-cell lineage markers (S100, SOX10), as well as loss of p16 immunoreactivity indicative of *CDKN2A* (Cyclin-dependent kinase inhibitor 2A) deletion or inactivation. These features support their classification as lesions at risk for malignant progression rather than overt sarcoma [20].

At the molecular level, the histological emergence of ANNUBPs marks a transition toward genomic instability, with recurrent *CDKN2A* (9p21) deletions frequently appearing early, often preceding clear definitive malignancy [21,22].

In contrast, high-grade MPNSTs display profound chromosomal instability, genome-wide CNVs, aneuploidy, and epigenetic deregulation [23–25]. Moreover, several studies in MPNST showed the inactivation of other additional tumor suppressor genes such as *RB1* (Retinoblastoma 1), *TP53* (Tumor protein p53), and *PTEN* (Phosphatase and Tensin homolog) in both NF1-associated and sporadic MPNSTs, highlighting a driving role of mutations in these genes in tumor malignancy [23].

Additionally, in malignant progression additional cooperating alterations amplify tumorigenic signaling such as the loss in the Polycomb Repressive Complex 2 (PRC2) which results in global depletion of the repressive histone mark H3K27me3 (trimethylation of lysine 27 on histone H3), enhancer reprogramming, and dedifferentiation of Schwann cells into invasive, therapy-resistant states, promoting malignant transformation [26].

From a diagnostic standpoint, taken together biallelic *NF1* loss and *CDKN2A/B* define the ANNUBP state, while PRC2 loss (±*TP53*) with widespread CNVs and other pathway rewiring (RTKs, WNT/HIPPO, and PI3K–mTOR) marks the malignant conversion to MPNST. Overall, this progression represents a stepwise molecular continuum driven by cumulative genetic, epigenetic, and microenvironmental alterations. Figure 1 schematically summarizes these events, illustrating the transition from PN to ANNUBP and finally to MPNST, along with the predominant pathways and cellular mechanisms involved. Regardless, there must be multiple genomic alterations before neurofibromas transform into malignant tumors; how molecular changes may drive the process of tumor deterioration is not fully clarified.

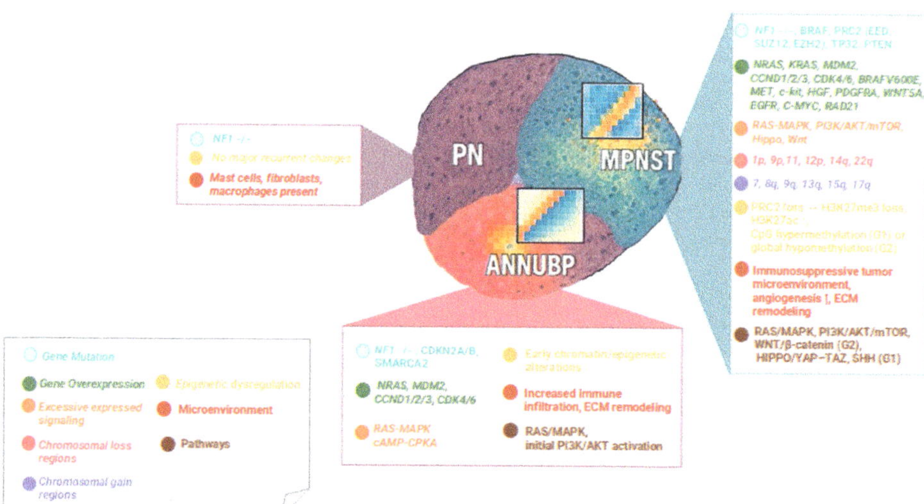

Figure 1. Molecular transition of PN–ANNUBP–MPNST in NF1-related tumors.

Stepwise model of tumor progression in NF1 associated peripheral nerve sheath tumors (PNSTs), showing the transition from plexiform neurofibroma (PN) to atypical neurofibromatous neoplasm of uncertain biological potential (ANNUBP) and malignant peripheral nerve sheath tumor (MPNST). Each stage displays progressive alterations. Color-coded boxes summarize the predominant alterations observed at each stage.

Symbol explanation:

The horizontal connector (→) indicates a sequential progression from one molecular alteration to the next within the same stage.

The upward arrow (↑) indicates an increased level or upregulation of the associated biological process or signaling pathway.

3. Omics Insights in NF1-Associated Tumors

3.1. Genomic Landscape and Evolution to MPNST

Whole exome sequencing (WES) and whole genome sequencing (WGS) have significantly advanced the understanding of cancer genomics and have been widely used to identify the characteristic mutational patterns of MPNSTs. Although the first studies on MPNST genomic landscape have been conducted in relatively small patients' cohorts, they allowed the detection of recurrent molecular events common to MPNSTs, without identifying uniform molecular markers for all tumors belonging to this specific histological group [27]. This gap largely stems from the low incidence of MPNST, which limits the availability of sufficient tumor samples for detailed investigation. These challenges led to the creation of the international consortiums such as the Genomics of MPNST (GeM), that aims at performing multi-omic analysis on MPNST samples to better clarify the time sequence and nature of genetic events associated with cancer onset and progression [27].

Although no recurrent genetic alterations have been detected in benign neurofibromas, except for the *NF1* gene variants, MPNST displays a diverse mutational spectrum including multiple gene mutations and DNA fragment deletions or duplications. As mentioned above other than *NF1* biallelic mutations, several other tumor suppressor genes have been detected as altered in MPNST tumors also in sporadic form, such as *CDKN2A*, *RB1*, *TP53*, and *PTEN*. Early inactivation of both *CDKN2A* copies appears to be a necessary condition for the formation of ANNUBP, as initially demonstrated by Beert et al. and later confirmed by Carrió et al. [28–31].

Several studies have shown that *RB1* loss is a central event driving uncontrolled Schwann cell proliferation and MPNST development. Under physiological conditions, RB1 restrains the G1/S transition by binding and inhibiting E2F transcription factors, thereby enforcing cell-cycle arrest and senescence. In Schwann cells, this RB1-dependent checkpoint is particularly important, as it prevents hyperproliferation of PNs and acts as a barrier to malignant progression [32,33].

In MPNSTs, the RB1 inactivation removes this checkpoint entirely, allowing continuous E2F activity, uncontrolled cell-cycle entry, and tumor growth. Importantly, the oncogenic driver *RABL6A*, which is highly expressed in MPNSTs, promotes tumorigenesis precisely by antagonizing the RB1 pathway, accelerating RB1 inactivation and thereby enabling persistent proliferation [32,33].

Moreover, the status of RB1 critically influences the efficacy of CDK4/6 inhibitors. These inhibitors function by preventing RB1 phosphorylation, thus keeping RB1 in its active, growth-suppressive form. Consequently, their efficacy depends on the presence of functional RB1. Tumors with complete RB1 loss are typically resistant to CDK4/6 blockade. However, in MPNSTs driven by RABL6A-mediated RB1 suppression, RB1 is not completely deleted; instead, its pathway is inhibited but not absent, which creates a therapeutic vulnerability. In this context, CDK4/6 inhibitors can restore RB1 activity, re-establishing cell-cycle arrest and reducing tumor growth, as demonstrated in RB1-dependent MPNST models [32].

Other alterations have been detected in the PTEN protein, a phosphatase responsible for inhibition of the PI3K/AKT signaling pathway. Indeed, *PTEN* mutations or loss led to hyperactivation of the PI3K/AKT pathway, promoting the survival and proliferation of MPNST cells [34]. Additionally, *PTEN* downregulation has been detected through promoter methylation to further reinforce PI3K/AKT/mTOR signaling [35].

Regardless of the mutational heterogeneity within these malignant tumors, inactivating alterations in the *TP53* gene are frequent changes detected in MPNST (up to 25%), which result in a loss of DNA damage response, increasing genomic instability and promoting tumor aggressiveness [36]. The *TP53* gene encodes the p53 protein, central tumor suppressor responsible for the surveillance of DNA damage and for promoting apoptosis. Peacock and colleagues analyzed longitudinal genomic evolution in clinical cases of NF1-associated MPNST, identifying early hemizygous microdeletions in the *NF1* and *TP53* genes. Furthermore, a nonsynonymous coding mutation in the *TP53* gene, present in the context of hemizygosity, was found. This suggests a mechanism where a functional alteration of *TP53* is accompanied by the loss of the normal allele, contributing to tumor progression through inactivation of the entire p53 pathway [37]. These recurrent genetic events suggest a fundamental role of these genes in the pathogenesis of MPNST. However, the non-universality of such alterations among all cases indicates that, despite being highly relevant from a biological perspective, they do not represent a unique genetic signature for a more accurate and generalizable molecular classification of MPNSTs.

Additional drivers accumulate, including receptor tyrosine kinase (RTK) amplifications, which involve key signaling receptors such as MET/HGF, EGFR, PDGFRA, and IGF1R [23,38], leading to constitutive activation of downstream proliferative and survival pathways and promoting aggressive growth, invasion, and therapeutic resistance. In NF1-associated MPNSTs, RTK activation often coexists with the loss of canonical tumor suppressors (such as *NF1*, *TP53*, and *CDKN2A*), generating a synergistic effect that drives cell-autonomous mitogenic signaling and enhances tumor progression. Importantly, these recurrent RTK amplification events may be fundamental to their potential as therapeutic targets, with ongoing efforts exploring multi-kinase inhibitors and RTK-directed combination therapies to overcome pathway redundancy and resistance mechanisms [39–41].

BRAF activating mutations or amplifications, such as *BRAF V600E* and *NRAS Q61* mutations, have been detected specifically in sporadic MPNST [42]. Less frequent changes, such as *AURKA* gain, *TYK2* activation, and *ATRX* alterations, are linked to maintenance of the alternative lengthening of telomeres as another mechanism of tumor survival [17,23].

In a large subset of cases, a distinctive defining event is the inactivation of PRC2, most often caused by mutations or deletions in *EZH2* (Enhancer of Zeste homolog 2), *SUZ12* (Suppressor of Zeste 12 homolog) or *EED* (Embryonic ectoderm development). This results in loss of histone H3 lysine 27 trimethylation (H3K27me3), an epigenetic change that leads to strong gene deregulations and serves as a useful diagnostic marker [43]. Several studies clearly highlight the critical role of the PRC2 loss in driving MPNST development and metastatic progression, comprising increased invasion, upregulation of matrix-remodeling enzymes, and elevated lung metastasis [44]. PRC2 somatic alterations are found in 70% of NF1-associated, 90% of sporadic and radiotherapy-associated MPNSTs, underscoring the critical role of the epigenetic dysregulation in MPNST pathogenesis [26,43]. Although the loss of *EZH2*, *SUZ12* and *EED* emerges as one of the most recurrent events, the frequencies and combinations of these alterations vary significantly across cohorts and models. In fact, exome sequencing of a large set of MPNST lines derived from primary tumor xenografts reported *SUZ12* loss in 62.5% of the samples, while the *TP53* loss was present in only 12.5% [45]. Similarly, another study observed loss of H3K27me3 in 55% of MPNST, with biallelic inactivation of *SUZ12* and *EED* in 28% and 17% of cases, respectively [46].

Consistent with this escalation in genomic complexity, longitudinal and cross-sectional datasets demonstrate that widespread chromosomal gains and losses emerge only at the MPNST stage, whereas earlier lesions such as ANNUBP show limited copy number changes (primarily *CDKN2A* loss) [22,23].

In 2015, Hirbe et al. performed analyses of matched samples from different disease stages, ranging from PN to primary and metastatic MPNSTs, showing a branched evolutionary pattern in which new driver events accumulate during malignant progression [47]. While pathogenic SNVs are enriched in primary tumors, metastatic lesions exhibit increased CNVs, reflecting increased genomic instability at later stages [46,48–50]. Notably, alterations in canonical MPNST-associated genes such as *TP53* and *SUZ12* were often confined to primary tumors, underscoring distinct molecular trajectories between primary and metastatic disease. Collectively, these findings suggest that metastatic MPNSTs evolve through divergent genetic mechanisms that only partially overlap with those driving primary transformation. This hypothesis was further supported by the study conducted by Godec et al. [47], which analyzed two MPNST-affected patients with multiple metastatic lesions to elucidate the genetic events involved in clonal progression and tumor spread. In both cases, metastases shared a common clonal origin with the primary tumor, maintaining distinctive genetic traits throughout the disease course. This suggests that cells with metastatic potential are already present within the primary neoplasm, and that dissemination results from the selection of specific adaptive subclones rather than the de novo acquisition of metastasis-specific mutations. However, the absence of shared point mutations across all samples highlights a pronounced genomic heterogeneity among tumor sites. In contrast, recurrent alterations in the *TRIM* gene family encoding E3-ubiquitin ligases involved in protein degradation and cell migration, were detected more frequently in metastatic than in primary tumors. Moreover, aberrant activation of additional signaling cascades beyond RAS has been increasingly recognized in MPNST pathogenesis. In particular, dysregulation of the Hippo and WNT pathways contributes to tumor growth and progression. Activation of the Hippo pathway effectors YAP and TAZ, characterized by their nuclear accumulation, has been documented both in patient-derived MPNST samples and in preclinical models, suggesting a role in promoting proliferation, stemness, and resistance to apoptosis. Similarly, altered WNT signaling, encompassing both canonical β-catenin dependent activation and non-canonical, context-dependent signaling mediated by Wnt5a, has been observed, further emphasizing the molecular complexity and crosstalk between oncogenic networks in MPNSTs [17].

Although the model has been largely elucidated by numerous studies highlighting key events such as (i) biallelic inactivation of *NF1*, as a common prerequisite; (ii) involvement of *TP53*; (iii) loss of function of PRC2 complex by mutations/deletions of *SUZ12* and *EED*, associated with global loss of H3K27me3; and (iv) progressive genomic complexification with large somatic CNVs in advanced stages, the precise molecular mechanisms determining the transformation of the PN, which is histologically classified as a benign tumor, are still largely unknown in MPNST.

3.2. Mutational Signatures and DNA Repair-Related Processes in MPNST

The complex mutational landscape of the MPNST may be characterized using COSMIC mutational signatures analysis [51] defining characteristic patterns of single base substitutions (SBS) to reveal the contributions of defective DNA repair mechanisms and other oncogenic processes.

In the GeM study, the single-base mutational load in MPNST was overall low, with no dominant exogenous signature comparable to UV or tobacco exposure, supporting a model in which chromosomal instability, rather than point mutations, drives tumorigenesis [30].

However, focused genomic analyses have begun to reveal discrete mutational patterns associated with specific DNA repair defects. In a recent sequencing comparison of superficial MPNST, deep MPNST, and desmoplastic/spindle melanomas, McAfee et al. [52] identified distinct COSMIC mutational signatures across these tumor types. While melanomas displayed UV-related SBS7a/b signatures, both superficial and deep MPNSTs clustered according to base-excision repair (BER)-associated signatures, specifically known as SBS30 and SBS36.

These signatures are linked to oxidative DNA damage and impaired repair of 8-oxoguanine lesions, commonly involving *MUTYH* or *OGG1* dysfunction [53]. The absence of UV-related signatures further supports a distinct etiology for MPNST and implicates endogenous oxidative stress [30] as a potential driver of Schwann cell transformation. According to the COSMIC database, SBS30 represents the canonical signature of defective BER associated with 8-oxo-dG processing, whereas SBS36 reflects a related pattern resulting from *MUTYH* deficiency [53]. Their presence in MPNST genomes suggests that sustained oxidative stress and inefficient repair of oxidative lesions may synergize with chromosomal instability to promote malignant progression.

Other mutational processes appear less prominent. Some MPNST tumors exhibit clock-like signatures (SBS1 and SBS5), which reflect the accumulation of spontaneous deamination [53] of 5-methylcytosine over time, a ubiquitous background process rather than an MPNST-specific mechanism. Evidence for homologous recombination deficiency (HRD)-associated signatures, such as SBS3, remains anecdotal [53] and has not been substantiated in larger MPNST cohorts. Notably, a study on malignant transformation of vestibular schwannomas [54] revealed extensive copy number alterations but no consistent radiation- or HRD-related mutational signatures, reinforcing the concept that copy number instability, rather than defective double-strand break repair, dominates the mutational landscape of nerve sheath tumors.

3.3. Copy Number Variation Analysis to Detect Chromosomal Aberrations

Genomic instability, characterized by large gains, losses, and chromosomal rearrangements, is the main feature of MPNST. These alterations not only fuel accelerated tumor growth and invasive capacity but also contribute to the acquisition of therapeutic resistance. Therefore, understanding the processes that generate and sustain genomic instability, as well as its consequences for neoplastic progression, constitutes a crucial area of research. Clarifying these dynamics could pave the way for new targeted therapeutic strategies and enhance the effectiveness of treatments already available [55].

In MPNSTs, chromosomal rearrangements result in recurrent patterns of losses and gains in specific genomic regions. The most frequent losses affect chromosomes 1p, 9p, 11q, 12p, 14q, 17q and 22q, while gains are mainly concentrated on chromosomal arms 7p, 8q, 9q, 13q, 15q and 17q [17,45,56,57]. Among these regions, CNVs targeting key genes such as *NF1*, *CDKN2A*, and *TP53* are those relevant [9].

Notably, duplication of the chromosomal region 8q has been associated with lower overall survival in soft tissue sarcomas [45]. This is probably related to the amplification and subsequent overexpression of two positive regulators of cell proliferation: the proto-oncogene *c-MYC* and the protein RAD21, which is involved in DNA double-strand break repair and chromatid cohesion during mitosis.

Co-loss of *NF1* and *SUZ12*, both located at 17q11.2, occurs frequently, particularly in *NF1* microdeleted tumors and correlates with loss of H3K27me3 expression. Likewise, *EED* alterations contribute to PRC2 inactivation and epigenetic deregulation in MPNST. *TP53* loss or deletion at 17p13.1 is present in a subset of tumors, consistent with its involvement in late-stage genomic instability events [58].

Among recurrent gains, broad 8q amplification emerges as a near-universal clonal CNV associated with poor overall survival in soft-tissue sarcomas and MPNSTs. Candidate effectors include *MYC* (8q24), *RAD21* (8q24.11), and *HEY1*, all of which show increased expression in MPNST compared with PN [45].

Additional receptor tyrosine kinase loci are affected by 7p/7q gains, notably *EGFR* (7p11.2) and *MET* (7q31)/*HGF* (7q21), which sustain mitogenic signaling and tumor aggressiveness [41].

Finally, LOH involving 5q, 11q, 7p, and 22q, as well as amplifications of 2q and 9q, have been correlated with adverse clinical outcomes in the GeM multi-omics cohort, reinforcing the prognostic relevance of CNV profiling in MPNST [9].

However, reported CNV profiles in MPNSTs remain heterogeneous and sometimes controversial. For instance, Szymanski et al. described gains in chromosomes 1q, 7p, 8q, 9q and 17q [59], while Suppiah et al. observed amplifications in chromosomes 13q, 17p and 18q associated with poor prognosis, but not in 7p [60]. In a study conducted by Cortes-Ciriano et al., LOH of chromosome 5q was also closely associated with reduced overall survival, followed by LOH of chromosomes 11q, 7p and 22q and amplifications of 2q and 9q [9]. Recently, a strong association between distinct CNV profiles and H3K27me3 methylation status has been detected, which remains under investigation [9].

Overall, a unique aberrant chromosomal pattern characterizing all MPNSTs has not yet been identified. Discrepancies between studies may reflect differences in the investigated cohorts (like NF1-associated vs. sporadic individuals), tumor grade, or the genomic platforms used.

3.4. Transcriptomics and Single-Cell Studies

Few recent studies have provided insights into the early transcriptional programs characterizing benign and malignant lesions [61].

Comprehensive gene expression and pathway analyses have revealed stage-specific dysregulation of both tumor-intrinsic programs and the surrounding microenvironment during MPNST development. A recent study applied spatial transcriptomics in distinct regions within individual tumor samples. The authors demonstrated that some of the molecular events driving the transition from PN to MPNST may arise before such alterations become histopathologically evident. By performing multi-regional and longitudinal profiling of human PN-MPNST samples (n = 35), they identified three molecularly distinct subclusters representing different stages in the PN–MPNST continuum. Cluster 1, predominantly composed of PNs, showed upregulation of *CDKN2A*, which was significantly reduced in both Cluster 2 (ANNUBP-predominant) and Cluster 3 (MPNST-predominant) [61]. Cluster 2 showed strong enrichment of pathways associated with immune system processes and antigen presentation (including *HLA-DQA1*, *HLA-DQB1*, and *HLA-DRB1*), indicating an "immune-active" microenvironment. Concurrently, pathways related to epigenetic regulation, interferon signaling, and hypoxia were also enriched, suggesting the onset of functional immunosuppression. Interestingly, previous studies have shown that hypoxia in the tumor microenvironment can drive epigenetic dysregulation, impair immune cell cytotoxicity, and reduce interferon-gamma signaling [62].

These findings support a potential role for impaired antitumor immune responses in PN evolution and transformation. In contrast, with ANNUBPs, MPNSTs displayed further disruptions in apoptotic and angiogenic pathways, as well as in genes involved in mitotic regulation and cell cycle integrity, including *MAPK*, *PI3K/AKT*, *Notch*, *WNT*, *TGF-β*, and *JAK/STAT*. ANNUBPs were also characterized by gene signatures associated with enhanced immune surveillance and T-cell infiltration, both of which were markedly diminished in MPNSTs. Finally, ANNUBPs exhibited heterogeneous distribution across all subclusters [61].

Spatial intratumoral heterogeneity has also been demonstrated through RNA sequencing of three spatially distinct regions from the same MPNST. Sixteen differentially expressed genes were identified among the three regions (such as *EEF1A1*, *RPS27*, *RPLP1*, *ATP5A1*, *HSPB1*, and *H3C3*) involved in protein synthesis and translation, energy metabolism, stress response, and epigenetic regulation [62,63]. In addition, distinct mutational landscapes were also observed, including missense, frameshift, and synonymous variants, as well as unique CNVs, indicating the coexistence of multiple tumor subclones. Notably, one of the three regions harbored a frameshift variant in *CSK* gene, encoding a C-terminal Src kinase that has previously been found to act as a tumor suppressor [63]. Alterations in *CSK* may provide another mechanism for disrupting the PRC2 complex in MPNSTs, similar to findings in breast cancer where *CSK* loss alters the expression of PRC2 subunits *EZH2* and *SUZ12* [64].

A recent study [65] exhibited a clear association between genomic and transcriptomic alterations, with copy number gains leading to increased activity of proliferative pathways and defining a transcriptomic subtype associated with poor prognosis. MPNSTs were stratified into two main transcriptomic subtypes. The "immune-active" subtype, which comprised approximately 44% of tumors, exhibited strong immune signaling, was more frequently low-grade, and correlated with a favorable prognosis. In contrast, the "immune-deficient" subtype, accounting for about 56% of tumors, was associated with aggressive disease, high proliferative activity, complex genomic alterations, PRC2 loss, and *TP53* aberrations. The immune-deficient subtype showed greater genomic instability, with a significantly higher burden of CNVs (notably 8q gains associated with PRC2 loss) and LOH compared with immune-active tumors. These tumors were often triploid, reflecting increased genomic complexity.

Approximately 29% of genes upregulated in immune-deficient tumors showed concurrent copy number gains, mainly affecting proliferative signaling pathways regulated by *E2F*, *MYC*, and the G2/M checkpoint, as well as oncogenes such as *EGFR*, *SMO*, *XPO1*, and *EZH2*. Similarly, about 20% of downregulated genes exhibited concurrent copy number losses, including key tumor suppressors such as *PTEN*, *RB1*, *JAK1*, *JAK2*, *CYLD*, *CBL*, *SDHB*, and *SDHD* [65]. In the same study, tumors with H3K27me3 loss were more aggressive, exhibiting a higher genomic mutation burden and lower immune activity. Instead, those with retained H3K27me3 exhibited stronger immune cell infiltration, suggesting a more favorable immune response and better clinical prognosis [9].

Moreover, numerous dysregulated long non-coding RNAs (lncRNAs) and microRNAs (miRNAs) have been identified in NF1-associated malignancies and are recognized as potential tumor biomarkers. miRNAs, which can act as either tumor suppressors or oncogenes (oncomiRs) in diverse human cancers, play a significant role in NF1 pathogenesis. Notably, miR-486-3p and miR-193a-5p, which target *PTEN* and *KRAS*, respectively, are upregulated in PN compared to dermal neurofibromas. MiR-486-3p may serve as a predictive marker for NF1 progression or as a discriminative marker between plexiform and dermal neurofibroma patients [66].

Moreover, upregulation of hsa-miR-100-5p, hsa-miR-16-2-3p, hsa-miR-4508, and hsa-miR-885-5p, along with downregulation of hsa-miR-107 and hsa-miR-4433b-5p, represent a specific NF1 signature. These six miRNAs regulate multiple genes involved in key cancer-related pathways such as ERK/MAPK and PI3K/AKT/mTOR, the main downstream pathways of neurofibromin [67].

Among lncRNAs implicated in NF1, *ANRIL* is the most studied. Located at chromosome 9p21.3, it plays a role in PN biology. The specific variant rs2151280-T has been associated with increased PN burden, reduced *ANRIL* expression, and a potential correlation with milder NF1 symptoms and optic glioma development. Another lncRNA, *H19* (11p15.5), has oncogenic roles in various cancers. It functions as a molecular sponge for miR-107, thereby regulating *NF1* expression and promoting tumor development [66].

Most neoplastic cells in MPNST lose Schwann cell markers, indicating dedifferentiation to a more primitive state. These cells also overexpress factors associated with early neural crest specification, including *TWIST1*, *SOX9*, *SNAI2*, *OTX2*, *PAX3*, and *PAX6*, which highlights developmental reprogramming during malignant transformation. Pseudotemporal trajectory analysis of tumor cells demonstrates a continuum from atypical neurofibroma (with a Schwann cell identity) to MPNST (with a neural crest-like cell identity), further supporting the hypothesis that these tumors follow developmental trajectories of the neural crest lineage [60].

3.5. Epigenomic Profiling in ANNUBP-to-MPNST Transition

The first genome-wide methylome profiling study, using pooled cohorts (10 MPNST, 10 neurofibromas, 6 normal Schwann cells), found no global hypomethylation in MPNST [68]. Instead, it identified focal, cancer-associated differentially methylated regions (DMRs) with distinctive repeat-element biases, such as hypomethylation at satellite (ARLα, SATR1) and SINE repeats, hypermethylation at LINEs, and strong enrichment of hypermethylated DMRs in CpG island (CGI) shores. Integration of methylation data with external expression datasets showed that genes linked to CGI-shore DMRs separate benign from malignant phenotypes, highlighting gene-level concordance, such as *SOX10* and *CDKN2A* promoter hypermethylation, with their reduced expression. Together, these findings support selective, functionally relevant epigenomic reprogramming in the Schwann-cell lineage, rather than a global methylation shift. They also suggest that repeat-element hypomethylation, especially at specific satellite subtypes, may occur early in the benign-to-malignant continuum [68].

Building on the genome-wide DNA methylation map defined by Feber et al. [68] which delineated focal and expression-linked DMRs rather than global hypomethylation, histone-modification profiling has revealed a complementary axis of epigenetic change, centered on PRC2 loss and H3K27me3 depletion. As noted previously, a critical step in the transition toward malignancy is disruption of the PRC2, most often through LOF mutations or deletions in *SUZ12*, *EED* and *EZH2*. This disruption marks a pivotal point in the progression from ANNUBP to MPNST. Rather than enforcing global chromatin repression, these alterations reshape the enhancer landscape and reprogram Schwann-cell differentiation states [26]. Functionally, PRC2 loss promotes a dedifferentiated, neural-crest-like phenotype associated with increased invasiveness and therapy resistance. From a diagnostic standpoint, the resulting loss of H3K27me3 immunostaining remains a practical marker of PRC2 deficiency, although its sensitivity and specificity are not absolute [25,69,70].

More recently, integrative methylation and transcriptomic profiling by Suppiah et al. [60] refined the MPNST landscape into two stable epigenetic subclasses, linked to distinct cell-state programs and signaling dependencies. This work bridges methylation-defined and transcriptional trajectories, emphasizing how PRC2-dependent and PRC2-independent chromatin remodeling jointly shape malignant progression and therapeutic response.

Although widely used, H3K27me3 immunohistochemistry may also exhibit reduced staining in fibrosarcomatous dermatofibrosarcoma protuberans, limiting its standalone specificity [25]. Integrating IHC results with methylation profiling or targeted sequencing improves diagnostic accuracy in such challenging cases [70].

Complementing this methylome-driven taxonomy, recent multi-omics maps comprising precursor lesions (e.g., ANNUBP) show that MPNSTs segregate into two biological trajectories defined by H3K27me3 status. PRC2-deficient/H3K27me3-loss cases undergo broad chromosomal losses that can culminate in near-haploidization, followed by whole-genome doubling with recurrent 8q amplification, and display an immune-depleted microenvironment. In contrast, H3K27me3-retained tumors follow alternative, non-haploid trajectories and are comparatively immune-enriched. Together, these profiling layers help position ANNUBP along the NF1 tumor continuum and provide a practical framework for monitoring progression [9].

At the DNA-methylation level, integrative analyses further link PRC2/H3K27me3 loss to a shift toward hypermethylation at defined CpG sets. This identifies significant signaling pathways, most prominently within the IL17 axis (e.g., *IL17D/IL17RD*), that correlate with progression, metastasis, and with H3K27me3 status across independent MPNST cohorts. These tissue-based signatures help discriminate benign from transformed lesions in NF1 and provide candidates for biomarker development [71].

Interestingly, integrated transcriptomic and epigenomic analyses revealed two distinct molecular MPNST subgroups with different biological characteristics and outcomes. MPNST-G1 is PRC2-deficient, exhibits CpG-island promoter hypermethylation and activation of the Sonic Hedgehog (SHH) pathway, which support tumor progression resulting in a worse prognosis. In contrast, MPNST-G2 is PRC2-intact and shows global hypomethylation and activation of the WNT/β-catenin/Cyclin-D1 signaling pathway, a specific hallmark of this subtype [60]. Mechanistically, WNT activation, driven, for instance, by the knockout of its negative regulator APC, drives malignant behavior in human Schwann cell models and sustains MPNST growth [72,73].

Additional networks implicated in MPNST pathogenesis include HIPPO/YAP-TAZ signaling pathway, whose activation has been documented in patient cohorts and functional models [72–74].

Moreover, methylation changes in key regulatory loci directly influence distinctive transcriptional programs. For instance, promoter hypermethylation of *SOX10* and *CDKN2A* correlates with their reduced expression, supporting their role as functional mediators of lineage reprogramming and cell-cycle escape [68].

Furthermore, epigenetic alterations and differential expressions have been observed in other genes, such as those in the IL17 pathway, where differentially methylated CpG sites have been associated with MPNST progression [71]. The *RASSF1A* gene has also been discussed in the study by Danielsen et al. which reported promoter hypermethylation in 60% of the analyzed samples. This epigenetic silencing correlates with an unfavorable prognosis in patients with NF1-associated MPNST, suggesting that *RASSF1A* may represent a potential prognostic marker [75].

3.6. Integrative Overview of Multi-Omics Findings

The multi-layered omics analyses presented in this section collectively outline a coherent molecular trajectory from PN to ANNUBP and, ultimately, to MPNST.

Despite heterogeneity across individual studies, several convergent principles emerge.

First, genomics remains the backbone of NF1-associated tumor evolution. Biallelic *NF1* loss serves as the initiating event, followed by early *CDKN2A/B* deletion, which defines ANNUBP. Subsequent widespread chromosomal instability and PRC2 inactivation culminate in MPNST. Together, these events drive the transition of Schwann cells from a proliferative but relatively stable state to a highly aneuploid, epigenetically deregulated, and malignant phenotype.

Second, transcriptomics and spatial omics data demonstrate that malignant progression is driven not only by genetic alterations but also by the rewiring of lineage identity, hypoxia-induced immune evasion, and remodeling of the tumor microenvironment. Immune-active versus immune-deficient transcriptomic subtypes, as along with PRC2-

dependent versus PRC2-independent regulatory programs, represent two biologically meaningful and prognostically significant classifications.

Third, epigenomic profiling provides another dimension, revealing distinct DNA methylation classes and H3K27me3-defined epigenetic trajectories.

Integration of methylation and expression data highlights key regulators, such as *SOX10, CDKN2A,* and genes in IL17-axis, whose altered chromatin states accompany lineage dedifferentiation, senescence escape, and metastatic behavior. PRC2 loss emerges as a central event that links genomic instability, epigenetic deregulation, and transcriptomic reprogramming.

Together, these multi-omics approaches offer a unified model of the stepwise, yet heterogeneous, evolution of NF1-associated tumors, a process shaped by both genetic mutations and environmental pressures. Table 1 provides an integrated overview of the major multi-omics studies discussed above, summarizing patient cohorts, technologies used, recurrently altered genes and pathways, and their diagnostic or prognostic relevance. Each study includes details on the analyzed patient cohort, reported in the cited references (NF1-associated or sporadic PN, ANNUBP, MPNST), the omics technology employed, the main findings encompassing identified mutations (e.g., *TP53, CDKN2A, SUZ12*), biomarkers, and dysregulated molecular pathways, as well as the corresponding clinical implications, including diagnostic and prognostic value and potential therapeutic targets. Abbreviations: ANNUBP, atypical neurofibromatous neoplasm of uncertain biological potential; cfDNA, circulating cell-free DNA; CNV, copy number variation; DNAm, DNA methylation; IHC, immunohistochemistry; MPNST, malignant peripheral nerve sheath tumor; PN, plexiform neurofibroma; PRC2, polycomb repressive complex 2; SNV, single nucleotide variant; ULP-WGS, ultra-low-pass whole-genome sequencing; WES, whole-exome sequencing; WGS, whole-genome sequencing; PNST, peripheral nerve sheath tumor; cNF, cutaneous neurofibroma; ANF, atypical neurofibroma [9,11,26,30,43,58,61,67,76–86].

Table 1. Summary of omics studies in NF1-related tumors (PN–ANNUBP–MPNST continuum).

Patients Cohort	Tested Omics Technology	Key Findings (Genes/Biomarkers/Pathways)	Clinical Implications (Diagnostic/Prognostic)	Ref.
NF1, cutaneous neurofibromas (cNF, benign): 11 patients (40 tumors)	WGS, RNAseq, SNP array	Biallelic *NF1*, low secondary drivers; baseline cNF transcriptome with ECM/immune signatures	–	[76]
NF1, plexiform neurofibroma derived Schwann cell models (PN): 7 donors, 11 cell lines (6 deeply profiled)	Targeted/WES, RNAseq, pharmacologic profiling	*NF1* loss: RAS-pathway activity; drug-response resource	Preclinical PN Schwann-cell panel for pharmacogenomic screening; supports testing MEK (selumetinib), mTOR, PI3K, RTK (EGFR/PDGFR), BET, and CDK4/6 inhibitors and combinations	[77]
ANNUBP/atypical neurofibromas (human): 16 ANF (WES); 26 ANF (CNV meta); 5 ANF (RNA-seq); comparators MPNST: 3 (WES), 28 (CNV), 5 (RNA-seq	WES, targeted seq, CNV, RNA-seq	Frequent *CDKN2A* and *SMARCA2* loss; PRC2 intact in ANNUBP; RAS/MAPK feature	–	[30]
ANNUBP vs. cNF/PN vs. MPNST: 40 ANNUBP	DNA methylation (EPIC array)	Distinct methylation class: ANNUBP clusters near benign PN; H3K27me3 largely retained	Diagnostic: methylation profiling aids classification/risk along cNF/PN, ANNUBP, MPNST	[78]
NF1-associated PNST spectrum (cNF/PN, ANNUBP, MPNST): 35 tumors	Spatial transcriptomics; RNA-seq	Early immuno-oncogenic programs at ANNUBP; progressive RAS/MAPK and microenvironment remodeling	–	[61]
MPNST (NF1-associated, sporadic, post-radiation): NF1-associated 27; sporadic 13; post-RT 9	WGS, WES, targeted seq, CNV; PRC2/IHC	Recurrent PRC2 loss (*EED, SUZ12*); frequent *NF1, TP53, CDKN2A*; RAS–MAPK activation	Diagnostic: H3K27me3 loss by IHC marks PRC2-deficient MPNST; Therapeutic: epigenetic vulnerabilities highlighted	[26]
MPNST 12	WES, SNP array	Recurrent *NF1, SUZ12/EED, TP53, CDKN2A*; broad CNV burden	–	[58]
NF1-associated and sporadic MPNST (GeM Consortium): 95 samples from 90 tumors (61 NF1-related/ 29 sporadic)	WGS, multi-regional WES, RNA-seq, DNAm, cfDNA	Evolutionary trajectories; CNV-driven progression; convergence on RAS/MAPK and PRC2-loss; cfDNA mirrors tumor alterations	–	[9]

Table 1. *Cont.*

Patients Cohort	Tested Omics Technology	Key Findings (Genes/Biomarkers/Pathways)	Clinical Implications (Diagnostic/Prognostic)	Ref.
NF1 PN vs. MPNST (liquid biopsy): 16 healthy, 23 PN, 14 MPNST	cfDNA ULP-WGS (fragmentomics and genome-wide aneuploidy profiling)	Plasma fragmentomics and genome-wide aneuploidy profiling distinguish MPNST from pNF and detect malignant transformation	Diagnostic/Prognostic: non-invasive classifier; enables longitudinal surveillance	[79]
883 healthy controls and 7 cNF, 9 PN, 12 MPNST	cfDNA genome-wide aneuploidy profiling and targeted mutation detection	cfDNA detects CNVs and tumor mutations associated with MPNST	Diagnostic: complementary assay for malignant transformation detection	[80]
MPNST (historical aCGH): 24 MPNST and 3 neurofibromas	aCGH (32K BAC)	Broad chromosomal gains/losses (incl. *CDKN2A* locus)	–	[81]
MPNST (n = 35; 15 treated and 10 on treatment), ANF (n = 17), PN (n = 69), and healthy controls (n = 21); 167 cfDNA libraries analyzed	cfDNA fragmentomics	cfDNA fragmentation profiling distinguishes PN–ANNUBP–MPNST; shorter fragments and altered ratios in MPNST; limited CNVs in ANNUBP vs. widespread losses (*SUZ12, SMARCA2, CDKN2A*) and gains (1q, 7p, 8q, 9q, 17q) in MPNST.	cfDNA fragmentomics enables non-invasive detection and monitoring of NF1 tumor progression.	[82]
42 tumors (37 patients): ANF (n = 5), MPNST (n = 27); 10 tumors: MPNST-like	DNA methylation (EPIC array), RNA-seq, Archer FusionPlex custom panel, Archer VariantPlex custom panel, and Illumina TruSight Oncology 500 panel (TSO500), CNV analysis	Distinct cfDNA fragmentation patterns across PN–ANNUBP–MPNST; shorter fragments and altered short/long ratios in MPNST; limited CNVs in ANNUBP, but extensive CNVs in MPNST (losses: *SUZ12, SMARCA2, CDKN2A*; gains: 1q, 7p, 8q, 9q, 17q).	DNAm profiling refines MPNST diagnosis, distinguishing low-grade TRK/EGFR-driven subtypes from high-grade PRC2/*CDKN2A*-deficient tumors, linked to aggressive behavior and poorer survival (p = 0.0024).	[83]
126 NF1 patients (G1–G5, mild to severe phenotypes) and 128 healthy controls	Small non-coding RNA-seq	Six-miRNA plasma signature identified (↑ miR-16-2-3p, miR-100-5p, miR-4508, miR-885-5p; ↓ miR-107, miR-4433b-5p), linked to RAS/MAPK, PI3K/AKT/mTOR, *PTEN*, *TP53*, and *NF1* pathways.	First serum miRNA panel distinguishing NF1 patients from controls; promising non-invasive biomarker for diagnosis and disease monitoring.	[67]
59 tumors from 55 NF1 patients (35 MPNSTs, 16 plexiform, 8 dermal neurofibromas	Targeted seq, aCGH	Recurrent deletions (*NF1, CDKN2A, TP53, RB1*) and amplifications (*MET, HGF, PDGFRA, EGFR*); co-amplification of *HGF/MET–PDGFRA* indicates activation of p70S6K/mTOR signaling.	Core CNV signature differentiating MPNSTs from benign NF1 tumors; highlights HGF/MET/PDGFRA–mTOR axis as therapeutic target; supports array-CGH for CNV-based diagnosis.	[84]
34 MPNSTs from 27 NF1 patients	*NF1* mutation screening used dHPLC, LOH, MLPA, array-CGH, and sequencing	Frequent *NF1* and *TP53* alterations; 7 novel *NF1* and 4 novel *TP53* mutations; combined *NF1–TP53* loss linked to higher tumor grade and aggressive MPNSTs.	*NF1–TP53* co-alterations confirm biallelic NF1 inactivation and cooperative role in MPNST progression; large deletions correlate with higher grade; MLPA/array-CGH improve detection and risk stratification.	[11]
88 MPNSTs (26 NF1-related, 62 sporadic) and 16 benign PN	Targeted seq	*TP53* mutations found in 24% of MPNSTs (mainly missense in exons 5–8); no mutations in benign PN. High p53 protein expression correlated with mutation status (p = 0.002). Mutations not enriched in NF1-related vs. sporadic MPNSTs	Demonstrated that *TP53* alterations are relatively rare in MPNSTs and not associated with NF1 status, indicating *TP53* plays a minor role in human tumorigenesis compared to mouse models.	[85]
50 MPNST, 11 NF	WGS, WES, Targeted seq	Identified recurrent *SUZ12* (26%) and *EED* loss-of-function mutations, mutually exclusive with other chromatin remodelers; correlated with H3K27me3 loss. Proposed the *NF1–SUZ12* "three-hit" model for malignant transformation	Established PRC2 loss as a hallmark of MPNST and H3K27me3 loss as a diagnostic and prognostic biomarker. Supported targeting epigenetic regulators in therapy.	[43]
8 MPNST, 1 pNF, 7 cNF	Exome seq, aCGH	Frequent biallelic loss of *SUZ12/EED*, *NF1* inactivation, and *CDKN2A* deletions; rare *TP53* mutations; novel *KDM2B* variant.	Confirmed PRC2 loss as MPNST hallmark and suggested KDM2B as a new chromatin regulator candidate.	[86]

Arrows indicate the direction of differential expression in the plasma miRNA signature: the upward arrow (↑) denotes miRNAs upregulated in NF1 patients compared with healthy controls, whereas the downward arrow (↓) denotes miRNAs downregulated in NF1 patients (small non-coding RNA-seq).

4. Liquid Biopsy: A Novel Approach for Early Detection and Disease Monitoring

4.1. Circulating Tumor DNA (ctDNA) and NF1-Specific Mutational Signatures

Circulating cell-free DNA (ccfDNA) was first described in 1948 by Mandel and Metais in both healthy subjects and patients. CcfDNA is normally present in blood at low concentrations (1–10 ng/mL), but its levels increase in various physiological and pathological conditions, including infections, trauma, and tumors. In 1994, tumor-specific DNA fragments, containing mutations identical to those found in tumor tissue (*K-RAS* gene), were identified for the first time in the plasma of patients with pancreatic cancer. This fraction was defined as circulating tumor DNA (ctDNA) [87]. As ctDNA is derived from tumors and released through apoptosis, necrosis, or extracellular vesicle release, researchers typically evaluate potential SNVs, structural variants, or epigenetic alterations using highly sensitive methods such as PCR, targeted NGS, or ultra-low pass whole genome sequencing (ULP-WGS). In addition, a particularly interesting aspect of ctDNA concerns the fragment length evaluation. The distribution of ctDNA fragment sizes constitutes a molecular signature, often defined as fragmentation signature, that can distinguish between different clinical states.

Integrating ctDNA analysis or ccfDNA fragmentomic approaches could be a valuable tool for improving the early diagnosis, risk stratification, and longitudinal monitoring of patients at risk of MPNST transformation [79,80,82]. For instance, patients with MPNST exhibit a higher proportion of shorter fragments compared to those with PN or healthy controls [82]. Recently, Taylor Sundby et al. analyzed plasma-derived fragment distributions and identified an altered fragmentation pattern characteristic of MPNST, which was absent in patients with only PN or ANNUBP.

In addition to fragment-length alterations, another analytical dimension of ctDNA involves studying the CNVs, which reflect the genomic instability characteristic of neoplastic transformation. Several studies [79,82,87] have demonstrated the ability to detect CNVs in cfDNA with high specificity in patients with MPNST, in some cases anticipating the radiological diagnosis of malignant transformation [80]. For example, Szymanski et al. used ULP-WGS at ~0.6× coverage, followed by in silico selection of 90–150 bp fragments, for quantifying the plasma tumor fraction and distinguish patients with MPNST from those with PN. The study achieved an area under the curve (AUC) of 0.83, with 75% sensitivity and 91% specificity at baseline, leading to an overall accuracy of 89% in serial sample analysis [79]. The plasma tumor fraction significantly correlated with tumor burden, as assessed by the standardized quantitative RECIST SLD (Response Evaluation Criteria In Solid Tumors as Sum of the Longest Diameters of the target lesions) method (Pearson correlation coefficient, $r = 0.39$), as well as with therapeutic response and minimal residual disease (MRD). This suggests that ctDNA changes may anticipate those observable by radiological imaging.

The copy number profile observed in ccfDNA mirrored that of the tumor, showing large chromosomal gains (1q, 7p, 8q, 9q, and 17q) and losses (6p and 9p), as well as focal deletions in the *CDKN2A*, *SUZ12*, and *SMARCA2* genes associated with the transition from PN to ANNUBP. Additionally, *NF1* loss was detected in the plasma of patients with PN and MPNST but not in healthy controls, confirming the tumor origin of ccfDNA and its potential as a non-invasive biomarker of progression [79].

Beyond the analysis of individual CNVs, a more comprehensive approach based on Genome-wide Aneuploidy Scoring (GAS) has been proposed [87]. GAS measures the overall degree of chromosomal instability in the ccfDNA. Specifically, GAS alone shows limited sensitivity (~33%) in detecting MPNSTs; on the other hand, combining it with focal subchromosomal events (e.g., loss of *TP53* or *SUZ12*) and/or specific mutations in ctDNA increases sensitivity to approximately 50%, while maintaining 97% specificity.

Notably, a distinctive loss of *SUZ12* was observed in the cfDNA derived from a PN patient, which was detected 25 months before the clinical diagnosis of MPNST, highlighting the predictive potential of liquid biopsies for identifying malignant transformation at early stages [80,87]. Another promising application of ctDNA analysis involves the study of epigenetic alterations, particularly DNA methylation patterns and histone modifications, which reflect transcriptional and structural changes associated with neoplastic progression [9]. Sundby et al. showed that combining CNV signals and methylation changes in ctDNA improves diagnostic sensitivity compared to methods based exclusively on genomic variations.

Furthermore, genome-wide methylation analysis by Tomczak et al. identified a panel of 53 specific, differentially methylated CpG sites associated with MPNST. These CpGs distinguish MPNST from PN or ANNUBP. The identified loci map to genes such as *OX9*, *RUNX1*, *PRDM16*, *PTPRN2*, and *COL23A1*, which are involved in transcriptional regulation and tumorigenesis. Therefore, this methylation classifier represents a non-invasive, functional diagnostic tool for early NF1-associated tumor diagnosis and screening [88].

Despite growing evidence supporting the utility of ctDNA in NF1-associated tumors, several limitations complicate its clinical implementation. The rarity of these neoplasms, particularly MPNSTs, combined with the low tumor burden in primary lesions, makes collecting sufficiently large patient cohorts challenging [80]. Furthermore, ctDNA concentrations in patients with NF1 are extremely low. Recent studies have shown only slightly increased ccfDNA levels compared to healthy controls, with ctDNA detectability limited to a few cases [87]. This scenario requires highly sensitive sequencing techniques and optimized bioinformatic pipelines to ensure reproducible results and reduce the risk of false negatives.

Technical variability in ccfDNA isolation, sequencing depth, and data processing remains a major challenge. To date, no plasma-based assay specific for NF1 detection has been clinically validated. Indeed, while several liquid biopsy panels, such as FoundationOne® Liquid CDx (Foundation Medicine, Inc., Cambridge, MA, USA), Guardant360® CDx (Guardant Health, Inc., Redwood City, CA, USA), PGDx elio™ Plasma Focus Dx (Personal Genome Diagnostics, Baltimore, MD, USA) and Shield® (Guardant Health, Inc., Redwood City, CA, USA), have been approved by the FDA for various solid tumors (e.g., lung, prostate and colorectal cancers), there are currently no clinically validated assays for ctDNA in MPNST or other NF1-associated tumors.

As highlighted by Sundby et al. [82] and Rahrmann et al. [88], approaches based on fragmentomics, copy number profiling, and methylation signatures have demonstrated high diagnostic potential. However, their integration into clinical practice requires prospective longitudinal studies in large cohorts to validate their sensitivity, specificity, and prognostic value.

Overall, ctDNA is a promising, noninvasive biomarker for early diagnosis and monitoring of malignant transformation in NF1, with potential to aid in addressing intra-tumor heterogeneity and supporting the search for therapeutic targets. However, further clinical validation and standardized protocols are necessary before ctDNA can be effectively integrated into clinical practice.

4.2. Circulating Cell-Free RNA (ccfRNA) and Gene Expression Profiling

Circulating cell-free RNA (ccfRNA) is an emerging analyte of great interest for monitoring various pathological conditions over time, including cancer. Present in plasma, ccfRNA provides complementary information to total RNA from blood cells, as it originates from both viable circulating cells and peripheral tissues via active secretion or apoptotic cell death processes. Due to these characteristics, ccfRNA is becoming a promising liquid biopsy tool capable of reflecting the body's physiological or pathological state in real time [89].

Alterations in miRNA profiles have been described in numerous pathological conditions, including various cancers, where they can act as oncogenes or tumor suppressors, influencing proliferation, apoptosis, and metastasis [90]. Consequently, quantifying miR-

NAs in plasma has been proposed as a non-invasive method for early cancer diagnosis and risk stratification.

In the context of NF1, available data on circulating microRNAs is limited but promising. One of the few systematic investigations to date was conducted by Napolitano et al. They analyzed a cohort of 126 NF1 patients with different phenotypes stratified into five phenotypic groups (G1–G5, in order of increasing aggressiveness), and compared them with 128 healthy subjects, aiming to outline a potential miRNA profile associated with the disease. They identified 87 differentially expressed miRNAs, selecting 37 primary candidates. Notably, miR-16-2-3p, miR-100-5p, miR-4508, and miR-885-5p were significantly overexpressed, while miR-107 and miR-4433b-5p were downregulated in NF1 patients compared to controls, suggesting a potential molecular signature of the disease. Although no significant differences were observed among NF1 phenotypic subgroups, but Ingenuity pathway analysis revealed a strong correlation between candidate miRNAs and pathways crucial in NF1-related tumorigenesis, including RAS/ERK/MAPK and PI3K/AKT/mTOR. Given that many of these miRNAs are already deregulated in other RAS-dependent cancers, their functional validation in NF1 could contribute to defining novel diagnostic or prognostic biomarkers and, potential new therapeutic targets [67].

In addition to miRNAs, several circulating coding RNA biomarkers have been proposed as potential indicators of malignant transformation in NF1 patients. Together with ccfRNA and ctDNA data, these biomarkers could represent reliable tools for longitudinal monitoring. For example, adrenomedullin levels are increased in patients with MPNST, suggesting a role in tumor angiogenesis. sAXL and melanoma inhibitory activity (MIA) correlate with tumor size and burden, while IGFBP-1 and RANTES are significantly overexpressed in MPNST compared to PN. Additionally, elevated levels of the pro-inflammatory cytokines IL-6, TNF-α, and IFN-γ indicate a state of systemic inflammation associated with tumor progression [87].

Further therapeutic targets in NF1-related tumors have been identified through gene expression profiling and phosphoproteomic screening studies. In particular, Aurora kinase A (*AURKA*) expression is 7.9-fold higher in human and murine MPNST samples than in healthy, and its pharmacological inhibition reduces tumor cell survival in vitro and in vivo [23]. Similarly, Polo-like kinase 1 (*PLK1*) has been identified as a crucial driver of proliferation in MPNST and Schwannoma cell lines. Like AURKA, PLK1acts at the G2/M transition of the cell cycle. PLK1 inhibitors such as BI6727 have been shown to stabilize tumor volume in MPNST xenografts, suggesting a potential therapeutic role, albeit within a limited therapeutic window [91].

Finally, the loss of the epigenetic marker H3K27me3, characteristic of MPNSTs as previously discussed, can result not only from genetic alterations or alternative epigenetic mechanisms affecting the PRC2 complex but also from microRNA-mediated regulation or *EZHIP* overexpression, as observed in other tumor types such as Merkel cell carcinoma [44].

These observations underscore the importance of integrating epigenetic, transcriptional, and proteomics data when studying NF1-associated tumor progression. Combining cfRNA and ctDNA analysis from the same sample increases diagnostic sensitivity by capturing both transcriptomic information and genomic instability.

5. Genomic Data Consortia in NF1: Collaborative Efforts in Data Sharing and Research Advancement

The rapid evolution of omics technologies and the development of high-throughput platforms have allowed high resolution study of genetic disorders such as NF1-associated disease. Advances in sequencing, including WES/WGS, RNA profiling and methylation analysis, have enabled deeper, multi-layered characterization of these disorders, consequently generating datasets, even for poorly characterized conditions like ANNUBP and MPNST. In the big-data era, however, the focus has moved from data generation to data sharing and analysis; this translated into the need for centralized and harmonized platforms.

Several collaborative initiatives have been proposed, aiming at collecting data, gathering resources, and sharing efforts and knowledge to advance our understanding of these conditions. Among the most widely used and data-richest platforms for NF1-related research are the Neurofibromatosis Therapeutic Acceleration Project (NTAP) [92], the Children's Tumor Foundation (CTF) Synodos [93], and the National Cancer Institute—Genomic Data Commons (NCI-GDC) [94]. NTAP is a collaborative action focused on leading and funding research in NF1-related plexiform and cutaneous neurofibromas. It aims to accelerate therapies development through a collaborative and transparent approach, covering multiple initiatives such as cell and tissue biobanks, animal and cell model systems, omics data generation and collection, and therapeutic screening. All data are accessible via the NF Data Portal (available online: https://nfdataportal.org/, accessed on 27 November 2025), an open repository with controlled access for NF1-related studies [95].

To further advance in NF-related research, NTAP has partnered with organizations such as the Children's Tumor Foundation CTF, a non-profit medical foundation dedicated to drug discovery for NF1 and Schwannomatosis. Recently, CTF launched CTF Synodos [96], a collaborative NF-centered consortium designed to accelerate discovery by sharing unpublished and curated data, knowledge, and workflows across participating institutions and research groups. Data openness and transparency are reached through online platforms, such as Synapse [95] available online: https://nf.synapse.org/ (accessed on 27 November 2025).

The third major resource is represented by NCI-GDC (available online: https://gdc.cancer.gov/, accessed on 27 November 2025), the genomic division of the NIH's Cancer Institute. NCI-GDC provides a large repository of multi-omics data, curated metadata, harmonized analysis pipelines, integrated computational tools, and interconnections with other platforms such as The Cancer Genome Atlas (TCGA) [97]. Although not exclusively focused on NF-related conditions, NCI-GDC comprises NF1 and MPNST samples along with molecular and omics profiles, offering valuable opportunities to advance NF1-related research.

In addition, the international GeM Consortium provides multi-omics datasets focused on MPNST evolution, comprising multi-regional WES and WGS, RNAseq, DNA methylation, and cfDNA data [9]. A summary of these resources is reported in Table 2.

Table 2. Overview of the major genomic consortia for NF1, ANNUBP, and MPNST research. The table shows the main collaborative consortia, displaying their name, content, available data type, access model, and key publications (PubMed ID). It summarizes institutional initiatives that generate or provide access to multi-omics data from NF1-associated tumors, including benign neurofibromas, ANNUBP, and MPNST, as well as large-scale repositories that integrate these datasets. bRNAseq: bulk RNA sequencing; cfDNA: cell free DNA; CTF: Children's Tumor Foundation; DNAm: DNA methylation; GeM: Genomics of MPNST; NCI-GDC: National Cancer Institute Genomic Data Commons; NTAP: Neurofibromatosis Therapeutic Acceleration Project; scRNAseq: single cell RNA sequencing; snRNAseq: single nucleus RNA sequencing; WES: Whole Exome Sequencing; WGS: Whole Genome Sequencing.

Consortium	Content	Data Type	Access Model	Key Publications
NTAP	NF1-derived ANNUBP and MPNST tumor samples; matched normal tissues; cell lines and preclinical models supporting translational studies	WES, WGS, RNAseq	Controlled access	[92,98]

Table 2. *Cont.*

Consortium	Content	Data Type	Access Model	Key Publications
CTF Synodos	Collaborative foundation-led program generating genomic and transcriptomic data from benign NF1 neurofibromas (cutaneous and plexiform) and patient-derived Schwann cell models	WES, WGS, snRNAseq	Controlled access (partially open)	[76,77,93]
NCI-GDC	Central NIH repository aggregating TCGA, TARGET, and sarcoma datasets, including NF1-associated tumors; harmonized data accessible through the GDC portal	WES, WGS, DNAm array, scRNAseq	Open access	[94]
GeM	International consortium investigating MPNSTs; integrates genomic, transcriptomic, methylation, and cfDNA analyses to define tumor evolution and therapeutic vulnerabilities	Multi-regional WES, WGS, RNAseq, DNAm, cfDNA	Controlled access	[9]

A relevant contribution to data sharing and integration for peripheral nerve tumors associated with NF1 is represented by the recently updated Johns Hopkins NF1 Biorepository [99]. This computational resource collects and harmonizes omics data (genomics, transcriptomics, and epigenomics) along with curated clinical information from numerous samples of PN, ANNUBP, and MPNST. This project serves as a centralized platform for translational research, promoting comparative and integrative multi-omics analysis, and supporting the definition of "evolutionary trajectories" that lead from benign lesions to malignant tumors.

Together, these efforts illustrate how strategic collaborative partnerships may accelerate disease characterization, empower basic research, and enable biomarkers discovery, mechanistic modelling, and variants prioritization that can be directly translated into personalized medical approaches. As omics technologies continue to advance, the values of such initiatives will depend not only on data generation but, crucially, on the creation of transparent, interoperable and curated repositories.

6. Conclusions and Future Perspectives

Research into the molecular and cellular mechanisms of MPNST pathogenesis in NF1 has been markedly refined through multi-omic analyses encompassing genomic, transcriptomic, and epigenomic profiling. Beyond *NF1* and *CDKN2A* inactivation, loss of PRC2 function and alterations in key signaling pathways such as RAS/MAPK, PI3K/AKT/mTOR, and Wnt/SHH, are now recognized as central drivers of tumor initiation and progression.

A multistep evolutionary trajectory from PN to ANNUBP and, ultimately, to MPNST has been proposed. Comprehensive multi-omic mapping has revealed two distinct evolutionary trajectories of MPNSTs distinguished by H3K27me3 status and PRC2 dependency. PRC2-deficient (H3K27me3-loss) tumors exhibit widespread chromosomal losses, near-haploidization followed by whole-genome doubling, recurrent 8q amplification, and an immune-depleted microenvironment. In contrast, PRC2-intact (H3K27me3-retained) tumors show non-haploid karyotypes and greater immune infiltration [9].

Moreover, transcriptomic and methylation-based subtyping have delineated biologically distinct MPNST classes, such as immune-active versus PRC2-deficient/proliferative subtypes, and SHH- versus WNT-driven mechanisms, which correlate with prognosis and therapeutic vulnerabilities.

Despite advances from genomic studies in identifying key events driving neurofibroma progression, major challenges remain in predicting malignant transformation potential. The rarity and heterogeneity of MPNST hinder biomarker validation and limit the power of therapeutic trials.

In parallel, liquid biopsy approaches based on cfDNA and cfRNA are emerging as powerful non-invasive tools for detection, monitoring and molecular stratification of NF1-associated tumors. However, greater standardization and validation in multicenter cohorts are urgently needed.

Future research should be focused on AI-based integration of multi-layered omics, spatial, transcriptomics, and single-cell analyses to more accurately map the tumor ecosystem, identify actionable dependencies, and track clonal evolution in real time. Such advances hold the potential to transform NF1 management and surveillance, paving the way toward precision oncology and improved patient outcomes.

Author Contributions: Conceptualization: V.B., S.B., I.R.C., V.U., D.M. and A.P.; data curation, literature search, figures, study design, data collection, data analysis, data interpretation, writing: S.B., I.R.C., A.L., A.T., B.M., E.A., S.C., M.T., C.A., L.B., D.C., V.U., D.M., V.B. and A.P.; funding acquisition: V.B. and A.P.; project administration: A.P., V.B., V.U., D.M. and V.B.; supervision, V.B. and A.P.; writing—original draft, S.B., I.R.C., A.L., A.T., B.M., V.B., D.M. and A.P.; BioRender.com (https://BioRender.com) and OpenAI ChatGPT (GPT-5) for figure creation and finalized by the authors. All authors have read and agreed to the published version of the manuscript.

Funding: This study was partially supported by the "Fondazione Emma ed Ernesto Rulfo per la Genetica Medica" and by the "FIL-BANDO DI ATENEO PER LA RICERCA 2022" from University of Parma. This study was funded by the European Union—Next Generation EU, PNRR-M4C2-I1.1—MUR Call for proposals n. 1409 del 14 September 2022—Bando PRIN 2022 PNRR—ERC sector LS2-, Project code P2022M9SRW—CUP Code D53D23016670001.

Institutional Review Board Statement: This study was conducted in accordance with the Declaration of Helsinki and in compliance with the local ethical guidelines.

Data Availability Statement: All relevant data are available from the corresponding author upon request.

Conflicts of Interest: The authors declare no conflicts of interest.

References

1. Hirbe, A.C.; Gutmann, D.H. Neurofibromatosis Type 1: A Multidisciplinary Approach to Care. *Lancet Neurol.* **2014**, *13*, 834–843. [CrossRef]
2. Friedman, J.M. *Neurofibromatosis 1*; Adam, M.P., Bick, S., Mirzaa, G.M., Pagon, R.A., Wallace, S.E., Amemiya, A., Eds.; University of Washington: Seattle, WA, USA, 2025.
3. Choi, J.; An, S.; Lim, S.Y. Current Concepts of Neurofibromatosis Type 1: Pathophysiology and Treatment. *Arch. Craniofacial Surg.* **2022**, *23*, 6–16. [CrossRef]
4. Evans, D.G.R.; Baser, M.E.; McGaughran, J.; Sharif, S.; Howard, E.; Moran, A. Malignant Peripheral Nerve Sheath Tumours in Neurofibromatosis 1. *J. Med. Genet.* **2002**, *39*, 311–314. [CrossRef] [PubMed]
5. Watson, K.L.; Al Sannaa, G.A.; Kivlin, C.M.; Ingram, D.R.; Landers, S.M.; Roland, C.L.; Cormier, J.N.; Hunt, K.K.; Feig, B.W.; Ashleigh Guadagnolo, B.; et al. Patterns of Recurrence and Survival in Sporadic, Neurofibromatosis Type 1–Associated, and Radiation-Associated Malignant Peripheral Nerve Sheath Tumors. *J. Neurosurg.* **2017**, *126*, 319–329. [CrossRef] [PubMed]
6. Saleh, M.; Dib, A.; Beaini, S.; Saad, C.; Faraj, S.; El Joueid, Y.; Kotob, Y.; Saoudi, L.; Emmanuel, N. Neurofibromatosis Type 1 System-Based Manifestations and Treatments: A Review. *Neurol. Sci.* **2023**, *44*, 1931–1947. [CrossRef] [PubMed]
7. Gutmann, D.H.; Ferner, R.E.; Listernick, R.H.; Korf, B.R.; Wolters, P.L.; Johnson, K.J. Neurofibromatosis Type 1. *Nat. Rev. Dis. Primers* **2017**, *3*, 17004. [CrossRef]
8. Gutmann, D.H.; Collins, F.S. Recent Progress toward Understanding the Molecular Biology of von Recklinghausen Neurofibromatosis. *Ann. Neurol.* **1992**, *31*, 555–561. [CrossRef]
9. Cortes-Ciriano, I.; Steele, C.D.; Piculell, K.; Al-Ibraheemi, A.; Eulo, V.; Bui, M.M.; Chatzipli, A.; Dickson, B.C.; Borcherding, D.C.; Feber, A.; et al. Genomic Patterns of Malignant Peripheral Nerve Sheath Tumor (MPNST) Evolution Correlate with Clinical Outcome and Are Detectable in Cell-Free DNA. *Cancer Discov.* **2023**, *13*, 654–671. [CrossRef]
10. Tucker, T.; Friedman, J. Pathogenesis of Hereditary Tumors: Beyond the "Two-hit" Hypothesis. *Clin. Genet.* **2002**, *62*, 345–357. [CrossRef]

11. Upadhyaya, M.; Kluwe, L.; Spurlock, G.; Monem, B.; Majounie, E.; Mantripragada, K.; Ruggieri, M.; Chuzhanova, N.; Evans, D.G.; Ferner, R.; et al. Germline and SomaticNF1 Gene Mutation Spectrum in NF1-Associated Malignant Peripheral Nerve Sheath Tumors (MPNSTs). *Hum. Mutat.* **2008**, *29*, 74–82. [CrossRef]
12. De Raedt, T.; Brems, H.; Wolkenstein, P.; Vidaud, D.; Pilotti, S.; Perrone, F.; Mautner, V.; Frahm, S.; Sciot, R.; Legius, E. Elevated Risk for MPNST in NF1 Microdeletion Patients. *Am. J. Hum. Genet.* **2003**, *72*, 1288–1292. [CrossRef]
13. Anastasaki, C.; Orozco, P.; Gutmann, D.H. RAS and beyond: The Many Faces of the Neurofibromatosis Type 1 Protein. *Dis. Model. Mech.* **2022**, *15*, dmm049362. [CrossRef] [PubMed]
14. Thomas, L.; Spurlock, G.; Eudall, C.; Thomas, N.S.; Mort, M.; Hamby, S.E.; Chuzhanova, N.; Brems, H.; Legius, E.; Cooper, D.N.; et al. Exploring the Somatic NF1 Mutational Spectrum Associated with NF1 Cutaneous Neurofibromas. *Eur. J. Hum. Genet.* **2012**, *20*, 411–419. [CrossRef]
15. Garcia-Linares, C.; Fernández-Rodríguez, J.; Terribas, E.; Mercadé, J.; Pros, E.; Benito, L.; Benavente, Y.; Capellà, G.; Ravella, A.; Blanco, I.; et al. Dissecting Loss of Heterozygosity (LOH) in Neurofibromatosis Type 1-Associated Neurofibromas: Importance of Copy Neutral LOH. *Hum. Mutat.* **2011**, *32*, 78–90. [CrossRef] [PubMed]
16. Gottfried, O.N.; Viskochil, D.H.; Couldwell, W.T. Neurofibromatosis Type 1 and Tumorigenesis: Molecular Mechanisms and Therapeutic Implications. *Neurosurg. Focus* **2010**, *28*, E8. [CrossRef]
17. Somatilaka, B.N.; Sadek, A.; McKay, R.M.; Le, L.Q. Malignant Peripheral Nerve Sheath Tumor: Models, Biology, and Translation. *Oncogene* **2022**, *41*, 2405–2421. [CrossRef]
18. Miettinen, M.M.; Antonescu, C.R.; Fletcher, C.D.M.; Kim, A.; Lazar, A.J.; Quezado, M.M.; Reilly, K.M.; Stemmer-Rachamimov, A.; Stewart, D.R.; Viskochil, D.; et al. Histopathologic Evaluation of Atypical Neurofibromatous Tumors and Their Transformation into Malignant Peripheral Nerve Sheath Tumor in Patients with Neurofibromatosis 1—A Consensus Overview. *Hum. Pathol.* **2017**, *67*, 1–10. [CrossRef]
19. Prudner, B.C.; Ball, T.; Rathore, R.; Hirbe, A.C. Diagnosis and Management of Malignant Peripheral Nerve Sheath Tumors: Current Practice and Future Perspectives. *Neurooncol Adv.* **2020**, *2*, i40–i49. [CrossRef]
20. Miyamoto, K.; Kobayashi, H.; Zhang, L.; Tsuda, Y.; Makise, N.; Yasunaga, Y.; Ikemura, M.; Nakai, Y.; Shibata, E.; Ushiku, T.; et al. Atypical Neurofibromatous Neoplasm with Uncertain Biologic Potential in the Posterior Mediastinum of a Young Patient with Neurofibromatosis Type 1: A Case Report. *Case Rep. Oncol.* **2022**, *15*, 988–994. [CrossRef]
21. González-Muñoz, T.; Kim, A.; Ratner, N.; Peinado, H. The Need for New Treatments Targeting MPNST: The Potential of Strategies Combining MEK Inhibitors with Antiangiogenic Agents. *Clin. Cancer Res.* **2022**, *28*, 3185–3195. [CrossRef] [PubMed]
22. Lucas, C.-H.G.; Gross, A.M.; Romo, C.G.; Dehner, C.A.; Lazar, A.J.; Miettinen, M.; Pekmezci, M.; Quezado, M.; Rodriguez, F.J.; Stemmer-Rachamimov, A.; et al. Consensus Recommendations for an Integrated Diagnostic Approach to Peripheral Nerve Sheath Tumors Arising in the Setting of Neurofibromatosis Type 1. *Neuro Oncol.* **2025**, *27*, 616–624. [CrossRef] [PubMed]
23. Lemberg, K.M.; Wang, J.; Pratilas, C.A. From Genes to -Omics: The Evolving Molecular Landscape of Malignant Peripheral Nerve Sheath Tumor. *Genes* **2020**, *11*, 691. [CrossRef]
24. Porter, D.E.; Prasad, V.; Foster, L.; Dall, G.F.; Birch, R.; Grimer, R.J. Survival in Malignant Peripheral Nerve Sheath Tumours: A Comparison between Sporadic and Neurofibromatosis Type 1-Associated Tumours. *Sarcoma* **2009**, *2009*, 756395. [CrossRef]
25. Cleven, A.H.G.; Sannaa, G.A.A.; Briaire-de Bruijn, I.; Ingram, D.R.; van de Rijn, M.; Rubin, B.P.; de Vries, M.W.; Watson, K.L.; Torres, K.E.; Wang, W.-L.; et al. Loss of H3K27 Tri-Methylation Is a Diagnostic Marker for Malignant Peripheral Nerve Sheath Tumors and an Indicator for an Inferior Survival. *Mod. Pathol.* **2016**, *29*, 582–590. [CrossRef] [PubMed]
26. Lee, W.; Teckie, S.; Wiesner, T.; Ran, L.; Prieto Granada, C.N.; Lin, M.; Zhu, S.; Cao, Z.; Liang, Y.; Sboner, A.; et al. PRC2 Is Recurrently Inactivated through EED or SUZ12 Loss in Malignant Peripheral Nerve Sheath Tumors. *Nat. Genet.* **2014**, *46*, 1227–1232. [CrossRef]
27. Miller, D.T.; Cortés-Ciriano, I.; Pillay, N.; Hirbe, A.C.; Snuderl, M.; Bui, M.M.; Piculell, K.; Al-Ibraheemi, A.; Dickson, B.C.; Hart, J.; et al. Genomics of MPNST (GeM) Consortium: Rationale and Study Design for Multi-Omic Characterization of NF1-Associated and Sporadic MPNSTs. *Genes* **2020**, *11*, 387. [CrossRef]
28. Beert, E.; Brems, H.; Daniëls, B.; De Wever, I.; Van Calenbergh, F.; Schoenaers, J.; Debiec-Rychter, M.; Gevaert, O.; De Raedt, T.; Van Den Bruel, A.; et al. Atypical Neurofibromas in Neurofibromatosis Type 1 Are Premalignant Tumors. *Genes Chromosomes Cancer* **2011**, *50*, 1021–1032. [CrossRef]
29. Carrió, M.; Gel, B.; Terribas, E.; Zucchiatti, A.C.; Moliné, T.; Rosas, I.; Teulé, Á.; Cajal, S.R.Y.; López-Gutiérrez, J.C.; Blanco, I.; et al. Analysis of Intratumor Heterogeneity in Neurofibromatosis Type 1 Plexiform Neurofibromas and Neurofibromas with Atypical Features: Correlating Histological and Genomic Findings. *Hum. Mutat.* **2018**, *39*, 1112–1125. [CrossRef]
30. Pemov, A.; Hansen, N.F.; Sindiri, S.; Patidar, R.; Higham, C.S.; Dombi, E.; Miettinen, M.M.; Fetsch, P.; Brems, H.; Chandrasekharappa, S.C.; et al. Low Mutation Burden and Frequent Loss of CDKN2A/B and SMARCA2, but Not PRC2, Define Premalignant Neurofibromatosis Type 1-Associated Atypical Neurofibromas. *Neuro Oncol.* **2019**, *21*, 981–992. [CrossRef]

31. Rhodes, S.D.; He, Y.; Smith, A.; Jiang, L.; Lu, Q.; Mund, J.; Li, X.; Bessler, W.; Qian, S.; Dyer, W.; et al. Cdkn2a (Arf) Loss Drives NF1-Associated Atypical Neurofibroma and Malignant Transformation. *Hum. Mol. Genet.* **2019**, *28*, 2752–2762. [CrossRef] [PubMed]
32. Kohlmeyer, J.L.; Kaemmer, C.A.; Pulliam, C.; Maharjan, C.K.; Samayoa, A.M.; Major, H.J.; Cornick, K.E.; Knepper-Adrian, V.; Khanna, R.; Sieren, J.C.; et al. RABL6A Is an Essential Driver of MPNSTs That Negatively Regulates the RB1 Pathway and Sensitizes Tumor Cells to CDK4/6 Inhibitors. *Clin. Cancer Res.* **2020**, *26*, 2997–3011. [CrossRef]
33. Kohlmeyer, J.L.; Kaemmer, C.A.; Umesalma, S.; Gourronc, F.A.; Klingelhutz, A.J.; Quelle, D.E. RABL6A Regulates Schwann Cell Senescence in an RB1-Dependent Manner. *Int. J. Mol. Sci.* **2021**, *22*, 5367. [CrossRef]
34. Keng, V.W.; Rahrmann, E.P.; Watson, A.L.; Tschida, B.R.; Moertel, C.L.; Jessen, W.J.; Rizvi, T.A.; Collins, M.H.; Ratner, N.; Largaespada, D.A. *PTEN* and *NF1* Inactivation in Schwann Cells Produces a Severe Phenotype in the Peripheral Nervous System That Promotes the Development and Malignant Progression of Peripheral Nerve Sheath Tumors. *Cancer Res.* **2012**, *72*, 3405–3413. [CrossRef]
35. Thomson, C.S.; Pundavela, J.; Perrino, M.R.; Coover, R.A.; Choi, K.; Chaney, K.E.; Rizvi, T.A.; Largaespada, D.A.; Ratner, N. WNT5A Inhibition Alters the Malignant Peripheral Nerve Sheath Tumor Microenvironment and Enhances Tumor Growth. *Oncogene* **2021**, *40*, 4229–4241. [CrossRef]
36. Legius, E.; Dierick, H.; Wu, R.; Hall, B.K.; Marynen, P.; Cassiman, J.; Glover, T.W. *TP53* Mutations Are Frequent in Malignant NFI Tumors. *Genes Chromosomes Cancer* **1994**, *10*, 250–255. [CrossRef] [PubMed]
37. Peacock, J.D.; Pridgeon, M.G.; Tovar, E.A.; Essenburg, C.J.; Bowman, M.; Madaj, Z.; Koeman, J.; Boguslawski, E.A.; Grit, J.; Dodd, R.D.; et al. Genomic Status of *MET* Potentiates Sensitivity to MET and MEK Inhibition in NF1-Related Malignant Peripheral Nerve Sheath Tumors. *Cancer Res.* **2018**, *78*, 3672–3687. [CrossRef] [PubMed]
38. Torres, K.E.; Liu, J.; Young, E.; Huang, K.-L.; Ghadimi, M.; Lusby, K.; Lazar, A.J.; Lev, D. Expression of 'Drugable' Tyrosine Kinase Receptors in Malignant Peripheral Nerve Sheath Tumour: Potential Molecular Therapeutic Targets for a Chemoresistant Cancer. *Histopathology* **2011**, *59*, 156–159. [CrossRef]
39. Bradford, D.; Kim, A. Current Treatment Options for Malignant Peripheral Nerve Sheath Tumors. *Curr. Treat. Options Oncol.* **2015**, *16*, 12. [CrossRef]
40. Torres, K.E.; Zhu, Q.-S.; Bill, K.; Lopez, G.; Ghadimi, M.P.; Xie, X.; Young, E.D.; Liu, J.; Nguyen, T.; Bolshakov, S.; et al. Activated MET Is a Molecular Prognosticator and Potential Therapeutic Target for Malignant Peripheral Nerve Sheath Tumors. *Clin. Cancer Res.* **2011**, *17*, 3943–3955. [CrossRef]
41. De Raedt, T.; Walton, Z.; Yecies, J.L.; Li, D.; Chen, Y.; Malone, C.F.; Maertens, O.; Jeong, S.M.; Bronson, R.T.; Lebleu, V.; et al. Exploiting Cancer Cell Vulnerabilities to Develop a Combination Therapy for Ras-Driven Tumors. *Cancer Cell* **2011**, *20*, 400–413. [CrossRef] [PubMed]
42. Kao, E.Y.; Wakeman, K.M.; Wu, Y.; Gross, J.M.; Chen, E.Y.; Ricciotti, R.W.; Liu, Y.J.; Mantilla, J.G. Prevalence and Detection of Actionable BRAF V600 and NRAS Q61 Mutations in Malignant Peripheral Nerve Sheath Tumor by Droplet Digital PCR. *Hum. Pathol.* **2022**, *129*, 90–97. [CrossRef]
43. Zhang, M.; Wang, Y.; Jones, S.; Sausen, M.; McMahon, K.; Sharma, R.; Wang, Q.; Belzberg, A.J.; Chaichana, K.; Gallia, G.L.; et al. Somatic Mutations of SUZ12 in Malignant Peripheral Nerve Sheath Tumors. *Nat. Genet.* **2014**, *46*, 1170–1172. [CrossRef]
44. Thangaiah, J.J.; Westling, B.E.; Roden, A.C.; Giannini, C.; Tetzlaff, M.; Cho, W.C.; Folpe, A.L. Loss of Dimethylated H3K27 (H3K27me2) Expression Is Not a Specific Marker of Malignant Peripheral Nerve Sheath Tumor (MPNST): An Immunohistochemical Study of 137 Cases, with Emphasis on MPNST and Melanocytic Tumors. *Ann. Diagn. Pathol.* **2022**, *59*, 151967. [CrossRef]
45. Dehner, C.; Moon, C.I.; Zhang, X.; Zhou, Z.; Miller, C.; Xu, H.; Wan, X.; Yang, K.; Mashl, J.; Gosline, S.J.; et al. Chromosome 8 Gain Is Associated with High-Grade Transformation in MPNST. *JCI Insight* **2021**, *6*, e146351. [CrossRef]
46. Magallón-Lorenz, M.; Fernández-Rodríguez, J.; Terribas, E.; Creus-Batchiller, E.; Romagosa, C.; Estival, A.; Perez Sidelnikova, D.; Salvador, H.; Villanueva, A.; Blanco, I.; et al. Chromosomal Translocations Inactivating CDKN2A Support a Single Path for Malignant Peripheral Nerve Sheath Tumor Initiation. *Hum. Genet.* **2021**, *140*, 1241–1252. [CrossRef]
47. Godec, A.; Jayasinghe, R.; Chrisinger, J.S.A.; Prudner, B.; Ball, T.; Wang, Y.; Srihari, D.; Kaushal, M.; Dietz, H.; Zhang, X.; et al. Whole Exome Sequencing Reveals the Maintained Polyclonal Nature from Primary to Metastatic Malignant Peripheral Nerve Sheath Tumor in Two Patients with NF1. *Neurooncol Adv.* **2020**, *2*, i75–i84. [CrossRef]
48. Hirbe, A.C.; Dahiya, S.; Miller, C.A.; Li, T.; Fulton, R.S.; Zhang, X.; McDonald, S.; DeSchryver, K.; Duncavage, E.J.; Walrath, J.; et al. Whole Exome Sequencing Reveals the Order of Genetic Changes during Malignant Transformation and Metastasis in a Single Patient with NF1-Plexiform Neurofibroma. *Clin. Cancer Res.* **2015**, *21*, 4201–4211. [CrossRef]
49. Brockman, Q.R.; Scherer, A.; McGivney, G.R.; Gutierrez, W.R.; Voigt, A.P.; Isaacson, A.L.; Laverty, E.A.; Roughton, G.; Knepper-Adrian, V.; Darbro, B.; et al. PRC2 Loss Drives MPNST Metastasis and Matrix Remodeling. *JCI Insight* **2022**, *7*, e157502. [CrossRef]

50. Cannizzaro, I.R.; Treccani, M.; Taiani, A.; Ambrosini, E.; Busciglio, S.; Cesarini, S.; Luberto, A.; De Sensi, E.; Moschella, B.; Gismondi, P.; et al. Proof of Concept for Genome Profiling of the Neurofibroma/Sarcoma Sequence in Neurofibromatosis Type 1. *Int. J. Mol. Sci.* **2024**, *25*, 10822. [CrossRef]
51. Tate, J.G.; Bamford, S.; Jubb, H.C.; Sondka, Z.; Beare, D.M.; Bindal, N.; Boutselakis, H.; Cole, C.G.; Creatore, C.; Dawson, E.; et al. COSMIC: The Catalogue Of Somatic Mutations In Cancer. *Nucleic Acids Res.* **2019**, *47*, D941–D947. [CrossRef]
52. McAfee, J.L.; Alban, T.J.; Makarov, V.; Rupani, A.; Parthasarathy, P.B.; Tu, Z.; Ronen, S.; Billings, S.D.; Diaz, C.M.; Chan, T.A.; et al. Genomic Landscape of Superficial Malignant Peripheral Nerve Sheath Tumor. *Lab. Investig.* **2025**, *105*, 102183. [CrossRef]
53. Alexandrov, L.B.; Kim, J.; Haradhvala, N.J.; Huang, M.N.; Tian Ng, A.W.; Wu, Y.; Boot, A.; Covington, K.R.; Gordenin, D.A.; Bergstrom, E.N.; et al. The Repertoire of Mutational Signatures in Human Cancer. *Nature* **2020**, *578*, 94–101. [CrossRef] [PubMed]
54. Håvik, A.L.; Bruland, O.; Miletic, H.; Poulsgaard, L.; Scheie, D.; Fugleholm, K.; Lund-Johansen, M.; Knappskog, P.-M. Genetic Alterations Associated with Malignant Transformation of Sporadic Vestibular Schwannoma. *Acta Neurochir.* **2022**, *164*, 343–352. [CrossRef]
55. Veschetti, L.; Treccani, M.; De Tomi, E.; Malerba, G. Genomic Instability Evolutionary Footprints on Human Health: Driving Forces or Side Effects? *Int. J. Mol. Sci.* **2023**, *24*, 11437. [CrossRef] [PubMed]
56. Mertens, F.; Rydholm, A.; Bauer, H.F.; Limon, J.; Nedoszytko, B.; Szadowska, A.; Willén, H.; Heim, S.; Mitelman, F.; Mandahl, N. Cytogenetic Findings in Malignant Peripheral Nerve Sheath Tumors. *Int. J. Cancer* **1995**, *61*, 793–798. [CrossRef]
57. Schmidt, H.; Taubert, H.; Würl, P.; Bache, M.; Bartel, F.; Holzhausen, H.J.; Hinze, R. Cytogenetic Characterization of Six Malignant Peripheral Nerve Sheath Tumors: Comparison of Karyotyping and Comparative Genomic Hybridization. *Cancer Genet. Cytogenet.* **2001**, *128*, 14–23. [CrossRef]
58. Brohl, A.S.; Kahen, E.; Yoder, S.J.; Teer, J.K.; Reed, D.R. The Genomic Landscape of Malignant Peripheral Nerve Sheath Tumors: Diverse Drivers of Ras Pathway Activation. *Sci. Rep.* **2017**, *7*, 14992. [CrossRef]
59. Banerjee, J.; Allaway, R.J.; Taroni, J.N.; Baker, A.; Zhang, X.; Moon, C.I.; Pratilas, C.A.; Blakeley, J.O.; Guinney, J.; Hirbe, A.; et al. Integrative Analysis Identifies Candidate Tumor Microenvironment and Intracellular Signaling Pathways That Define Tumor Heterogeneity in NF1. *Genes* **2020**, *11*, 226. [CrossRef] [PubMed]
60. Suppiah, S.; Mansouri, S.; Mamatjan, Y.; Liu, J.C.; Bhunia, M.M.; Patil, V.; Rath, P.; Mehani, B.; Heir, P.; Bunda, S.; et al. Multiplatform Molecular Profiling Uncovers Two Subgroups of Malignant Peripheral Nerve Sheath Tumors with Distinct Therapeutic Vulnerabilities. *Nat. Commun.* **2023**, *14*, 2696. [CrossRef]
61. Mitchell, D.K.; Burgess, B.; White, E.E.; Smith, A.E.; Sierra Potchanant, E.A.; Mang, H.; Hickey, B.E.; Lu, Q.; Qian, S.; Bessler, W.; et al. Spatial Gene-Expression Profiling Unveils Immuno-Oncogenic Programs of NF1-Associated Peripheral Nerve Sheath Tumor Progression. *Clin. Cancer Res.* **2024**, *30*, 1038–1053. [CrossRef]
62. Ma, S.; Zhao, Y.; Lee, W.C.; Ong, L.-T.; Lee, P.L.; Jiang, Z.; Oguz, G.; Niu, Z.; Liu, M.; Goh, J.Y.; et al. Hypoxia Induces HIF1α-Dependent Epigenetic Vulnerability in Triple Negative Breast Cancer to Confer Immune Effector Dysfunction and Resistance to Anti-PD-1 Immunotherapy. *Nat. Commun.* **2022**, *13*, 4118. [CrossRef] [PubMed]
63. Moon, C.-I.; Tompkins, W.; Wang, Y.; Godec, A.; Zhang, X.; Pipkorn, P.; Miller, C.A.; Dehner, C.; Dahiya, S.; Hirbe, A.C. Unmasking Intra-Tumoral Heterogeneity and Clonal Evolution in NF1-MPNST. *Genes* **2020**, *11*, 499. [CrossRef]
64. Smith, H.W.; Hirukawa, A.; Sanguin-Gendreau, V.; Nandi, I.; Dufour, C.R.; Zuo, D.; Tandoc, K.; Leibovitch, M.; Singh, S.; Rennhack, J.P.; et al. An ErbB2/c-Src Axis Links Bioenergetics with PRC2 Translation to Drive Epigenetic Reprogramming and Mammary Tumorigenesis. *Nat. Commun.* **2019**, *10*, 2901. [CrossRef]
65. Høland, M.; Berg, K.C.G.; Eilertsen, I.A.; Bjerkehagen, B.; Kolberg, M.; Boye, K.; Lingjærde, O.C.; Guren, T.K.; Mandahl, N.; van den Berg, E.; et al. Transcriptomic Subtyping of Malignant Peripheral Nerve Sheath Tumours Highlights Immune Signatures, Genomic Profiles, Patient Survival and Therapeutic Targets. *EBioMedicine* **2023**, *97*, 104829. [CrossRef]
66. Khosravi, T.; Oladnabi, M. The Role of MiRNAs and LncRNAs in Neurofibromatosis Type 1. *J. Cell Biochem.* **2023**, *124*, 17–30. [CrossRef]
67. Napolitano, F.; Abbadessa, G.; Dell'Aquila, M.; Ravo, M.; Ventola, G.M.; Marchese, G.; Miele, G.; Franzese, G.; De Blasiis, P.; Palomba, N.P.; et al. Serum MiRNAs as Biomarkers in Neurofibromatosis 1: New Promising Findings. *J. Neurol. Sci.* **2025**, *476*, 123643. [CrossRef]
68. Feber, A.; Wilson, G.A.; Zhang, L.; Presneau, N.; Idowu, B.; Down, T.A.; Rakyan, V.K.; Noon, L.A.; Lloyd, A.C.; Stupka, E.; et al. Comparative Methylome Analysis of Benign and Malignant Peripheral Nerve Sheath Tumors. *Genome Res.* **2011**, *21*, 515–524. [CrossRef] [PubMed]
69. Prieto-Granada, C.N.; Wiesner, T.; Messina, J.L.; Jungbluth, A.A.; Chi, P.; Antonescu, C.R. Loss of H3K27me3 Expression Is a Highly Sensitive Marker for Sporadic and Radiation-Induced MPNST. *Am. J. Surg. Pathol.* **2016**, *40*, 479–489. [CrossRef] [PubMed]
70. Pekmezci, M.; Cuevas-Ocampo, A.K.; Perry, A.; Horvai, A.E. Significance of H3K27me3 Loss in the Diagnosis of Malignant Peripheral Nerve Sheath Tumors. *Mod. Pathol.* **2017**, *30*, 1710–1719. [CrossRef] [PubMed]

71. Brockman, Q.R.; Rytlewski, J.D.; Milhem, M.; Monga, V.; Dodd, R.D. Integrated Epigenetic and Transcriptomic Analysis Identifies Interleukin 17 DNA Methylation Signature of Malignant Peripheral Nerve Sheath Tumor Progression and Metastasis. *JCO Precis. Oncol.* **2024**, *8*, e2300325. [CrossRef]
72. Isfort, I.; Elges, S.; Cyra, M.; Berthold, R.; Renner, M.; Mechtersheimer, G.; Åman, P.; Larsson, O.; Ratner, N.; Hafner, S.; et al. Prevalence of the Hippo Effectors YAP1/TAZ in Tumors of Soft Tissue and Bone. *Sci. Rep.* **2019**, *9*, 19704. [CrossRef]
73. Huang, P.-Y.; Shih, I.-A.; Liao, Y.-C.; You, H.-L.; Lee, M.-J. A Novel HDAC11 Inhibitor Potentiates the Tumoricidal Effects of Cordycepin against Malignant Peripheral Nerve Sheath Tumor through the Hippo Signaling Pathway. *Am. J. Cancer Res.* **2022**, *12*, 873–892.
74. Wu, L.M.N.; Deng, Y.; Wang, J.; Zhao, C.; Wang, J.; Rao, R.; Xu, L.; Zhou, W.; Choi, K.; Rizvi, T.A.; et al. Programming of Schwann Cells by Lats1/2-TAZ/YAP Signaling Drives Malignant Peripheral Nerve Sheath Tumorigenesis. *Cancer Cell* **2018**, *33*, 292–308.e7. [CrossRef] [PubMed]
75. Danielsen, S.A.; Lind, G.E.; Kolberg, M.; Høland, M.; Bjerkehagen, B.; Sundby Hall, K.; van den Berg, E.; Mertens, F.; Smeland, S.; Picci, P.; et al. Methylated RASSF1A in Malignant Peripheral Nerve Sheath Tumors Identifies Neurofibromatosis Type 1 Patients with Inferior Prognosis. *Neuro Oncol.* **2015**, *17*, 63–69. [CrossRef] [PubMed]
76. Gosline, S.J.C.; Weinberg, H.; Knight, P.; Yu, T.; Guo, X.; Prasad, N.; Jones, A.; Shrestha, S.; Boone, B.; Levy, S.E.; et al. A High-Throughput Molecular Data Resource for Cutaneous Neurofibromas. *Sci. Data* **2017**, *4*, 170045. [CrossRef]
77. Ferrer, M.; Gosline, S.J.C.; Stathis, M.; Zhang, X.; Guo, X.; Guha, R.; Ryman, D.A.; Wallace, M.R.; Kasch-Semenza, L.; Hao, H.; et al. Pharmacological and Genomic Profiling of Neurofibromatosis Type 1 Plexiform Neurofibroma-Derived Schwann Cells. *Sci. Data* **2018**, *5*, 180106. [CrossRef]
78. Kresbach, C.; Dottermusch, M.; Eckhardt, A.; Ristow, I.; Paplomatas, P.; Altendorf, L.; Wefers, A.K.; Bockmayr, M.; Belakhoua, S.; Tran, I.; et al. Atypical Neurofibromas Reveal Distinct Epigenetic Features with Proximity to Benign Peripheral Nerve Sheath Tumor Entities. *Neuro Oncol.* **2023**, *25*, 1644–1655. [CrossRef] [PubMed]
79. Szymanski, J.J.; Sundby, R.T.; Jones, P.A.; Srihari, D.; Earland, N.; Harris, P.K.; Feng, W.; Qaium, F.; Lei, H.; Roberts, D.; et al. Cell-Free DNA Ultra-Low-Pass Whole Genome Sequencing to Distinguish Malignant Peripheral Nerve Sheath Tumor (MPNST) from Its Benign Precursor Lesion: A Cross-Sectional Study. *PLoS Med.* **2021**, *18*, e1003734. [CrossRef]
80. Mattox, A.K.; Douville, C.; Silliman, N.; Ptak, J.; Dobbyn, L.; Schaefer, J.; Popoli, M.; Blair, C.; Judge, K.; Pollard, K.; et al. Detection of Malignant Peripheral Nerve Sheath Tumors in Patients with Neurofibromatosis Using Aneuploidy and Mutation Identification in Plasma. *Elife* **2022**, *11*, e74238. [CrossRef]
81. Mantripragada, K.K.; de Ståhl, T.D.; Patridge, C.; Menzel, U.; Andersson, R.; Chuzhanova, N.; Kluwe, L.; Guha, A.; Mautner, V.; Dumanski, J.P.; et al. Genome-wide High-resolution Analysis of DNA Copy Number Alterations in NF1-associated Malignant Peripheral Nerve Sheath Tumors Using 32K BAC Array. *Genes Chromosomes Cancer* **2009**, *48*, 897–907. [CrossRef]
82. Sundby, R.T.; Szymanski, J.J.; Pan, A.C.; Jones, P.A.; Mahmood, S.Z.; Reid, O.H.; Srihari, D.; Armstrong, A.E.; Chamberlain, S.; Burgic, S.; et al. Early Detection of Malignant and Premalignant Peripheral Nerve Tumors Using Cell-Free DNA Fragmentomics. *Clin. Cancer Res.* **2024**, *30*, 4363–4376. [CrossRef] [PubMed]
83. Patrizi, S.; Miele, E.; Falcone, L.; Vallese, S.; Rossi, S.; Barresi, S.; Giovannoni, I.; Pedace, L.; Nardini, C.; Masier, I.; et al. Malignant Peripheral Nerve Sheath Tumor (MPNST) and MPNST-like Entities Are Defined by a Specific DNA Methylation Profile in Pediatric and Juvenile Population. *Clin. Epigenetics* **2024**, *16*, 9. [CrossRef]
84. Mantripragada, K.K.; Spurlock, G.; Kluwe, L.; Chuzhanova, N.; Ferner, R.E.; Frayling, I.M.; Dumanski, J.P.; Guha, A.; Mautner, V.; Upadhyaya, M. High-Resolution DNA Copy Number Profiling of Malignant Peripheral Nerve Sheath Tumors Using Targeted Microarray-Based Comparative Genomic Hybridization. *Clin. Cancer Res.* **2008**, *14*, 1015–1024. [CrossRef]
85. Verdijk, R.M.; den Bakker, M.A.; Dubbink, H.J.; Hop, W.C.J.; Dinjens, W.N.M.; Kros, J.M. *TP53* Mutation Analysis of Malignant Peripheral Nerve Sheath Tumors. *J. Neuropathol. Exp. Neurol.* **2010**, *69*, 16–26. [CrossRef]
86. Sohier, P.; Luscan, A.; Lloyd, A.; Ashelford, K.; Laurendeau, I.; Briand-Suleau, A.; Vidaud, D.; Ortonne, N.; Pasmant, E.; Upadhyaya, M. Confirmation of Mutation Landscape of NF1-associated Malignant Peripheral Nerve Sheath Tumors. *Genes Chromosomes Cancer* **2017**, *56*, 421–426. [CrossRef]
87. Jones, J.; Cain, S.; Pesic-Smith, J.; Choong, P.F.M.; Morokoff, A.P.; Drummond, K.J.; Dabscheck, G. Circulating Tumor DNA for Malignant Peripheral Nerve Sheath Tumors in Neurofibromatosis Type 1. *J. Neurooncol* **2021**, *154*, 265–274. [CrossRef]
88. Tomczak, K.; Patel, M.S.; Bhalla, A.D.; Peterson, C.B.; Landers, S.M.; Callahan, S.C.; Zhang, D.; Wong, J.; Landry, J.P.; Lazar, A.J.; et al. Plasma DNA Methylation-Based Biomarkers for MPNST Detection in Patients With Neurofibromatosis Type 1. *Mol. Carcinog.* **2025**, *64*, 44–56. [CrossRef] [PubMed]
89. Loy, C.; Ahmann, L.; De Vlaminck, I.; Gu, W. Liquid Biopsy Based on Cell-Free DNA and RNA. *Annu. Rev. Biomed. Eng.* **2024**, *26*, 169–195. [CrossRef]
90. Hussen, B.M.; Hidayat, H.J.; Salihi, A.; Sabir, D.K.; Taheri, M.; Ghafouri-Fard, S. MicroRNA: A Signature for Cancer Progression. *Biomed. Pharmacother.* **2021**, *138*, 111528. [CrossRef] [PubMed]

91. Guo, J.; Chaney, K.E.; Choi, K.; Witek, G.; Patel, A.V.; Xie, H.; Lin, D.; Whig, K.; Xiong, Y.; Schultz, D.C.; et al. Polo-like Kinase 1 as a Therapeutic Target for Malignant Peripheral Nerve Sheath Tumors (MPNST) and Schwannomas. *Am. J. Cancer Res.* **2020**, *10*, 856–869.
92. Allaway, R.J.; La Rosa, S.; Verma, S.; Mangravite, L.; Guinney, J.; Blakeley, J.; Bakker, A.; Gosline, S.J.C. Engaging a Community to Enable Disease-Centric Data Sharing with the NF Data Portal. *Sci. Data* **2019**, *6*, 319. [CrossRef]
93. Allaway, R.; Angus, S.P.; Beauchamp, R.L.; Blakeley, J.O.; Bott, M.; Burns, S.S.; Carlstedt, A.; Chang, L.-S.; Chen, X.; Clapp, D.W.; et al. Traditional and Systems Biology Based Drug Discovery for the Rare Tumor Syndrome Neurofibromatosis Type 2. *PLoS ONE* **2018**, *13*, e0197350. [CrossRef]
94. Heath, A.P.; Ferretti, V.; Agrawal, S.; An, M.; Angelakos, J.C.; Arya, R.; Bajari, R.; Baqar, B.; Barnowski, J.H.B.; Burt, J.; et al. The NCI Genomic Data Commons. *Nat. Genet.* **2021**, *53*, 257–262. [CrossRef]
95. Synapse. NF Data Portal. Available online: https://nf.synapse.org/ (accessed on 27 November 2025).
96. Angus, S.P.; Oblinger, J.L.; Stuhlmiller, T.J.; DeSouza, P.A.; Beauchamp, R.L.; Witt, L.; Chen, X.; Jordan, J.T.; Gilbert, T.S.K.; Stemmer-Rachamimov, A.; et al. EPH Receptor Signaling as a Novel Therapeutic Target in NF2-Deficient Meningioma. *Neuro Oncol.* **2018**, *20*, 1185–1196. [CrossRef]
97. Weinstein, J.N.; Collisson, E.A.; Mills, G.B.; Shaw, K.R.M.; Ozenberger, B.A.; Ellrott, K.; Shmulevich, I.; Sander, C.; Stuart, J.M. The Cancer Genome Atlas Pan-Cancer Analysis Project. *Nat. Genet.* **2013**, *45*, 1113–1120. [CrossRef] [PubMed]
98. Pollard, K.; Banerjee, J.; Doan, X.; Wang, J.; Guo, X.; Allaway, R.; Langmead, S.; Slobogean, B.; Meyer, C.F.; Loeb, D.M.; et al. A Clinically and Genomically Annotated Nerve Sheath Tumor Biospecimen Repository. *Sci. Data* **2020**, *7*, 184. [CrossRef] [PubMed]
99. Banerjee, J.; Lyu, Y.; Makri, S.C.; Scott, A.J.; Zhang, L.; Calizo, A.; Pollard, K.; Yang, K.; Gross, J.M.; Lucas, C.-H.G.; et al. Integrated Genomic Analysis of NF1-Associated Peripheral Nerve Sheath Tumors: An Updated Biorepository Dataset. *Sci. Data* **2025**, *12*, 1229. [CrossRef] [PubMed]

cancers

MDPI

Article

The RXR Agonist MSU-42011 Reduces Tumor Burden in a Murine Preclinical NF1-Deficient Model

Pei-Yu Hung [1], Jessica A. Moerland [2,3], Ana S. Leal [4,*], Bilal Aleiwi [3], Edmund Ellsworth [3], D. Wade Clapp [2,5,6,7], Verena Staedtke [8], Renyuan Bai [9,10] and Karen T. Liby [3,4]

1 Department of Physiology, Michigan State University, East Lansing, MI 48824, USA; hungpeiy@msu.edu
2 Department of Pediatrics and Herman B Wells Center for Pediatric Research, Indiana University School of Medicine, Indianapolis, IN 46202, USA; jamoerla@iu.edu (J.A.M.); dclapp@iu.edu (D.W.C.)
3 Department of Pharmacology and Toxicology, Michigan State University, East Lansing, MI 48824, USA; aleiwibi@msu.edu (B.A.); ellswo59@msu.edu (E.E.); ktliby@iu.edu (K.T.L.)
4 Department of Medicine, Divisions of Hematology/Oncology, Indiana University School of Medicine, Indianapolis, IN 46202, USA
5 Department of Microbiology and Immunology, Indiana University School of Medicine, Indianapolis, IN 46202, USA
6 Department of Biochemistry and Molecular Biology, Indiana University School of Medicine, Indianapolis, IN 46202, USA
7 Department of Medical and Molecular Genetics, Indiana University School of Medicine, Indianapolis, IN 46202, USA
8 Department of Neurology, Johns Hopkins University, Baltimore, MD 21287, USA; vstaedt1@jhmi.edu
9 Kennedy Krieger Institute, Baltimore, MD 21205, USA; rbai1@jhmi.edu
10 Department of Neurosurgery, Johns Hopkins University, Baltimore, MD 21287, USA
* Correspondence: anmendes@iu.edu

Simple Summary: Neurofibromatosis type 1 (NF1) is a genetic disorder that leads to the formation of plexiform neurofibromas (PNFs), which can progress to malignant peripheral nerve sheath tumors (MPNSTs), a major cause of death in individuals with NF1. Current treatments, like the MEK inhibitor selumetinib, are limited to PNFs and have significant side effects, highlighting the urgent need for more effective therapies. Our research identified MSU-42011, a retinoid X receptor (RXR) agonist, as a promising candidate in preclinical NF1-deficient models. MSU-42011 reduced tumor growth, pERK levels, and tumor-promoting immune cells, while increasing activated T cells; further tumor reduction was observed when combined with selumetinib. The combination therapy also suppressed pro-tumor cytokine signaling, suggesting potential for immune modulation. These findings highlight RXR agonists as an effective therapeutic strategy for NF1, with combination therapy offering a promising treatment option.

Abstract: Background/Objectives: Neurofibromatosis type 1 (NF1) is a prevalent inherited disorder, with approximately 50% of affected individuals developing plexiform neurofibromas (PNFs), which can progress to highly aggressive malignant peripheral nerve sheath tumors (MPNSTs). While selumetinib is FDA-approved for PNFs, its efficacy in MPNSTs is limited and associated with dose-limiting toxicities. *NF1* deficiency drives tumorigenesis and alters immune dynamics via RAS hyperactivation. Given the substantial macrophage infiltration in NF1 lesions and its association with disease progression, we hypothesized that targeting tumor-promoting immune cells with the retinoid X receptor (RXR) agonist MSU-42011 could be an alternative therapeutic strategy, as it has shown promise in KRAS-driven cancers by decreasing pERK levels and reducing tumor-promoting immune cells. **Methods:** We examined the effects of MSU-42011 and selumetinib, alone and in combination, on NF1-deficient cells and in a syngeneic MPNST model. **Results:** In vivo, the combination of MSU-42011 and selumetinib significantly reduced tumor growth, pERK

https://doi.org/10.3390/cancers17121920

levels, and tumor-promoting macrophages and increased activated CD8+ T cells in syngeneic MPNST models. In NF1-deficient cells, MSU-42011 or selumetinib reduced pERK levels, with combination treatment achieving greater reductions. Conditioned media (CM) from NF1-deficient cells increased the protein and mRNA levels of several cytokines and chemokines in human THP1 cells and bone marrow-derived macrophages (BMDMs). MSU-42011 and selumetinib, alone or in combination, partially reversed this induction. **Conclusions:** These findings suggest RXR agonists may have therapeutic potential against NF1, and their combination with MEK inhibitors could represent a promising strategy for NF1-associated tumors. Further studies are needed to validate these results and assess their translational relevance.

Keywords: neurofibromatosis type 1; plexiform neurofibromas (PNFs); malignant peripheral nerve sheath tumors (MPNSTs); retinoid X receptor (RXR) agonist; selumetinib

1. Introduction

Neurofibromatosis type 1 (NF1) is an autosomal dominant genetic disease with an incidence of 1 in 3000 individuals [1]. It is caused by germline mutations of the *NF1* tumor suppressor gene, which encodes neurofibromin, a GTPase-activating protein (GAP) for p21RAS [2–4]. Loss of *NF1* results in a hyperactive RAS signaling pathway and its downstream cascades, including the MAPK pathway (RAF/MEK/ERK), which promotes abnormal cell proliferation and neoplasia [2–4]. Plexiform neurofibromas (PNFs), a hallmark manifestation of *NF1* loss, are benign nerve and soft tissue tumors that develop in about 20–50% of patients [5]. These tumors can arise in various locations, including the eyes and skin. While these lesions are typically not medically serious, PNFs can significantly impact the patient's quality of life due to disfigurement, pain, and functional impairment [6]. Although PNFs are among the most recognizable features of NF1, more clinically severe tumors in neurofibromatosis include trigeminal and vestibular schwannomas, as well as high-grade IDH-mutant astrocytomas in the posterior cranial fossa. These tumors present major therapeutic challenges due to their complex locations and risk of neurological deficits, as highlighted in a recent clinical series emphasizing long-term functional outcomes and recurrence risks following surgical and multimodal interventions [7,8]. Additionally, about 10% of PNFs can progress to highly aggressive malignant peripheral nerve sheath tumors (MPNSTs), a leading cause of death in patients with *NF1* loss [5]. Currently, no effective drugs are available to treat MPNSTs; moreover, these tumors respond poorly to chemotherapy and exhibit high rates of recurrence [9,10]. Consequently, the prognosis for patients with MPNST remains poor, with a 5-year survival rate of approximately 20% to 50% [11,12]. The malignant transformation of PNF often occurs through intermediate lesions known as atypical neurofibroma or atypical neurofibromatous neoplasms of uncertain biological potential (ANF/ANNUBP), which are characterized by distinct histopathologic features and *CDKN2A* copy number loss, serving as a critical transition step between PNFs and MPNSTs [13,14]. While surgical resection can partially remove tumors, complete resection is rarely possible due to the infiltrative nature of these tumors [9].

Currently, selumetinib is an FDA-approved MEK1/2 inhibitor for treating symptomatic, inoperable PNF in pediatric patients with NF1 [15]. Oral administration of selumetinib inhibits ERK phosphorylation and reduces the number, volume, and proliferation of PNFs [16,17]. However, some patients either do not respond to MEK inhibitor monotherapy, including selumetinib, binimetinib, and trametinib [18–20], or eventually develop MPNST within a few months of treatment, indicating that MEK inhibitor monotherapy may be insufficient to prevent malignant transformation [21]. Moreover, selumetinib has toxic effects, including acneiform rash, gastrointestinal disturbance, and asymptomatic creatine kinase elevation [16]. As such, there remains an unmet need for new NF1 treatment strategies that bypass resistance or reduce toxicity.

Deficiency of the *NF1* gene not only promotes tumorigenesis but also has broad effects on the immune cells and cytokine signaling driven by the hyperactive RAS signaling pathway [22–24]. Although immune cells are rare in healthy peripheral nerves, up to 30% of the cells in PNF and 50% of the cells in MPNST are macrophages [24], with macrophage recruitment correlating with disease progression [25,26]. These neurofibroma-associated macrophages play a key role in shaping the tumor microenvironment (TME) by recruiting T cells and other immune cells, contributing to an immunosuppressive milieu [24]. While the direct role of T cells in neurofibromatosis has yet to be fully explored, recent studies demonstrate that T cells are important for sustaining macrophage recruitment within the TME, promoting NF1 tumor initiation and growth [27]. Preclinical studies have shown that the combination of cyclin-dependent kinase 4/6 (CDK4/6) and MEK inhibitors can improve the responsiveness of MPNST to anti-PD-L1 immune checkpoint blockade (ICB) [28]. And several clinical trials of ICB in MPNSTS are currently underway, including a phase I study (NCT04465643) assessing the use of neoadjuvant nivolumab (PD-1 inhibitor) in combination with ipilimumab (CTLA-4 inhibitor) in patients with newly diagnosed ANNUBP and MPNST. These studies demonstrate the potential of immunotherapy in a subset of NF1-associated MPNSTs, and the combination treatment offers a promising approach to address some of these gaps, providing more effective and comprehensive solutions compared to existing therapies.

Several retinoid X receptor (RXR) agonists modulate immune cells in the TME and reduce tumor growth in *Kras*-mutated cancers [29,30]. As with *NF1* mutations [23,24], *KRAS* mutations increase tumor-promoting immune cell function in the TME [31,32], which suggests these compounds offer a promising new therapeutic strategy for PNF and MPNST [33]. RXR agonists are ligands that bind to and activate retinoid X receptors. Upon binding, RXR dimerizes with various receptors, acting as transcription factors for genes involved in several biological processes, including immune regulation [34]. In a carcinogenesis-induced Kras-driven lung cancer, the novel RXR agonist MSU-42011 decreased tumor burden by reducing tumor-promoting $CD206^+$ macrophages, immunosuppressive CD4-FOXP3 (Tregs), which led to increasing activated cytotoxic T cells [29]. Furthermore, MSU-42011 decreased pERK levels within the lung tumors [29]. The immunomodulatory and anti-tumor effects of MSU-42011 were also found in a $HER2^+$ breast cancer model [29]. Despite the efficacy of RXR agonists for the reduction of tumor-promoting immune cells in the TME and inhibition of tumor progression [29,30,33,35], no RXR agonist has been directly tested in clinical trials or preclinical studies for PNFs or MPNSTs. Due to the similarities between NF1- and Kras-driven cancers, including a hyperactive RAS signaling pathway and aberrant inflammatory signaling, we tested MSU-42011 in relevant preclinical models of NF1.

In this study, we assessed the effects of MSU-42011, selumetinib, and combinations using in vitro, ex vivo, and in vivo models of NF1. In murine and human NF1-deficient cells, combination treatment with MSU-42011 and selumetinib decreased pERK levels. It also partially inhibited the elevated cytokine and chemokine levels in macrophages treated with conditioned media (CM) from NF1-deficient cells. Moreover, in an immunocompetent mouse model of MPNST, the combination treatment of MSU-42011 and selumetinib reduced pERK levels, $CD206^+$ cells, and tumor growth, further than single treatments. These data demonstrate the immunomodulatory and anti-tumor effects of MSU-42011 alone or in combination with selumetinib and support their potential use as a combination therapy for the treatment of PNFs and MPNSTs in patients with NF1.

2. Materials and Methods

2.1. Drugs

MSU-42011 was synthesized (>95% purity) as described [30]. Selumetinib (>99% purity) and bexarotene (>99% purity) were purchased from LC Laboratories (Woburn, MA, USA).

2.2. Cell Culture

2.2.1. Culture of Human Immortalized NF1$^{-/-}$ Schwann Cells, Murine Nf1-Related MPNSTs, and Murine Lewis Lung Carcinoma Cells (LL2)

Human immortalized normal Schwann cells (ipn02.3 2λ), non-tumor Schwann cells with *NF1* mutation (ipnNF95.11c) and PNF cells (ipNF95.11bC and ipNF95.6), and murine LL2 lung cancer cells, a Kras/Nras mutant lung cancer model [36], were purchased from ATCC (Manassas, VA, USA). The human immortalized NF1$^{-/-}$ Schwann cells were used in the preclinical evaluation of targeted therapies for NF1-associated PNF, including selumetinib [37,38]. Primary murine Nf1-related MPNSTs from a *cis* Nf1;Tp53 C57BL/6 mice were provided by Verena Staedtke and Renyuan Bai lab (Baltimore, MD, USA) [39]. The addition of heterozygous Tp53 knockout accelerates cancer development, mimicking mutations required for malignant transformation, and has been used to study Nf1-related MPNSTs [39]. Cells were cultured at 37 °C and 5% CO_2 in DMEM media (Corning Cellgro, Manassas, VA, USA) containing FBS (10%, Corning Cellgro) and penicillin/streptomycin (1%, Corning Cellgro). Trypsin-EDTA (0.25%, Corning Cellgro) was used to dissociate cells for passaging upon reaching confluence.

2.2.2. Culture of Primary Murine Nf1 Cdkn2a$^{-/-}$ and Nf1$^{-/-}$ DNSCs

Primary murine dorsal root ganglia (DRG)/neurosphere cells (DNSCs) isolated from Nf1$^{flox/flox}$ and Nf1$^{flox/flox}$ Cdkn2a$^{flox/flox}$ genotypes were obtained from Wade Clapp lab (Indianapolis, IN, USA) [13,40]. These cells contain the neural crest-derived tumorigenic cell of origin for PNFs [41] and have been used in multiple studies modeling PNF initiation, malignant progression, and the molecular mechanisms driving NF1-related tumorigenesis [13,40]. Cells were cultured at 37 °C and 5% CO_2 in DNSC complete media. DNSC complete media was made with serum-free DMEM/F12 media (Gibco) containing HEPES (1 M, Gibco, Grand Island, NY, USA), heparin (0.2%, StemCell, Vancouver, BC, Canada), glucose (30%, Sigma, St. Louis, MO, USA), sodium bicarbonate (7.5%, Gibco), N2 supplement (1%, Gibco), glutamine (1%, Gibco), sodium pyruvate (1%, Gibco), B27 (without vitamin A, 2%, Gibco), epidermal growth factor (20 ng/mL, Sigma), basic fibroblast growth factor (40 ng/mL, PeproTech, Cranbury, NJ, USA), penicillin/streptomycin (1%, Corning Cellgro), and amphotericin B/fungizone (1 µg/mL, Gibco). Nf1$^{flox/flox}$ DNSCs were transiently infected with a GFP-Cre adenovirus (1:500, University of Iowa) for 24 h to delete the Nf1 floxed alleles (served as PNF precursor; Nf1$^{f/f}$ Cre+) or GFP adenovirus (1:500, University of Iowa, Iowa City, IA, USA) as a control (DNSC without *Nf1* mutation; Nf1$^{f/f}$ Cre-). Fluorescence microscopy was used to observe the efficiency of virus transduction (Figure S1A). Efficient Cre-mediated excision of floxed Nf1 alleles and the corresponding loss of neurofibromin expression were confirmed by Western blot (Figure S1B). Unlike Nf1$^{flox/flox}$ DNSCs, Nf1$^{flox/flox}$ Cdkn2a$^{flox/flox}$ DNSCs were already infected with Cre recombinase (served as MPNST precursors) and confirmed by polymerase chain reaction (PCR) in the Clapp lab before we obtained the cells [13]. TrypLE express enzyme (1×, Gibco) was used to dissociate cells for passaging upon reaching confluence.

2.2.3. Culture and Differentiation of Human THP1 Cells and BMDMs

A human THP1 monocyte was purchased from ATCC. Bone marrow-derived macrophages (BMDMs) were isolated from C57BL/6 mice. THP1 and BMDMs were cultured at 37 °C and 5% CO_2 in DMEM media (Corning Cellgro) containing FBS (10%, Corning Cellgro) and penicillin/streptomycin (1%, Corning Cellgro). THP1 monocytes were treated with PMA (phorbol 12-myristate 13-acetate; 50 ng/mL, Sigma) for 3 days to differentiate into THP1 macrophages. BMDMs were differentiated with M-CSF (macrophage colony-stimulating factor; 20 ng/mL, Sigma) for 5 days.

2.3. Conditioned Medium (CM) Collection

Cells were seeded at the following optimized densities: human immortalized NF1$^{-/-}$ Schwann cells (5×10^5/mL), primary murine Nf1$^{-/-}$ DNSCs (5×10^5/mL), and human THP1 cells (1×10^6/mL) in DMEM media with 1% FBS. After 24 h, the media was collected, centrifuged at 1500 rpm for 10 min, and the supernatant was removed for experimental treatment.

2.4. Cytokine Production

Culture supernatants from BMDMs treated with 50% CM from primary murine Nf1$^{-/-}$ DNSCs for 24 h were collected and analyzed using the ProcartaPlex™ Mouse Immune Monitoring Panel (48plex, EPX480-20834-901, Thermo Fisher Scientific, Grand Island, NY, USA), following the manufacture protocol. Samples were measured by Luminex 200 (Luminex Corporation, Austin, TX, USA), and data analysis was performed using the ProcartaPlex Analysis App (Thermo Fisher Scientific). To account for cytokines present in the CM, parallel control CM from Nf1$^{-/-}$ DNSCs were incubated without BMDMs for the same duration and analyzed. Baseline cytokine levels were subtracted from the CM samples that had been incubated with BMDMs, and data were further normalized to CM-untreated BMDMs (treated with standard media) to ensure changes reflected macrophage activation.

Culture supernatants from human THP1 cells treated with 50% CM from human immortalized NF1$^{-/-}$ Schwann cells for 24 h were collected and analyzed using human IL-6 ELISA Kit (KHC0061, Thermo Fisher Scientific), human TNFα ELISA Kit (KAC1751, Thermo Fisher Scientific), and human CCL2 (MCP-1) ELISA Kit (BMS281, Thermo Fisher Scientific), following the manufacture protocol. Samples were measured using a VersaMax Microplate Reader (Molecular Devices, San Jose, CA, USA). Absorbance was read at 450 nm, and data analysis was performed using SoftMax Pro 5.4.1 software (Molecular Devices). For these experiments, control CM incubated without THP1 cells was similarly processed and subtracted to account for baseline cytokine levels.

2.5. Western Blot

Treated cells were lysed in RIPA buffer (1 M Tris-Cl, pH 7.4, 0.5 M EDTA, 5 M NaCl, 1% triton-X, 25 mM sodium deoxycholate, 0.1% SDS) with protease inhibitors (1% PMSF, 0.5% apoprotein, 0.1% leupeptin). xTractor Buffer (Takara Bio, San Jose, CA, USA) was used to extract high-molecular-weight proteins, such as NF1, using the same protease inhibitors described above. Lysis buffer was added to each sample, followed by sonication and vortexing three times and centrifugation for 10 min at 13,000 rpm. Protein concentrations of the supernatants were determined using a BCA assay (Sigma). Isolated proteins were fractionated using 10% SDS-PAGE gels or 4–20% precast polyacrylamide gels (Bio-Rad, Hercules, CA, USA) and transferred to polyvinylidene difluoride (PVDF) membranes. Membranes were incubated with pERK (RRID:AB_2315112), ERK (RRID:AB_330744), and vinculin (RRID:AB_2728768) (1:1000, all from Cell Signaling, Danvers, MA, USA), NF1 (1:1000, Abcam, Cambridge, MA, USA, RRID:AB_444142), and GAPDH (1:2000, Santa Cruz, Dallas,

TX, USA, RRID:AB_627678) primary antibodies. Following incubation with the appropriate anti-rabbit or anti-mouse secondary antibodies conjugated to HRP (Cell Signaling), a signal was detected using the ECL Western Blotting Substrate (GE Healthcare, Chicago, IL, USA), and protein levels were quantified using ImageJ 5.2 (NIH, RRID:SCR_003070) and statistically analyzed using GraphPad Prism v10 (RRID:SCR_002798).

2.6. Cell Viability

Human immortalized NF1$^{-/-}$ Schwann cells and primary murine Nf1$^{-/-}$ DNSCs were plated at a density of 1500 cells per well in 96-well plates and allowed to adhere overnight. The following day, cells were treated with increasing concentrations of drugs (0–1000 nM selumetinib, 0–2000 nM MSU-42011, or the combination) or 200 nM MSU-42011, 50 nM selumetinib, and the combination with or without 50% CM from human THP1 cells. At 72 h post-treatment, 50 µL MTT (3-[4,5-dimethylthiazol-2-yl]-2,5-diphenyltetrazolium bromide; Sigma) was added, and plates were incubated at 37 °C for approximately 4 h. Supernatant was then removed, and 100 µL developing solution (0.04 N HCl in isopropanol) was added. Samples were measured by a VersaMax Microplate Reader (Molecular Devices). Absorbance was read at 570 nm, and data analysis was performed using SoftMax Pro 5.4.1 software (Molecular Devices).

2.7. Real Time-PCR

Flash-frozen tumors were processed for total RNA extraction using the RNeasy Mini Kit (Qiagen, Germantown, MD, USA), and RNA from treated cells was isolated with TRIzol (Invitrogen, Waltham, MA, USA), both per the manufacturer's instructions. RNA purity and quality were assessed by Nanodrop. Two micrograms of RNA were reverse transcribed to cDNA with the High-Capacity cDNA Reverse Transcription Kit (Thermo Fisher Scientific), following optimized thermal cycling conditions (10 min at 25 °C, 2 h at 37 °C, 5 min at 85 °C, and storage at 4 °C). For real-time PCR, the Fast SYBR™ Green Master Mix (Thermo Fisher Scientific) was used with template cDNA and optimized forward and reverse primers ordered from IDT (Supplemental Table S1). The QuantStudio 7 Flex Real-Time PCR system (Thermo Fisher Scientific) was used with the optimized qPCR conditions (20 s at 95 °C, followed by 40 cycles of 1 s at 95 °C and 20 s at 60 °C, with a final step of 1 s at 95 °C, 20 s at 60 °C, and 1 s at 95 °C). Fold change in mRNA expression was quantified using the $^{\Delta\Delta}$Ct method, normalized to the control as indicated in the respective figure legends.

2.8. In Vivo Experiments

Murine LL2 lung cancer cells (1×10^6 cells/mouse) or murine Nf1-related MPNST cells (3×10^5 cells/mouse) were injected into the flank of male and female C57BL/6 mice. Mice were age-matched (7–8 weeks old, average weight 20–25 g) and excluded if they exhibited signs of illness or abnormal physiology before tumor implantation. Once the tumors reached 3–4 mm in diameter, mice were randomized into groups and treated as indicated in the respective figure legends. Dosing solutions for treatment were prepared on the first day of dosing. The test substances were dissolved in a mixture of DMSO (10%), Cremophor (10%), and PBS (80%) and administered via intraperitoneal injection. The required volume of vehicle or drug solution for each mouse was calculated based on the most recent individual body weight. Tumors were measured by calipers twice per week (LL2) or every two days (MPNST), and body weight was measured once per week to monitor tumor growth and toxicity during the treatment period. At the time of necropsy, mice were euthanized using carbon dioxide. Tumors were harvested, weighed, and divided into two pieces. One piece was fixed in formalin for immunohistochemical analysis, while the other was flash-frozen and stored for RT-PCR. Blood samples were collected by cardiac puncture into tubes containing heparin as an anticoagulant and centrifuged at 5000 rpm for 5 min to separate plasma for triglyceride assay. To minimize bias, investigators were blinded to the treatment groups during data collection and analysis.

2.9. Immunohistochemistry

Harvested tumors were fixed in 10% phosphate-buffered formalin for at least 48 h, embedded in paraffin blocks, and sectioned. Endogenous peroxidase activity was quenched using hydrogen peroxide. Sections were then immunostained with antibodies against CD206 (1:200, Abcam, RRID:AB_1523910), FOXP3 (1:50, Cell Signaling, RRID:AB_2797979), and pERK (1:50, Cell Signaling, RRID:AB_2315112) and visualized with biotinylated anti-rabbit secondary antibodies (Cell Signaling). A signal was detected using a DAB substrate (Cell Signaling), following the manufacturer's recommendations. Sections were counterstained with hematoxylin (Vector Labs, Burlingame, CA, USA). The positive staining signals were quantified using ImageJ 5.2 (NIH, RRID:SCR_003070), and the data were statistically analyzed with GraphPad Prism v10 (RRID:SCR_002798).

2.10. Flow Cytometry

Flank tumors and spleens were harvested from the MPNST mouse model treated as described in the 'In Vivo Experiments' section above. Samples were dissociated using the gentleMACS™ Dissociator (Miltenyi Biotec, Gaithersburg, MD, USA) with the 37C_m_TDK_1 program and a digestion medium containing collagenase (300 U/mL, Sigma), dispase (1 U/mL, Worthington, Lakewood, NJ, USA), and DNAse (2 U/mL, Calbiochem, Burlington, MA, USA). Cells were passed through a 40 μm cell strainer (BD Falcon, Glendale, AZ, USA), and red blood cells were removed using a lysis solution. The resulting single cells were resuspended in Brilliant Buffer (BD Biosciences, Sparks Glencoe, MD, USA) and stained at 4 °C for 30 min with the following antibodies: CD4-BV750 (1:100, Biolegend, San Diego, CA, USA, GK1.5), CD25-PE (0.5:100, Biolegend, 3C7), CD8-BV605 (1:100, Biolegend, 104732), FOXP3-PE-Cy5 (1:100, eBioscience, FJK-16s), CD206-BV421 (1:100, Biolegend, C068C2), F4/80-APC-Fire 750 (1:100, Biolegend, BM8), IA-IE-BV650 (0.5:100, Biolegend, M5/114.15.2), CD163-APC (1:100, Biolegend, S15049F), CD45-PerCP-Cy5.5 (0.5:100, Biolegend, 30-F11), CD11b-FITC (1:100, Miltenyi Biotec, M1/70.15.11.5), CD11c-BV510 (1:100, Biolegend, M1/70), CD19-BV570 (0.5:100, Biolegend, 6D5), CD3-Vioblue (5:100, Miltenyi Biotec, 17A2), Viability–LIVE-DEAD Far Red (0.5:100, Thermo Fisher Scientific), and 5 μg/mL anti-mouse CD16/CD32 antibody (Biolegend) to reduce antibody binding to Fc receptors. Cells were analyzed using Cytek Aurora and FlowJo v10.0.7r2 software (Tree Star). The gating strategy used is shown in Figure S2.

2.11. Triglyceride Assay

Triglyceride levels in plasma were quantified using the Triglyceride Quantification Assay Kit (Abcam, ab65336), following the recommended protocol supplied by the manufacturer for colorimetric readout.

2.12. Statistical Analysis

GraphPad Prism v10 (RRID:SCR_002798) was used for all data analysis. Data are presented as the mean ± standard deviation or the mean ± standard error as indicated in the respective figure legends. The in vitro and ex vivo experiments were performed in triplicate for each treatment (cell viability and real-time PCR), and independent experiments were repeated at least three times. Data from in vitro and ex vivo experiments followed normal distributions and were analyzed using one-way ANOVA, with significant differences between groups assessed by the Tukey HSD multiple comparison method. For in vivo experiments, data were analyzed using SigmaStat 3.5, applying one-way ANOVA followed by the Holm–Sidak test for multiple comparisons when the data were normally distributed. For non-normally distributed data, the Kruskal–Wallis one-way ANOVA on ranks was used, followed by the Dunn test for multiple comparisons. Statistical significance was defined as $p < 0.05$ for all analyses.

3. Results

3.1. MSU-42011 Reduced Tumor Burden, pERK Levels, and Tumor-Promoting CD206⁺ Macrophages in a Subcutaneous Kras-Driven Lung Cancer Model

In our previously published studies, the RXR agonist MSU-42011 can prevent or treat carcinogenesis in a Kras-driven lung cancer model [29,30]. In this model, the anti-tumor effects of MSU-42011 are due to its ability to reduce tumor-promoting $CD206^+$ macrophages and $FOXP3^+$ Tregs and increase tumor-killing cells [29,30]. Moreover, MSU-42011 reduces the level of pERK in both lung and mammary murine tumors [29]. Therefore, to test if MSU-42011 can enhance the effects of a clinically approved MEK inhibitor, selumetinib [15], we implanted murine LL2 lung cancer cells, a *Kras/Nras* mutant cell line [36], into the flank of C57BL/6 mice (1×10^6 cells/mouse). Once the tumors reached 3–4 mm in diameter, mice were randomized into groups and treated intraperitoneally (i.p.) once per day, five days per week, for 14 days with a vehicle, MSU-42011 (12.5–100 mg/kg or 25 mg/kg), selumetinib (10 mg/kg) [42], or the combination. The FDA-approved synthetic RXR agonist, bexarotene (Targretin$^{(R)}$, 30 mg/kg), used for treating cutaneous T-cell lymphoma [43], was also evaluated. Tumors were measured twice per week. MSU-42011, but not bexarotene, significantly (on day 11, 25–100 mg/kg, $p < 0.0001$; on day 14, 12.5 mg/kg, $p = 0.023$ and 25–100 mg/kg, $p < 0.0001$) reduced tumor volume in a dose-dependent manner compared to the vehicle treatment (Figure 1A). Increasing concentrations of MSU-42011 were well tolerated, did not cause body weight loss (Figure S3A), and did not increase plasma triglycerides (Figure S3B). An increase in triglycerides was observed with bexarotene (Figure S3B), as previously reported [44].

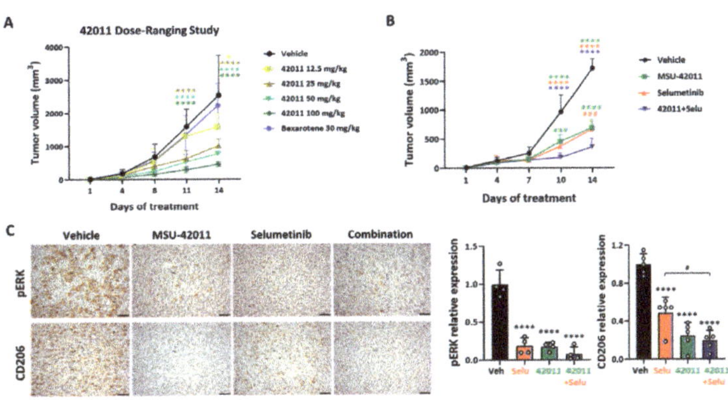

Figure 1. MSU-42011, alone or in combination with selumetinib, suppressed tumor growth and reduced pERK and $CD206^+$ levels in an immunocompetent LL2 model of lung cancer. Mouse LL2 lung cancer cells were injected into the flank of male C57BL/6 mice. Once the tumors reached 3–4 mm in diameter, mice were treated i.p. once per day, 5 days per week for 14 days with (**A**) vehicle, MSU-42011 (12.5–100 mg/kg), or bexarotene (30 mg/kg) or with (**B**,**C**) vehicle, 25 mg/kg MSU-42011 (42011), 10 mg/kg selumetinib (Selu), or the combination. (**A**,**B**) Tumor volumes were measured by calipers twice per week. Data represent means ± standard deviations (n = 7–9). * $p < 0.05$, **** $p < 0.0001$ vs. treated group; ### $p < 0.001$, #### $p < 0.0001$ vs. combination. (**C**) Tumors were harvested at the time of necropsy for immunohistochemical detection of pERK and CD206. Data represent means ± standard deviations (n = 4–5). Scale bar = 60 microns. **** $p < 0.0001$ vs. vehicle; # $p < 0.05$.

The 25 mg/kg dose provided significant biological effects without elevating triglyceride levels, and it was the optimal dose where we saw a strong therapeutic response for combination therapy [29,30], making it suitable for subsequent studies. Treatment with 25 mg/kg MSU-42011 (458 mm^3, $p < 0.0001$) or 10 mg/kg selumetinib (373 mm^3, $p < 0.0001$), and the combination (182 mm^3, $p < 0.0001$), significantly reduced tumor volume after 10 days compared to the vehicle (964 mm^3) (Figure 1B). Moreover, by day 10, the combination treatment showed a 60.3% greater inhibition of tumor volume compared to MSU-42011 alone (MSU-42011, 458 mm^3 vs. combination, 182 mm^3, $p = 0.0003$) but not with selumetinib. By day 14, at the end of treatment, the combination significantly reduced tumor volume by 47.8% compared to MSU-42011 alone and by 45.5% compared to selumetinib alone (MSU-42011, 695 mm^3, $p < 0.0001$; selumetinib, 666 mm^3, $p = 0.0007$ vs. combination, 363 mm^3) (Figure 1B). No differences were observed in body weight between the treatment groups (Figure S3C). After 14 days of treatment, tumors were harvested for immunohistochemical (IHC) staining to assess the levels of pERK and CD206 (tumor-promoting macrophage marker). Both selumetinib and MSU-42011 alone significantly reduced pERK levels by 81.44% ($p < 0.0001$) and 82.51% ($p < 0.0001$), respectively, and decreased the number of $CD206^+$ macrophages by 51.46% ($p < 0.0001$) and 75.41% ($p < 0.0001$) compared to vehicle treatment. The combination treatment resulted in a greater reduction, lowering pERK levels to 92.13% ($p < 0.0001$) and $CD206^+$ macrophages to 78.35% ($p < 0.0001$) compared to vehicle treatment within the tumors. However, the difference relative to single-agent treatments was modest, with only the selumetinib-treated group showing a significant difference in $CD206^+$ macrophages when compared to the combination treatment (Figure 1C).

3.2. MSU-42011, Selumetinib, and the Combination Suppressed Tumor Growth, Reduced pERK Levels, and Modulated the Tumor Microenvironment in a Mouse Model of MPNST

Due to the importance of immune cells in the progression of neurofibromas [24,25] and the in vivo efficacy of MSU-42011 in Kras-driven lung cancer (Figure 1) [29,30], which shares similarities with NF1 models, immunocompetent C57BL/6 mice were used to evaluate the immunomodulatory and anti-tumor effects of MSU-42011 in vivo in MPNST. Selumetinib has been tested in clinical trials for MPNST treatment, primarily focusing on developing effective combination strategies with the mTOR inhibitor sirolimus (NCT03433183) or the bromodomain inhibitor AZD5153 plus the programmed death-ligand 1 (PD-L1) antibody durvalumab (NCT05253131) [45]. Murine Nf1-related MPNST cells, which harbor both *Nf1* and *Tp53* mutations that enhance aggressiveness and promote tumor formation [39] were injected into the flank of C57BL/6 mice (3×10^5 cells/mouse). Due to the high aggressiveness of this cell, a continuous 10-day treatment regimen was used to prevent ulceration from treatment gaps. Once the tumors reached 3–4 mm in diameter, the mice were treated i.p. once daily for 10 days with the vehicle, 25 mg/kg MSU-42011, 10 mg/kg selumetinib, or the combination. Tumor growth was monitored every two days during the treatment period. MSU-42011 (139 mm^3, $p = 0.0072$) and selumetinib (99 mm^3, $p = 0.0009$), either alone or in combination (40 mm^3, $p < 0.0001$), significantly reduced tumor volume after 7 days compared to the vehicle treatment (419 mm^3) (Figure 2A). At the 10-day end point, the combination treatment showed a greater reduction in tumor volume compared to each single-agent treatment (vehicle, 1260 mm^3, $p < 0.0001$; MSU-42011, 377 mm^3, $p = 0.0115$; selumetinib, 365 mm^3, $p = 0.0277$ vs. combination, 95 mm^3). Additionally, at the 10-day end point, tumor weights were also significantly reduced compared to vehicle treatment (MSU-42011, 0.46 g; selumetinib, 0.35 g; combination, 0.18 g vs. vehicle, 1.30 g, $p < 0.0001$) (Figure 2B). No differences in body weight were observed among the groups (Figure S4A), similar to what we observed in the LL2 model (Figure S3C). In contrast, bexarotene, the FDA-approved RXR agonist, in the same mouse model of MPNST, showed no effects on tumor burden (Figure S5).

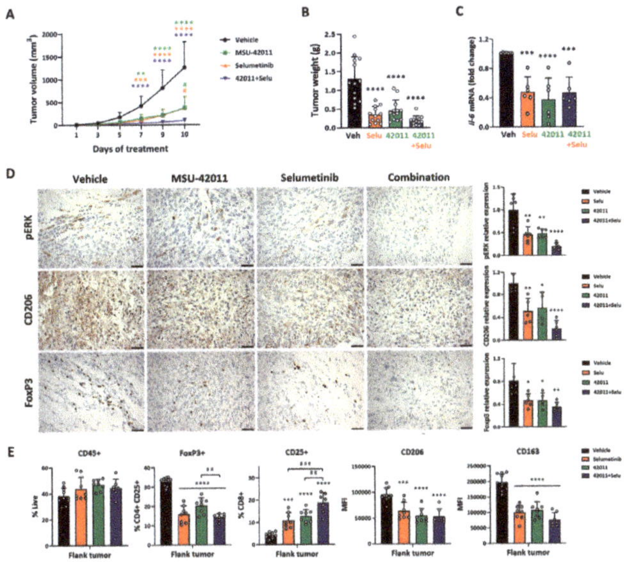

Figure 2. MSU-42011, selumetinib, and the combination reduced tumor growth, pERK levels, tumor-promoting macrophages, FOXP3^{+} Treg, and *Il6* mRNA expression, while increasing activated CD8^{+} T cells in an immunocompetent mouse model of MPNST. Mouse Nf1-related MPNST cells (mMPNST) were injected into the flank of both male and female C57BL/6 mice. Once the tumors reached 3–4 mm in diameter, mice were treated i.p. once per day for 10 days with vehicle, 25 mg/kg MSU-42011, 10 mg/kg selumetinib, or the combination. (**A**) Tumor volumes were measured by calipers every two days. Data represent means ± standard deviations (n = 12–13). ** $p < 0.01$, *** $p < 0.001$, **** $p < 0.0001$ vs. treated group; # $p < 0.05$ vs. combination. (**B**) Tumor weights were recorded at the time of necropsy (n = 12–13). (**C**) Tumors were harvested for *Il6* mRNA expression analysis by qPCR (n = 6) (**D**) for immunohistochemical detection of pERK, CD206, and FOXP3 (n = 6). Scale bar = 60 microns or (**E**) for flow cytometry analysis of immune cell populations using whole tumor lysates (n = 8–10). Data represent means ± standard deviations. * $p < 0.05$, ** $p < 0.01$, *** $p < 0.001$, **** $p < 0.0001$ vs. vehicle; ## $p < 0.01$, ### $p < 0.001$.

MEK inhibitors have been shown to decrease long-chain fatty acids, reducing lipid oxidation, which was accompanied by an increase in triacylglycerides in some patients with NF1-associated PNF [46]. In the LL2 lung cancer model, we observed higher plasma triglyceride levels in the selumetinib-treated group but not in the MSU-42011-treated group (Figure S3D). In the mouse model of MPNST, selumetinib and bexarotene increased plasma levels of triglycerides, but no increase was observed in MSU-42011-treated mice (Figure S4B,C). The increase observed in the combination treatment may be due to selumetinib (Figures S3D and S4B). These data point out that MSU-42011, unlike selumetinib and bexarotene, did not induce triglyceride accumulation, indicating a potentially safer metabolic profile for use in cancer treatment.

Schwannomatosis (SWN), a distinct NF-related disorder, often causes severe chronic pain leading to disability [47,48]. Studies in SWN cell lines show that macrophages trigger pain responses through IL-6 overproduction, with a fourteen-fold increase in secretion observed in mouse peritoneal macrophages stimulated by SWN-conditioned medium [49]. Moreover, IL-6 blockade significantly reduces pain in orthotopic sciatic nerve and spine patient-derived xenograft (PDX) models [49]. Notably, both selumetinib and MSU-42011, alone and in combination, reduced *Il-6* mRNA expression by 52.76% ($p = 0.0007$), 63.12% ($p < 0.0001$), and 54.26% ($p = 0.0005$) compared with vehicle treatment, as measured in tumor lysates (Figure 2C). Since IL-6 overproduction in NF1-deficient models is mostly associated with increased infiltration and activation of myeloid-derived suppressor cells (MDSCs) [22], and previous observations that MSU-42011 reduced expression of CD206 tumor-promoting macrophage marker (Figure 1C) [29,30], we analyzed the levels of CD206 in MPNST flank tumors by IHC staining. Selumetinib and MSU-42011 reduced CD206 expression by approximately 49% ($p = 0.0043$) and 44% ($p = 0.0172$), respectively; the combination was greatly effective, with an 80% ($p < 0.0001$) reduction compared with vehicle treatment (Figure 2D). High numbers of $FOXP3^+$ Tregs in tumors are generally associated with worse overall survival in breast cancer [50]. As observed in the $HER2^+$ breast cancer and Kras-driven lung cancer models [29,30], MSU-42011 (~43%, $p = 0.0246$) and selumetinib (~43%, $p = 0.0175$) alone or in combination (~57%, $p = 0.0016$) reduced the expression of $FOXP3^+$ in the flank tumors of MPNST compared with vehicle treatment. Moreover, despite not carrying an *RAS* mutation, MSU-42011 (~52%, $p = 0.0018$), selumetinib (~55%, $p = 0.0010$), and the combination (~81%, $p < 0.0001$) reduced the expression of pERK compared with vehicle treatment (Figure 2D). To complement IHC analysis, we performed flow cytometry on whole tumor lysates to further characterize the immune landscape of MPNST tumors. Drug treatments did not affect the total $CD45^+$ immune cell population (Figure 2E). Selumetinib, MSU-42011, and the combination significantly reduced the percentage of $FOXP3^+CD25^+CD4^+$ Treg (~52%; ~38%; ~56% vs. vehicle, $p < 0.0001$) and decreased the mean fluorescence intensity (MFI) of $CD206^+$ (~33%, $p = 0.0004$; ~43%, $p < 0.0001$; ~45%, $p < 0.0001$ vs. vehicle) and $CD163^+$ tumor-promoting macrophages (~49%; ~46%; ~62% vs. vehicle, $p < 0.0001$) (Figure 2E), in agreement with the reduction in FOXP3 and CD206 expressions observed by IHC analysis (Figure 2D). Furthermore, selumetinib and MSU-42011 increased the percentage of activated $CD25^+CD8^+$ T cells (2.5X, $p = 0.0007$; 3.0X, $p < 0.0001$ vs. vehicle), and the combination enhanced this response to a 4.4-fold increase compared with the vehicle ($p < 0.0001$). No alterations in the percentage or MFI of the aforementioned immune cell populations were observed in the spleen from the same cohort of mice (Figure S6). The combination treatment demonstrated superior efficacy in reducing the tumor burden and modulating the tumor microenvironment, highlighting its potential as a therapeutic strategy for aggressive MPNSTs.

3.3. Selumetinib Reduced pERK Levels in NF1-Deficient Tumor Cells, While MSU-42011 Showed Limited Effects In Vitro

To understand the potential mechanisms underlying the anti-tumor effects of MSU-42011 in NF1, we used several mouse and human NF1-deficient cell lines to perform in vitro studies. These included human immortalized $NF1^{-/-}$ Schwann cells [37,38], murine Nf1-related MPNSTs (referred to as mMPNST) [39], and primary murine Nf1 $Cdkn2a^{-/-}$ and $Nf1^{-/-}$ DNSCs (referred to as mSC, $Nf1^{f/f}$ Cre-; mPNF, $Nf1^{f/f}$ Cre+; mMPNST precursor, $Nf1^{f/f}$ $Cdkn2a^{f/f}$ Cre+) [41]. pERK is elevated in these human and mouse cells due to both a germline and somatic mutation in *NF1/Nf1*, which activates RAS and the downstream MAPK signaling pathway [37,39,41].

In human PNF cells (hPNF95.6), treatment with MSU-420011 at 200 nM reduced the levels of pERK starting at 0.5 h, reaching peak reduction at 3 h, but this reduction was lost at 6 and 24 h. In contrast, 50 nM selumetinib reduced pERK levels from 0.5 to 24 h (Figure S7A). Based on the maximum reduction in pERK by MSU-42011 at 3 h, this time point was selected as the optimal treatment time for pERK level analysis. After 3 h of treatment, selumetinib significantly reduced pERK levels in human PNF cells, mouse MPNST precursor cells, and mouse MPNST cells by approximately 77% ($p < 0.0001$), 63% ($p = 0.0031$), and 66% ($p = 0.0036$), respectively, compared with vehicle-treated cells (Figure 3). MSU-42011 alone reduced pERK levels in human PNF cells by about 33% ($p = 0.0016$ vs. vehicle-treated cells) (Figure 3A). MSU-42011 was ineffective in reducing pERK in mouse MPNST precursor cells and mouse MPNST cells (Figure 3B,C). The combination treatment reduced pERK levels by 83% ($p < 0.0001$), 77% ($p = 0.0009$), and 75% ($p = 0.0017$) in human PNF cells, mouse MPNST precursor cells, and mouse MPNST cells but showed no additive effect compared to single-agent treatment (Figure 3). Additionally, human PNF cells and mouse MPNST precursor cells were treated with increasing concentrations of MSU-42011 and selumetinib for 72 h, alone or in combination, and cell viability was measured using the MTT assay. A trend of reduced cell viability was observed with increasing concentrations of the combination in both cell lines, though the reduction in mouse MPNST precursor cells may be primarily attributed to selumetinib. MPNST precursor cells did not respond to MSU-42011 alone (Figure S7B). These findings suggest that the combination of MSU-42011 and selumetinib reduced pERK levels. However, the reduction in viability of NF1-deficient cells is most likely due to selumetinib.

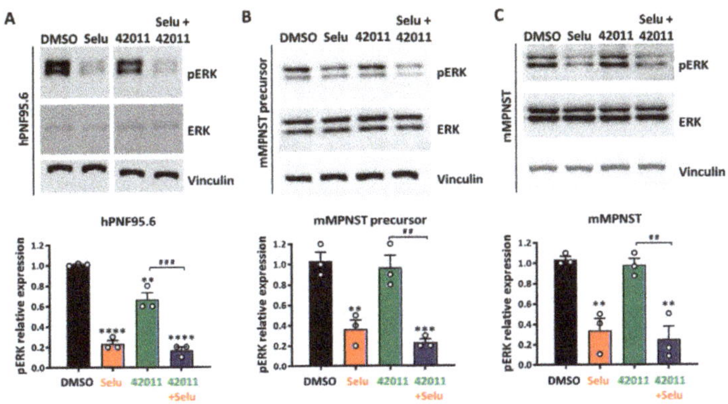

Figure 3. Selumetinib reduced pERK levels in NF1-deficient cells, while MSU-42011 had a limited effect alone and no additive effect in combination. (**A**) ipNF95.6 human PNF cells (hPNF95.6), (**B**) mouse MPNST precursor cells (Nf1$^{f/f}$ Cdkn2a$^{f/f}$ Cre+), and (**C**) mouse Nf1-related MPNST cells (mMPNST) were treated with 50 nM selumetinib (Selu), 200 nM MSU-42011 (42011), or the combination for 3 h. The level of pERK was evaluated by Western blotting. Data represent means ± standard deviations ($n = 3$). ** $p < 0.01$, *** $p < 0.001$, **** $p < 0.0001$ vs. DMSO; ## $p < 0.01$, ### $p < 0.001$. The uncropped blots are shown in File S1.

In Nf1-deficient mice, increased macrophage infiltration correlates with disease severity [25], and to mimic the communication between tumor-associated macrophages (TAMs) and tumor cells, conditioned media (CM) from macrophages and NF1-deficient cells were used to model this interaction. CM from macrophages were collected after a 24 h incubation with 1×10^6/mL human THP1 monocytes (CM) or THP1 macrophages (PMA-CM) differentiated with 50 ng/mL PMA for 3 days [51]. The 50% CM were subsequently added to human PNF cells, with treatments administered simultaneously with the vehicle, 200 nM MSU-42011, 50 nM selumetinib, or the combination for either 3 h (to assess pERK levels) or 72 h (to assess cell viability). In a similar study using MCF7 breast cancer cells, CM from macrophages was reported to induce ERK signaling that can be inhibited by MEK inhibitor PD98059 [52]. Contrary to the increase in pERK observed in MCF7 cells, human PNF cells stimulated with CM from both THP1 monocytes or THP1 macrophages showed modestly reduced pERK levels ($p > 0.05$) (Figure S8A). Although MSU-42011 alone had no impact on pERK, its combination with selumetinib in the presence of CM led to a further reduction in pERK levels, an effect likely driven primarily by selumetinib (Figure S8A). Cell viability, assessed using an MTT assay and normalized to control without CM treatment , revealed that CM from THP1 monocytes and macrophages reduced the viability of human PNF cells by approximately 20%. Moreover, the combination treatment further reduced the cell viability (Figure S8B).

3.4. NF1-Deficient Cells Increased the Secretion and Expression of Cytokine and Chemokine in Macrophages, and Treatment with MSU-42011 and Selumetinib Partially Reduced the Increase

NF1 mutations have broad effects on immune cells and cytokine signaling, driven by a hyperactive MAPK signaling pathway [22,53], leading to elevated levels of inflammatory signals such as IL-6, VEGF, and CCL2 in patients with NF1 [22,24,49,54]. To assess the impact of NF1-deficient cells on macrophage activation, CM were collected after a 24 h incubation with 5×10^5/mL murine and human NF1-deficient cells. The collected CM were then added at 50% to murine primary bone marrow-derived macrophages (BMDMs) and human THP1 cells, respectively, with treatments administered simultaneously for 24 h. BMDMs were isolated from C57BL/6 mice and differentiated with 20 ng/mL M-CSF for 5 days [55]. After a 24 h CM stimulation and treatment, the expression and secretion of cytokines and chemokines in macrophages (BMDMs and THP1 cells) were analyzed by RT-PCR, ELISA, and multiplex assay.

The heatmap from the cytokine/chemokine multiplex assay visually represented the relative concentrations of multiple cytokines and chemokines (Figure 4A). These concentrations were measured in the supernatants of BMDMs treated with CM from both mouse Schwann cells and PNF cells and normalized to BMDMs without CM treatment. CM treatment induced upregulation in the secretion of BAFF, betacellulin (BTC), ENA-78 (CXCL5), G-CSF (CSF-3), GM-CSF, GRO alpha (CXCL1), IL-1 alpha, IL-1 beta, IL-2, IL-3, IL-4, IL-5, IL-6, IL-7R alpha, IL-10, IL-12p70, IL-13, IL-19, IL-22, IL-27, IL-31, IL-33, M-CSF, MCP-1 (CCL2), MIP-1 alpha (CCL3), MIP-1 beta (CCL4), MIP-2 alpha (CXCL2), RANKL, RANTES (CCL5), TNF alpha, and VEGF-A in BMDMs exposed to the CM from both mouse Schwann cells and PNF cells (Figure 4A). Additionally, the bar graph illustrated the concentration levels of the factors in the supernatants of BMDMs exposed to CM from mouse Schwann cells, PNF cells (Figure 4B), and MPNST precursor cells (Figure S9A). Although not statistically significant, CM from PNF cells showed a trend toward increased levels of secretions compared to normal Schwann cells, including betacellulin (BTC), G-CSF (CSF-3), GRO alpha (CXCL1), IL-1 alpha, IL-1 beta, IL-3, IL-5, IL-6, IL-7R alpha, IL-9, IL-13, IL-27, IL-31, IL-33, MCP-1 (CCL2), MIP-1 beta (CCL4), RANTES (CCL5), and TNF alpha (Figure 4B). mRNA expression levels of key cytokines and chemokines were used to confirm the observations made on the multiplex assay. *Ccl2*, *Tnfα*, and *Il-6* mRNA expression increased by approximately 12X ($p = 0.0026$), 2.7X ($p = 0.0119$), and 7X ($p < 0.0001$), respectively, in BMDMs treated with CM from PNF cells compared to non-CM-treated groups. In contrast, MPNST precursor cells also increased *Ccl2* mRNA expression by about 15X ($p = 0.0005$) but did not significantly alter *Tnfα* or *Il-6* levels compared to non-CM-treated groups (Figure 5A). Importantly, the increased *Ccl2* mRNA expression induced by CM from both mouse PNF and MPNST precursor cells was effectively inhibited by 200 nM MSU-42011 (PNF, $p = 0.0007$; MPNST precursor, $p < 0.0001$) and 50 nM selumetinib (PNF, $p = 0.0012$; MPNST precursor, $p < 0.0001$) and further reduced by their combination (PNF and MPNST precursor, $p < 0.0001$) compared to the vehicle treatment. Additionally, the combination treatment reduced *Tnfα* expression in BMDMs exposed to CM from both mouse PNF cells ($p = 0.0005$) and MPNST precursor cells ($p < 0.0001$) (Figure 5B).

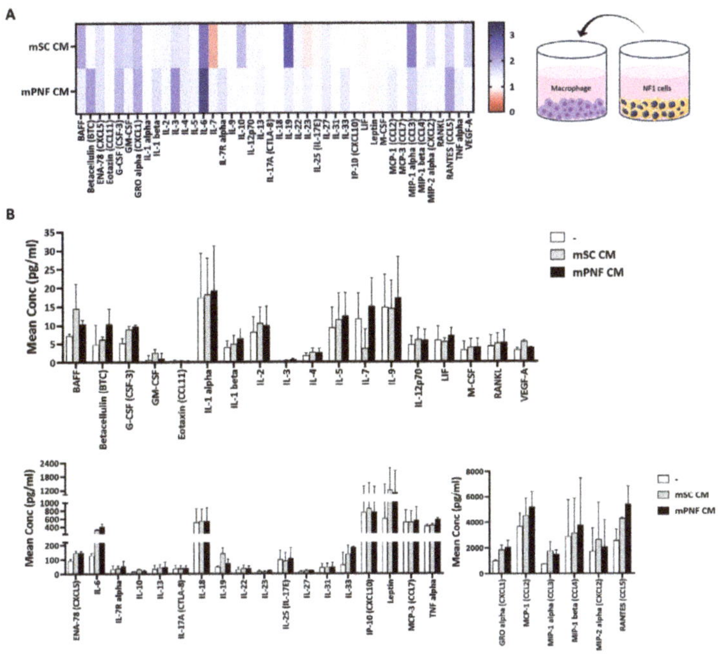

Figure 4. Conditioned media (CM) from murine Schwann cells and PNF cells increased cytokine and chemokine secretion in bone marrow-derived macrophages (BMDMs). Supernatants from BMDMs, differentiated with 20 ng/mL M-CSF for 5 days and then treated with 50% CM from mouse normal Schwann cells ($Nf1^{f/f}$ Cre-) and PNF cells ($Nf1^{f/f}$ Cre+) for 24 h, were analyzed by a multiplex assay. (**A**) The heat map illustrated the relative analyte concentrations, normalized to the BMDMs without CM treatment. (**B**) The mean concentrations were categorized as low (<20 pg/mL), medium (<1400 pg/mL), and high (<5000 pg/mL). Data were averaged across two replicates.

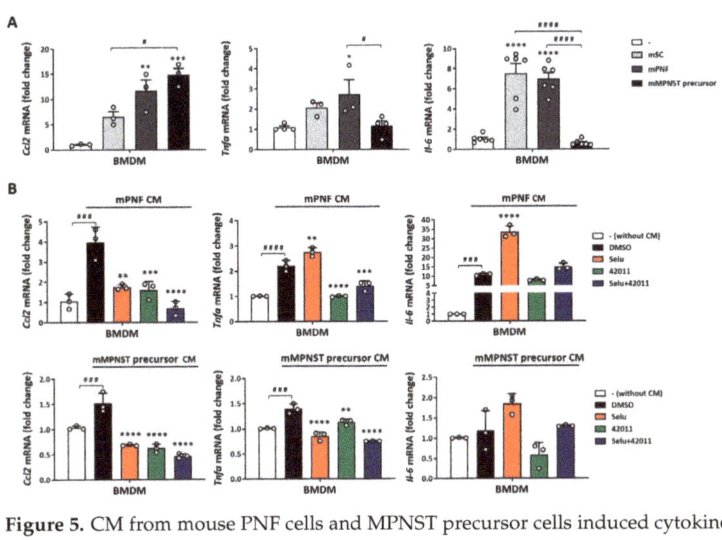

Figure 5. CM from mouse PNF cells and MPNST precursor cells induced cytokine mRNA expression in BMDMs, which was reduced by combination treatment with MSU-42011 and selumetinib. (**A**) BMDMs differentiated with 20 ng/mL M-CSF for 5 days were treated with 50% CM from mouse

Schwann cells ($Nf1^{f/f}$ Cre-), PNF cells ($Nf1^{f/f}$ Cre+), and MPNST precursor cells ($Nf1^{f/f}$ $Cdkn2a^{f/f}$ Cre+) for 24 h. Data represent means ± standard deviations (n = 3–6). (**B**) Differentiated BMDMs were treated with 50% CM from mouse PNF cells (mPNF CM), MPNST precursor cells (mMPNST precursor CM), and drugs (50 nM selumetinib, 200 nM MSU-42011, or the combination) for 24 h. mRNA expression was evaluated by qPCR and normalized to the BMDMs without CM and drug treatment. Data are representative of three independent experiments. * $p < 0.05$, ** $p < 0.01$, *** $p < 0.001$, **** $p < 0.0001$ vs. BMDMs without CM treatment (**A**) or vs. DMSO (**B**); # $p < 0.05$, ### $p < 0.001$, #### $p < 0.0001$.

Macrophages are broadly categorized as classically activated type 1 (M1) and alternatively activated type 2 (M2) [56,57]. TAMs typically exhibit an M2-like phenotype promoting tumor progression and resistance to chemotherapy [58,59]. While it is well established that many tumors recruit monocytes from circulation and transform them into immunosuppressive M2-like subsets [60], our data showed that mouse PNF cells induced higher expression of both M1 (*iNOS*, 39X, $p = 0.0026$) and M2 (*Arg1*, 12X, $p = 0.0044$) macrophage markers compared to non-CM-treated groups. In contrast, mouse MPNST precursor cells only induced *Arg1* mRNA expression (9X, $p = 0.0374$) in BMDMs, without affecting *iNOS* expression (Figure S9B).

The results observed in murine cells were also confirmed in human NF1-deficient cells and human THP1 monocytes or THP1 macrophages differentiated as described above. CM from PNF cells (ipNF95.11bC) increased CCL2 secretion in THP1 monocytes ($p = 0.0019$) compared to non-CM-treated groups. Additionally, CM from PNF cells (ipNF95.6) elevated IL-6 secretion in both THP1 monocytes ($p = 0.0011$) and macrophages ($p = 0.0006$), and CM from NF1-mutant non-tumor Schwann cells (ipnNF95.11c, $p = 0.0196$) and PNF cells (ipNF95.11bC, $p = 0.0026$; ipNF95.6, $p = 0.0431$) induced TNFα secretion in THP1 macrophages compared to non-CM-treated groups (Figure 6A). Furthermore, *CCL2* mRNA expression was upregulated 1.5-2.5X in THP1 macrophages treated with CM from PNF cells (ipNF95.11bC, $p < 0.0001$; ipNF95.6, $p = 0.0018$) compared to non-CM-treated groups (Figure 6C). The combination treatment reduced the secretion of CCL2 and TNFα by about 43% ($p = 0.0288$ vs. DMSO) and 89% ($p = 0.0004$ vs. DMSO) in THP1 monocytes and macrophages, respectively (Figure 6B), as well as the mRNA expression of *CCL2* and *TNFα* by about 68% ($p = 0.0121$ vs. DMSO) and 73% ($p < 0.0001$ vs. DMSO) in THP1 macrophages stimulated with CM from PNF cells (Figure 6D). The reductions were also observed in TNFα secretion by selumetinib alone (~87%, $p = 0.0006$ vs. DMSO) (Figure 6B) and in *TNFα* expression by MSU-42011 (~27%, $p = 0.0165$ vs. DMSO) and selumetinib alone (~70%, $p < 0.0001$ vs. DMSO) (Figure 6D) in THP1 macrophages stimulated with CM from PNF cells. Though selumetinib may be the main driver, only the combination treatment reached statistical significance in inhibiting CCL2 protein and mRNA levels. These findings support the hypothesis that NF1 deficiency enhances the activation of inflammatory pathways by increasing both protein and mRNA levels of cytokines and chemokines. Additionally, the combination of MSU-42011 and selumetinib partially reversed these effects, highlighting its potential as a therapeutic intervention.

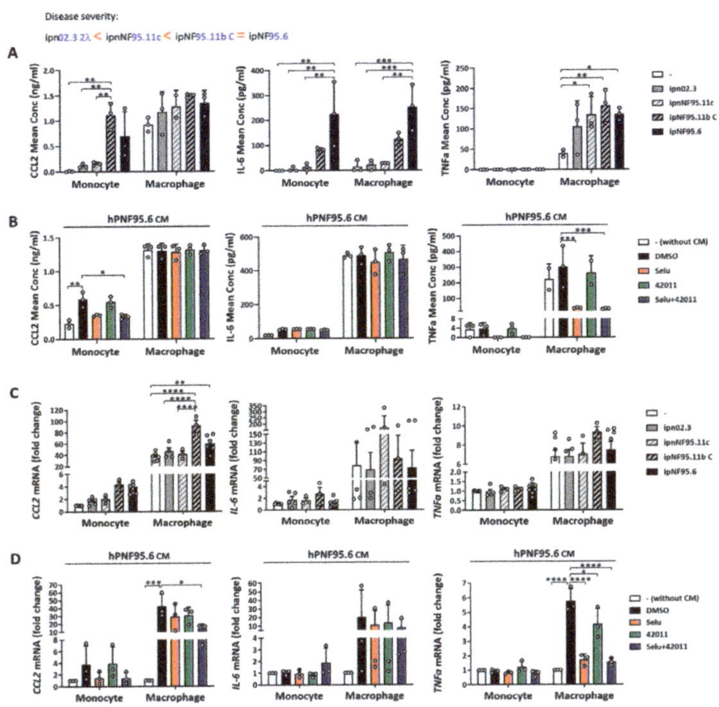

Figure 6. CM from human PNF cells increased cytokine secretion and mRNA expression in THP1 cells, which was reduced by combination treatment with MSU-42011 and selumetinib. THP1 monocytes or macrophages (THP1 cells differentiated with 50 ng/mL PMA for 3 days) were treated with (**A**,**C**) 50% CM from human Schwann cells (ipn02.3 2λ), non-tumor Schwann cells with an *NF1* mutation (ipnNF95.11c), and PNF cells (ipNF95.11bC and ipNF95.6) or with (**B**,**D**) 50% CM from ipNF95.6 human PNF cells (hPNF95.6 CM) and drugs (50 nM selumetinib, 200 nM MSU-42011, or the combination) for 24 h. (**A**,**B**) IL-6, TNFα, and CCL2 secretion in the supernatants were measured by ELISAs. (**C**,**D**) mRNA expression was evaluated by qPCR and normalized to the monocyte without CM treatment. Data represent means ± standard deviations (n = 3–8). * $p < 0.05$, ** $p < 0.01$, *** $p < 0.001$, **** $p < 0.0001$.

4. Discussions

In this study, we tested the potential of MSU-42011, alone or in combination with selumetinib, to reduce tumor growth in neurofibromatosis, and evaluated the mechanistic effects of this combination. The RAS signaling pathway is constitutively activated in both the LL2 lung cancer model, through an activating *RAS* mutation [36], and the MPNST model, by the loss of *NF1* [2–4]. As a result, ERK phosphorylation is highly expressed in both models. MSU-42011 reduced the levels of pERK in both murine models, alone or in combination with selumetinib (Figures 1C and 2D). Targeting RAS or its downstream effectors, such as the MAPK signaling pathway, has been a longstanding goal in cancer research, and recent progress has been made with the development of MAPK and KRAS G12C small-molecule inhibitors [61,62]. However, MPNST cells, in particular, exhibit low responsiveness to MEK inhibition [42], and clinical applicability is limited due to toxicity and resistance [63]. Interestingly, pERK reduction by MSU-42011 was observed exclusively in in vivo models (Figures 1C and 2D). In vitro, the effects of MSU-42011 on pERK reduction and cell viability were limited compared to selumetinib (Figures 3 and S7). This suggests that the primary effects of MSU-42011 may not directly target tumor cells but instead involve alternative mechanisms, such as modulating the TME. Supporting the hypothesis that MSU-42011 modulated inflammatory mediators and immune cell populations in tumors with *KRAS* mutations (Figure 1) or RAS signaling pathway activation (Figure 2). Specifically, the IHC staining showed the ability of MSU-42011 to reduce the expression of CD206 and FOXP3 (Figure 2D), and this was confirmed by flow cytometry, which showed that MSU-42011 reduced tumor-promoting macrophages (low CD206 and CD163), $FOXP3^+$ Treg, and increased the presence of activated $CD8^+$ T cells in the flank tumors of MPNST (Figure 2E). The immune-modulating properties of MSU-42011 were also evident by using conditioned media (CM) from NF1-deficient cells in BMDMs or THP1 cells, where it reduced the expression and secretion of pro-inflammatory cytokines and chemokines (Figures 5 and 6). Moreover, MSU-42011 showed no anti-tumor efficacy in an athymic A549 lung cancer xenograft mode, further validating the dependency on an intact immune system [29]. This creates a limitation for using MSU-42011 as a standalone therapy in such models, and its application may need to be considered alongside other strategies or in models with an intact immune response.

The RXR agonist MSU-42011 has been shown to reduce $FOXP3^+$ Treg and increase activated cytotoxic T cells in several tumor murine models [29], including in MPNST (Figure 2D,E). While the role of T cells in NF1 is poorly understood, their distribution across different tumor stages suggests a dynamic involvement in disease progression. Activated and effector T cells are elevated in patients with a low PNF tumor burden compared to those without PNFs, but these levels decline as the tumor burden increases [64], suggesting a muted T-cell response with a greater tumor burden. Moreover, ANNUBP tumors show enriched immune surveillance and infiltration by $CD4^+FOXP3^-$ and $CD8^+FOXP3^-$ T cells. However, these T cells are significantly diminished in MPNSTs and are replaced by an increase in $FOXP3^+$ Tregs [65]. PD-L1, a marker of immune exhaustion, is also significantly enriched in MPNST [66]. Thus, the role of MSU-42011 in reducing $FOXP3^+$ Tregs and increasing activated $CD8^+$ T cells in the MPNST model is particularly intriguing (Figure 2D,E), potentially alleviating immune suppression and enhancing anti-tumor immunity. These immunological changes by MSU-42011 are highly beneficial for cancer treatment but were not observed with bexarotene [35]. Given the enrichment of PD-L1 in MPNSTs and the ability of MSU-42011 to modulate the immune landscape, combining MSU-42011 with immune checkpoint inhibitors such as anti-PD-1 or anti-PD-L1 may further enhance anti-tumor immunity. Further characterization of the T cell population infiltrating into the flank tumors of MPNST and the role of MSU-42011 in modulating these populations is warranted and currently underway at our laboratory.

Macrophages are one of the dominant immune cell populations in neurofibromas and have long been hypothesized to contribute to neurofibromas development [24]. Studies in mouse models of PNF indicated that neurofibroma-associated macrophages have both anti-tumor and pro-tumor roles at different disease stages, initially inhibiting PNF development and later promoting the growth of established PNF [25]. However, the relative contributions of macrophages to neurofibromas, and specific macrophage functions or subtypes, remain unclear. TAMs typically exhibit an M2-like phenotype that supports tumor progression [58,59]. Yet, in the $Nf1^{fl/fl}$; DhhCre mouse model, macrophages exhibited mixed M1/M2 profiles, expressing M1 markers without clear M2 sub-population clustering in benign neurofibromas [67]. These observations align with our findings that CM from mouse PNF cells induced both M1 (*iNOS*) and M2 (*Arg1*) marker expression in macrophages, while more aggressive tumors, like MPNST precursor cells, skewed macrophages toward an M2-like phenotype, characterized by the increase in only *Arg1* expression (Figure S9B). This mix phenotype is also consistent with the cytokine levels measured by RT-PCR in this report, as mouse PNF cells induced higher pro-inflammatory *Tnfα* or *Il-6* RNA expression compared to MPNST precursor cells (Figure 5A). The ability of PNF cells to drive heightened inflammatory responses in macrophages is further supported by Figure 4B, which shows that CM from PNF cells enhanced cytokine and chemokine secretion in BMDMs compared to normal Schwann cells. Additionally, Figure 6A,C indicates a correlation between NF1 deficiency and increased secretion (CCL2, IL-6, and TNFα) and mRNA expression (*CCL2*), progressing from normal Schwann cells to NF1-mutant non-tumor Schwann cells to PNF cells. These data support the hypothesis that neurofibroma-associated macrophages may help sustain the pro-inflammatory state within the benign neurofibroma microenvironment, contributing to prolonged chronic inflammation that is critical for neurofibroma development and disease progression [25,67]. However, as tumors progress, it remains to be determined whether macrophages become increasingly polarized toward an M2-like phenotype or another tumor-promoting subtype to support tumor growth and how pharmacological intervention with MSU-42011 can intercept this progression.

Bexarotene, the FDA-approved RXR agonist, used for the treatment of cutaneous T-cell lymphoma [43], increased survival in a subset of lung cancer patients [68–70] but was not approved, likely due to toxicity and limited potency as a single agent [33]. Despite these challenges, these trials support the potential of RXR agonists for cancer treatment. RXR agonists were initially developed to reduce cancer cell proliferation and induce apoptosis or differentiation [71,72]. However, their immune regulatory effects are particularly significant in diseases with strong inflammatory components, such as cancer, neurodegenerative diseases, and viral infections [73–75]. RXRs likely exert immune regulatory effects through multiple immune cell types, including macrophages, dendritic cells, and $CD8^+$ T cells [34]. RXRα is highly expressed in macrophages and regulates inflammatory responses via PPARγ and LXR signaling. In dendritic cells, RXR agonists enhance antigen presentation and cell survival. RXR activation also promotes $CD8^+$ T cell infiltration, while its disruption impairs T cell proliferation, particularly in $CD8^+$ subsets [44]. These findings support the involvement of these immune cells as key mediators of RXR-targeted effects. Despite this, compared to bexarotene [76], MSU-42011 has significant advantages: (1) it does not elevate triglycerides (Figures S3 and S4), (2) it is more potent as a single agent (EC50 for RXR activation: 30 nM for MSU-42011 vs. 55 nM for bexarotene) [30], and (3) it has a stronger immune-modulatory profile [29,30,33]. The differences in efficacy observed between MSU-42011 and bexarotene in the MPNST model, including triglyceride levels and tumor burden (Supplemental Table S2), may be attributed to their distinct mechanisms of action. Bexarotene off-target signaling through RAR can lead to various adverse effects, including triglyceride elevation [44]. In contrast, MSU-42011 is specifically selective for RXR, without induction of other nuclear receptors [44].

While our findings support the therapeutic potential of RXR agonists in NF1-associated models, several limitations should be noted. First, NF1 is a complex genetic disorder characterized by diverse mutation combinations, and our model, NF1-deficient cells with *CDKN2A* and *TP53* deletions, represents only a subset of mutation profiles. Thus, the results may not fully capture the heterogeneity observed in patients. Additionally, the rapid tumor growth in syngeneic mouse models fails to recapitulate the natural progression and complexity of the TME, lacking immune-editing stages seen in patients. To address these issues, we are currently testing MSU-42011 in additional NF1 models (e.g., transgenic mice) to evaluate its interactions with specific pathways, immune cells, and cancer progression, providing insights into its mechanisms of action. We are also conducting intensive immune profiling of the tumors using RNA sequencing to assess other immune populations, including not only tumor-promoting immune cells but also mast cells and cytotoxic T cells, given its previously observed role in increasing activated cytotoxic T cells in other models [29,30]. Further studies are also needed to evaluate the translational relevance of these findings. The combination of the present study and future proposed experiments will enable future clinical trials of MSU-42011 as a single agent or in combination with other current or future therapeutic options, such as MEK inhibitors or immunotherapy.

5. Conclusions

In summary, we described the efficacy of MSU-42011 in preclinical NF1-deficient models, its ability to reduce pERK levels and tumor-promoting immune cell populations (CD206/CD163 macrophages and FOXP3$^+$ Tregs) and increase activated CD8$^+$ T cells within the tumor and its potential to further decrease tumor burden when combined with an MEK inhibitor, selumetinib.

Supplementary Materials: The following supporting information can be downloaded at: https://www.mdpi.com/article/10.3390/cancers17121920/s1, Figure S1. Knockdown efficiency of adenovirus-mediated Cre recombinase targeting Nf1 in DRG/nerve root neurosphere cells (DNSCs). Figure S2. Gating strategy used for flow cytometry analysis of myeloid and T cell populations. Figure S3. Triglyceride levels increased in the bexarotene and selumetinib-treated groups, but not in the MSU-42011-treated group in an immunocompetent LL2 model of lung cancer. Figure S4. Triglyceride levels increased in the 10-day bexarotene and selumetinib-treated groups, but not in the MSU-42011-treated group in a mouse model of MPNST. Figure S5. Bexarotene had no effect in an immunocompetent mouse model of MPNST. Figure S6. Immune cell populations in the spleen. Figure S7. Effects of MSU-42011 and selumetinib on pERK levels and cell viability in NF1-deficient cells. Figure S8. Conditioned media (CM) from human THP1 monocytes or macrophages did not alter pERK levels or cell viability in human PNF cells. Figure S9. CM from murine MPNST precursor cells increased cytokine and chemokine secretion, while CM from murine PNF cells enhanced *Arg1* and *iNOS* mRNA expression in bone marrow-derived macrophages (BMDMs). Table S1: Primer sequences used in qPCR experiments. Table S2: Comparison of MSU-42011 and bexarotene in mouse models of MPNST and LL2 lung cancer. File S1: Western blot information.

Author Contributions: Conceptualization: P.-Y.H. and K.T.L.; conducting experiments: P.-Y.H. and J.A.M.; writing the original manuscript: P.-Y.H.; review and editing the manuscript: P.-Y.H., A.S.L. and K.T.L.; funding acquisition: K.T.L.; cell line provision: D.W.C., V.S. and R.B.; RXR agonist provision: B.A. and E.E. All authors have read and agreed to the published version of the manuscript.

Funding: This research was funded by a Michigan State University (MSU) grant/contract and the Falk Medical Research Trust Catalyst Award (4487555). Additional support was provided by Akeila Bio, Inc., where one author serves as the founding scientist and Chief Scientific Officer.

Institutional Review Board Statement: Animal studies conducted at Michigan State University followed animal protocol (201800050), approved by the Institutional Animal Care and Use Committee (IACUC) at MSU, and complied with AAALAC-accredited standards for laboratory animal management. Similarly, studies conducted at Indiana University adhered to protocol (23143), approved by the IACUC at Indiana University, and were performed in accordance with institutional guidelines.

Informed Consent Statement: Not applicable.

Data Availability Statement: The data generated in this study are available within the article and its supplementary data files.

Acknowledgments: We thank Jamie Bernard from the Department of Pharmacology and Toxicology at Michigan State University for valuable comments and feedback on the initial draft of this manuscript.

Conflicts of Interest: A.S.L., B.A., E.E. and K.T.L. are named inventors on a patent filed on the novel RXR agonist and owned by MSU. The other authors have no potential conflicts of interest.

References

1. Evans, D.G.; Howard, E.; Giblin, C.; Clancy, T.; Spencer, H.; Huson, S.M.; Lalloo, F. Birth Incidence and Prevalence of Tumor-prone Syndromes: Estimates from a UK Family Genetic Register Service. *Am. J. Med. Genet. A* **2010**, *152*, 327–332. [CrossRef] [PubMed]
2. Gottfried, O.N.; Viskochil, D.H.; Couldwell, W.T. Neurofibromatosis Type 1 and Tumorigenesis: Molecular Mechanisms and Therapeutic Implications. *Neurosurg. Focus* **2010**, *28*, E8. [CrossRef] [PubMed]
3. Le, L.Q.; Parada, L.F. Tumor Microenvironment and Neurofibromatosis Type I: Connecting the GAPs. *Oncogene* **2007**, *26*, 4609–4616. [CrossRef]
4. DeClue, J.E.; Papageorge, A.G.; Fletcher, J.A.; Diehl, S.R.; Ratner, N.; Vass, W.C.; Lowy, D.R. Abnormal Regulation of Mammalian P21ras Contributes to Malignant Tumor Growth in von Recklinghausen (Type 1) Neurofibromatosis. *Cell* **1992**, *69*, 265–273. [CrossRef]
5. Korf, B.R. Plexiform Neurofibromas. *Am. J. Med. Genet.* **1999**, *89*, 31–37. [CrossRef]
6. Prada, C.E.; Rangwala, F.A.; Martin, L.J.; Lovell, A.M.; Saal, H.M.; Schorry, E.K.; Hopkin, R.J. Pediatric Plexiform Neurofibromas: Impact on Morbidity and Mortality in Neurofibromatosis Type 1. *J. Pediatr.* **2012**, *160*, 461–467. [CrossRef]
7. Choucha, A.; Troude, L.; Morin, L.; Fernandes, S.; Baucher, G.; De Simone, M.; Lihi, A.; Mazen, K.; Alseirihi, M.; Passeri, T.; et al. Management of Large Trigeminal Schwannoma: Long-Term Oncologic and Functional Outcome from a Multicentric Retrospective Cohort. *Acta Neurochir* **2024**, *166*, 440. [CrossRef]
8. De Simone, M.; Choucha, A.; Ranalli, C.; Pecoraro, G.; Appay, R.; Chinot, O.L.; Dufour, H.; Iaconetta, G. Astrocytomas IDH-Mutant of Posterior Cranial Fossa, Clinical Presentation, Imaging Features and Onco-Functional Balance in Surgical Management. *Neurosurg. Rev.* **2025**, *48*, 271. [CrossRef]
9. Rabab'h, O.; Gharaibeh, A.; Al-Ramadan, A.; Ismail, M.; Shah, J. Pharmacological Approaches in Neurofibromatosis Type 1-Associated Nervous System Tumors. *Cancers* **2021**, *13*, 3880. [CrossRef]
10. Natalie Wu, L.M.; Lu, Q.R. Therapeutic Targets for Malignant Peripheral Nerve Sheath Tumors. *Future Neurol.* **2019**, *14*, FNL7. [CrossRef]
11. Reilly, K.M.; Kim, A.; Blakely, J.; Ferner, R.E.; Gutmann, D.H.; Legius, E.; Miettinen, M.M.; Randall, R.L.; Ratner, N.; Jumbé, N.L.; et al. Neurofibromatosis Type 1–Associated MPNST State of the Science: Outlining a Research Agenda for the Future. *JNCI J. Natl. Cancer Inst.* **2017**, *109*, djx124. [CrossRef] [PubMed]
12. Kim, A.; Stewart, D.R.; Reilly, K.M.; Viskochil, D.; Miettinen, M.M.; Widemann, B.C. Malignant Peripheral Nerve Sheath Tumors State of the Science: Leveraging Clinical and Biological Insights into Effective Therapies. *Sarcoma* **2017**, *2017*, 1–10. [CrossRef]
13. Rhodes, S.D.; He, Y.; Smith, A.; Jiang, L.; Lu, Q.; Mund, J.; Li, X.; Bessler, W.; Qian, S.; Dyer, W.; et al. Cdkn2a (Arf) Loss Drives NF1-Associated Atypical Neurofibroma and Malignant Transformation. *Hum. Mol. Genet.* **2019**, *28*, 2752–2762. [CrossRef]
14. Miettinen, M.M.; Antonescu, C.R.; Fletcher, C.D.M.; Kim, A.; Lazar, A.J.; Quezado, M.M.; Reilly, K.M.; Stemmer-Rachamimov, A.; Stewart, D.R.; Viskochil, D.; et al. Histopathologic Evaluation of Atypical Neurofibromatous Tumors and Their Transformation into Malignant Peripheral Nerve Sheath Tumor in Patients with Neurofibromatosis 1—A Consensus Overview. *Hum. Pathol.* **2017**, *67*, 1–10. [CrossRef] [PubMed]
15. U.S. Food and Drug Administration. FDA Approves Selumetinib for Neurofibromatosis Type 1 with Symptomatic, Inoperable Plexiform Neurofibromas. 2020. Available online: https://www.fda.gov/drugs/resources-information-approved-drugs/fda-approves-selumetinib-neurofibromatosis-type-1-symptomatic-inoperable-plexiform-neurofibromas. (accessed on 13 March 2025).
16. Dombi, E.; Baldwin, A.; Marcus, L.J.; Fisher, M.J.; Weiss, B.; Kim, A.; Whitcomb, P.; Martin, S.; Aschbacher-Smith, L.E.; Rizvi, T.A.; et al. Activity of Selumetinib in Neurofibromatosis Type 1–Related Plexiform Neurofibromas. *N. Engl. J. Med.* **2016**, *375*, 2550–2560. [CrossRef]
17. U.S. Food and Drug Administration. KOSELUGO Safely and Effectively. 2020. Available online: https://www.accessdata.fda.gov/drugsatfda_docs/label/2020/213756s000lbl.pdf. (accessed on 13 March 2025).
18. Gross, A.M.; Wolters, P.L.; Dombi, E.; Baldwin, A.; Whitcomb, P.; Fisher, M.J.; Weiss, B.; Kim, A.; Bornhorst, M.; Shah, A.C.; et al. Selumetinib in Children with Inoperable Plexiform Neurofibromas. *N. Engl. J. Med.* **2020**, *382*, 1430–1442. [CrossRef] [PubMed]
19. Mueller, S.; Reddy, A.T.; Dombi, E.; Allen, J.; Packer, R.; Clapp, W.; Goldman, S.; Schorry, E.; Tonsgard, J.; Blakeley, J.; et al. NFB-17. Mek Inhibitor Binimetinib Shows Clinical Activity in Children with Neurofibromatosis Type 1-Associated Plexiform Neurofibromas: A Report from Pnoc and the NF Clinical Trials Consortium. *Neuro Oncol.* **2020**, *22*, iii420–iii421. [CrossRef]
20. McCowage, G.B.; Mueller, S.; Pratilas, C.A.; Hargrave, D.R.; Moertel, C.L.; Whitlock, J.; Fox, E.; Hingorani, P.; Russo, M.W.; Dasgupta, K.; et al. Trametinib in Pediatric Patients with Neurofibromatosis Type 1 (NF-1)–Associated Plexiform Neurofibroma: A Phase I/IIa Study. *J. Clin. Oncol.* **2018**, *36*, 10504. [CrossRef]
21. Fasih, S.; Suppiyah, S.; Barron, J.; Barnett-Tapia, C.; Avery, R.; Dickson, B.; Ferguson, P.; Swallow, C.; Zadeh, G.; Gupta, A.A. Malignant Transformation of Plexiform Neurofibroma to MPNST While on MEK Inhibitor. *Neuro-Oncol. Adv.* **2021**, *3*, vdab033. [CrossRef]
22. Karmakar, S.; Reilly, K.M. The Role of the Immune System in Neurofibromatosis Type 1-Associated Nervous System Tumors. *CNS Oncol.* **2017**, *6*, 45–60. [CrossRef]

23. Wei, C.-J.; Gu, S.-C.; Ren, J.-Y.; Gu, Y.-H.; Xu, X.-W.; Chou, X.; Lian, X.; Huang, X.; Li, H.-Z.; Gao, Y.-S.; et al. The Impact of Host Immune Cells on the Development of Neurofibromatosis Type 1: The Abnormal Immune System Provides an Immune Microenvironment for Tumorigenesis. *Neuro-Oncol. Adv.* **2020**, *2*, i33–i39. [CrossRef]
24. Fletcher, J.S.; Pundavela, J.; Ratner, N. After Nf1 Loss in Schwann Cells, Inflammation Drives Neurofibroma Formation. *Neuro-Oncol. Adv.* **2020**, *2*, i23–i32. [CrossRef]
25. Prada, C.E.; Jousma, E.; Rizvi, T.A.; Wu, J.; Dunn, R.S.; Mayes, D.A.; Cancelas, J.A.; Dombi, E.; Kim, M.-O.; West, B.L.; et al. Neurofibroma-Associated Macrophages Play Roles in Tumor Growth and Response to Pharmacological Inhibition. *Acta Neuropathol.* **2013**, *125*, 159–168. [CrossRef] [PubMed]
26. Patwardhan, P.P.; Surriga, O.; Beckman, M.J.; de Stanchina, E.; Dematteo, R.P.; Tap, W.D.; Schwartz, G.K. Sustained Inhibition of Receptor Tyrosine Kinases and Macrophage Depletion by PLX3397 and Rapamycin as a Potential New Approach for the Treatment of MPNSTs. *Clin. Cancer Res.* **2014**, *20*, 3146–3158. [CrossRef] [PubMed]
27. Fletcher, J.S.; Wu, J.; Jessen, W.J.; Pundavela, J.; Miller, J.A.; Dombi, E.; Kim, M.-O.; Rizvi, T.A.; Chetal, K.; Salomonis, N.; et al. Cxcr3-Expressing Leukocytes Are Necessary for Neurofibroma Formation in Mice. *JCI Insight* **2019**, *4*, e98601. [CrossRef] [PubMed]
28. Kohlmeyer, J.L.; Lingo, J.J.; Kaemmer, C.A.; Scherer, A.; Warrier, A.; Voigt, E.; Raygoza Garay, J.A.; McGivney, G.R.; Brockman, Q.R.; Tang, A.; et al. CDK4/6-MEK Inhibition in MPNSTs Causes Plasma Cell Infiltration, Sensitization to PD-L1 Blockade, and Tumor Regression. *Clin. Cancer Res.* **2023**, *29*, 3484–3497. [CrossRef]
29. Leal, A.S.; Moerland, J.A.; Zhang, D.; Carapellucci, S.; Lockwood, B.; Krieger-Burke, T.; Aleiwi, B.; Ellsworth, E.; Liby, K.T. The RXR Agonist MSU42011 Is Effective for the Treatment of Preclinical HER2+ Breast Cancer and Kras-Driven Lung Cancer. *Cancers* **2021**, *13*, 5004. [CrossRef]
30. Moerland, J.A.; Zhang, D.; Reich, L.A.; Carapellucci, S.; Lockwood, B.; Leal, A.S.; Krieger-Burke, T.; Aleiwi, B.; Ellsworth, E.; Liby, K.T. The Novel Rexinoid MSU-42011 Is Effective for the Treatment of Preclinical Kras-Driven Lung Cancer. *Sci. Rep.* **2020**, *10*, 22244. [CrossRef]
31. Hamarsheh, S.; Groß, O.; Brummer, T.; Zeiser, R. Immune Modulatory Effects of Oncogenic KRAS in Cancer. *Nat. Commun.* **2020**, *11*, 5439. [CrossRef]
32. Pereira, F.; Ferreira, A.; Reis, C.A.; Sousa, M.J.; Oliveira, M.J.; Preto, A. KRAS as a Modulator of the Inflammatory Tumor Microenvironment: Therapeutic Implications. *Cells* **2022**, *11*, 398. [CrossRef]
33. Liby, K.T.; Sporn, M.B. Rexinoids for Prevention and Treatment of Cancer: Opportunities and Challenges. *Curr. Top. Med. Chem.* 2016, *Epub ahead of print*.
34. Leal, A.S.; Hung, P.-Y.; Chowdhury, A.S.; Liby, K.T. Retinoid X Receptor Agonists as Selective Modulators of the Immune System for the Treatment of Cancer. *Pharmacol. Ther.* **2023**, *252*, 108561. [CrossRef] [PubMed]
35. Leal, A.S.; Zydeck, K.; Carapellucci, S.; Reich, L.A.; Zhang, D.; Moerland, J.A.; Sporn, M.B.; Liby, K.T. Retinoid X Receptor Agonist LG100268 Modulates the Immune Microenvironment in Preclinical Breast Cancer Models. *NPJ Breast Cancer* **2019**, *5*, 39. [CrossRef]
36. He, Q.; Sun, C.; Pan, Y. Whole-exome Sequencing Reveals Lewis Lung Carcinoma Is a Hypermutated Kras/Nras–Mutant Cancer with Extensive Regional Mutation Clusters in Its Genome. *Sci. Rep.* **2024**, *14*, 100. [CrossRef]
37. Li, H.; Chang, L.-J.; Neubauer, D.R.; Muir, D.F.; Wallace, M.R. Immortalization of Human Normal and NF1 Neurofibroma Schwann Cells. *Lab. Investig.* **2016**, *96*, 1105–1115. [CrossRef]
38. Tian, Z.; You, Y.; Xiao, M.; Liu, J.; Xu, G.; Ma, C.; Du, Z.; Wang, Y. Inhibition of YAP Sensitizes the Selumetinib Treatment for Neurofibromatosis Type 1 Related Plexiform Neurofibroma. *Int. J. Med. Sci.* **2023**, *20*, 125–135. [CrossRef]
39. Staedtke, V.; Gray-Bethke, T.; Riggins, G.J.; Bai, R.-Y. Preventative Effect of Mebendazole against Malignancies in Neurofibromatosis 1. *Genes* **2020**, *11*, 762. [CrossRef]
40. Flint, A.C.; Mitchell, D.K.; Angus, S.P.; Smith, A.E.; Bessler, W.; Jiang, L.; Mang, H.; Li, X.; Lu, Q.; Rodriguez, B.; et al. Combined CDK4/6 and ERK1/2 Inhibition Enhances Antitumor Activity in NF1-Associated Plexiform Neurofibroma. *Clin. Cancer Res.* **2023**, *29*, 3438–3456. [CrossRef] [PubMed]
41. Chen, Z.; Liu, C.; Patel, A.J.; Liao, C.-P.; Wang, Y.; Le, L.Q. Cells of Origin in the Embryonic Nerve Roots for NF1-Associated Plexiform Neurofibroma. *Cancer Cell* **2014**, *26*, 695–706. [CrossRef]
42. Jessen, W.J.; Miller, S.J.; Jousma, E.; Wu, J.; Rizvi, T.A.; Brundage, M.E.; Eaves, D.; Widemann, B.; Kim, M.-O.; Dombi, E.; et al. MEK Inhibition Exhibits Efficacy in Human and Mouse Neurofibromatosis Tumors. *J. Clin. Investig.* **2013**, *123*, 340–347. [CrossRef]
43. Qu, L.; Tang, X. Bexarotene: A Promising Anticancer Agent. *Cancer Chemother. Pharmacol.* **2010**, *65*, 201–205. [CrossRef] [PubMed]
44. Leal, A.S.; Reich, L.A.; Moerland, J.A.; Zhang, D.; Liby, K.T. Potential Therapeutic Uses of Rexinoids. *Adv. Pharmacol.* **2021**, *91*, 141–183. [CrossRef]
45. Millesi, E.; Rechberger, J.S.; Wang, H.; Mardini, S.; Spinner, R.J.; Daniels, D.J. Advancements in Therapeutic Approaches for Malignant Peripheral Nerve Sheath Tumor. *Ther. Deliv.* **2023**, *14*, 385–389. [CrossRef] [PubMed]

46. U.S. Food and Drug Administration. Multi-Disciplinary Review and Evaluation NDA 213756 Koselugo (Selumetinib). 2019. Available online: https://www.accessdata.fda.gov/drugsatfda_docs/nda/2020/213756Orig1s000MultidisciplineR.pdf. (accessed on 13 March 2025).
47. MacCollin, M.; Chiocca, E.A.; Evans, D.G.; Friedman, J.M.; Horvitz, R.; Jaramillo, D.; Lev, M.; Mautner, V.F.; Niimura, M.; Plotkin, S.R.; et al. Diagnostic Criteria for Schwannomatosis. *Neurology* **2005**, *64*, 1838–1845. [CrossRef] [PubMed]
48. Merker, V.L.; Esparza, S.; Smith, M.J.; Stemmer-Rachamimov, A.; Plotkin, S.R. Clinical Features of Schwannomatosis: A Retrospective Analysis of 87 Patients. *Oncologist* **2012**, *17*, 1317–1322. [CrossRef]
49. Yin, Z.; Wu, L.; Zhang, Y.; Sun, Y.; Chen, J.W.; Subudhi, S.; Ho, W.; Lee, G.Y.; Wang, A.; Gao, X.; et al. Co-Targeting IL-6 and EGFR Signaling for the Treatment of Schwannomatosis and Associated Pain. *bioRxiv* **2023**. [CrossRef]
50. Shou, J.; Zhang, Z.; Lai, Y.; Chen, Z.; Huang, J. Worse Outcome in Breast Cancer with Higher Tumor-Infiltrating FOXP3+ Tregs: A Systematic Review and Meta-Analysis. *BMC Cancer* **2016**, *16*, 687. [CrossRef]
51. Pinto, S.M.; Kim, H.; Subbannayya, Y.; Giambelluca, M.S.; Bösl, K.; Ryan, L.; Sharma, A.; Kandasamy, R.K. Comparative Proteomic Analysis Reveals Varying Impact on Immune Responses in Phorbol 12-Myristate-13-Acetate-Mediated THP-1 Monocyte-to-Macrophage Differentiation. *Front. Immunol.* **2021**, *12*, 679458. [CrossRef]
52. Kundu, P.; Shankar, B.S. Macrophage Induced ERK-TGF-B1 Signaling in MCF7 Breast Cancer Cells Result in Reversible Cancer Stem Cell Plasticity and Epithelial Mesenchymal Transition. *Biochim. Biophys. Acta (BBA) General. Subj.* **2022**, *1866*, 130215. [CrossRef]
53. Kumar, S.; Principe, D.R.; Singh, S.K.; Viswakarma, N.; Sondarva, G.; Rana, B.; Rana, A. Mitogen-Activated Protein Kinase Inhibitors and T-Cell-Dependent Immunotherapy in Cancer. *Pharmaceuticals* **2020**, *13*, 9. [CrossRef]
54. Fletcher, J.S.; Springer, M.G.; Choi, K.; Jousma, E.; Rizvi, T.A.; Dombi, E.; Kim, M.-O.; Wu, J.; Ratner, N. STAT3 Inhibition Reduces Macrophage Number and Tumor Growth in Neurofibroma. *Oncogene* **2019**, *38*, 2876–2884. [CrossRef]
55. Mendoza, R.; Banerjee, I.; Manna, D.; Reghupaty, S.C.; Yetirajam, R.; Sarkar, D. *Mouse Bone Marrow Cell Isolation and Macrophage Differentiation*; Humana: New York, NY, USA, 2022; Volume 2455, pp. 85–91. [CrossRef]
56. Martinez, F.O. Macrophage Activation and Polarization. *Front. Biosci.* **2008**, *13*, 453. [CrossRef] [PubMed]
57. Yunna, C.; Mengru, H.; Lei, W.; Weidong, C. Macrophage M1/M2 Polarization. *Eur. J. Pharmacol.* **2020**, *877*, 173090. [CrossRef]
58. Mantovani, A.; Sozzani, S.; Locati, M.; Allavena, P.; Sica, A. Macrophage Polarization: Tumor-Associated Macrophages as a Paradigm for Polarized M2 Mononuclear Phagocytes. *Trends Immunol.* **2002**, *23*, 549–555. [CrossRef] [PubMed]
59. Larionova, I.; Cherdyntseva, N.; Liu, T.; Patysheva, M.; Rakina, M.; Kzhyshkowska, J. Interaction of Tumor-Associated Macrophages and Cancer Chemotherapy. *Oncoimmunology* **2019**, *8*, e1596004. [CrossRef]
60. Qian, B.-Z.; Pollard, J.W. Macrophage Diversity Enhances Tumor Progression and Metastasis. *Cell* **2010**, *141*, 39–51. [CrossRef] [PubMed]
61. Drosten, M.; Barbacid, M. Targeting the MAPK Pathway in KRAS-Driven Tumors. *Cancer Cell* **2020**, *37*, 543–550. [CrossRef]
62. Bar-Sagi, D.; Knelson, E.H.; Sequist, L.V. A Bright Future for KRAS Inhibitors. *Nat. Cancer* **2020**, *1*, 25–27. [CrossRef]
63. Kitajima, S.; Thummalapalli, R.; Barbie, D.A. Inflammation as a Driver and Vulnerability of KRAS Mediated Oncogenesis. *Semin. Cell Dev. Biol.* **2016**, *58*, 127–135. [CrossRef]
64. Farschtschi, S.; Park, S.-J.; Sawitzki, B.; Oh, S.-J.; Kluwe, L.; Mautner, V.F.; Kurtz, A. Effector T Cell Subclasses Associate with Tumor Burden in Neurofibromatosis Type 1 Patients. *Cancer Immunol. Immunother.* **2016**, *65*, 1113–1121. [CrossRef]
65. Mitchell, D.K.; Burgess, B.; White, E.E.; Smith, A.E.; Sierra Potchanant, E.A.; Mang, H.; Hickey, B.E.; Lu, Q.; Qian, S.; Bessler, W.; et al. Spatial Gene-Expression Profiling Unveils Immuno-Oncogenic Programs of NF1-Associated Peripheral Nerve Sheath Tumor Progression. *Clin. Cancer Res.* **2024**, *30*, 1038–1053. [CrossRef] [PubMed]
66. Shurell, E.; Singh, A.S.; Crompton, J.G.; Jensen, S.; Li, Y.; Dry, S.; Nelson, S.; Chmielowski, B.; Bernthal, N.; Federman, N.; et al. Characterizing the Immune Microenvironment of Malignant Peripheral Nerve Sheath Tumor by PD-L1 Expression and Presence of CD8+ Tumor Infiltrating Lymphocytes. *Oncotarget* **2016**, *7*, 64300–64308. [CrossRef] [PubMed]
67. Choi, K.; Komurov, K.; Fletcher, J.S.; Jousma, E.; Cancelas, J.A.; Wu, J.; Ratner, N. An Inflammatory Gene Signature Distinguishes Neurofibroma Schwann Cells and Macrophages from Cells in the Normal Peripheral Nervous System. *Sci. Rep.* **2017**, *7*, 43315. [CrossRef]
68. Ramlau, R.; Zatloukal, P.; Jassem, J.; Schwarzenberger, P.; Orlov, S.V.; Gottfried, M.; Pereira, J.R.; Temperley, G.; Negro-Vilar, R.; Rahal, S.; et al. Randomized Phase III Trial Comparing Bexarotene (L1069-49)/Cisplatin/Vinorelbine With Cisplatin/Vinorelbine in Chemotherapy-Naïve Patients With Advanced or Metastatic Non–Small-Cell Lung Cancer: SPIRIT I. *J. Clin. Oncol.* **2008**, *26*, 1886–1892. [CrossRef]
69. Blumenschein, G.R.; Khuri, F.R.; von Pawel, J.; Gatzemeier, U.; Miller, W.H.; Jotte, R.M.; Le Treut, J.; Sun, S.-L.; Zhang, J.K.; Dziewanowska, Z.E.; et al. Phase III Trial Comparing Carboplatin, Paclitaxel, and Bexarotene With Carboplatin and Paclitaxel in Chemotherapy-Naïve Patients With Advanced or Metastatic Non–Small-Cell Lung Cancer: SPIRIT II. *J. Clin. Oncol.* **2008**, *26*, 1879–1885. [CrossRef]

70. Dragnev, K.H.; Ma, T.; Cyrus, J.; Galimberti, F.; Memoli, V.; Busch, A.M.; Tsongalis, G.J.; Seltzer, M.; Johnstone, D.; Erkmen, C.P.; et al. Bexarotene Plus Erlotinib Suppress Lung Carcinogenesis Independent of *KRAS* Mutations in Two Clinical Trials and Transgenic Models. *Cancer Prev. Res.* **2011**, *4*, 818–828. [CrossRef]
71. Li, Y.; Zhang, Y.; Hill, J.; Kim, H.-T.; Shen, Q.; Bissonnette, R.P.; Lamph, W.W.; Brown, P.H. The Rexinoid, Bexarotene, Prevents the Development of Premalignant Lesions in MMTV-ErbB2 Mice. *Br. J. Cancer* **2008**, *98*, 1380–1388. [CrossRef]
72. Li, Y.; Shen, Q.; Kim, H.-T.; Bissonnette, R.P.; Lamph, W.W.; Yan, B.; Brown, P.H. The Rexinoid Bexarotene Represses Cyclin D1 Transcription by Inducing the DEC2 Transcriptional Repressor. *Breast Cancer Res. Treat.* **2011**, *128*, 667–677. [CrossRef] [PubMed]
73. Rőszer, T.; Menéndez-Gutiérrez, M.P.; Cedenilla, M.; Ricote, M. Retinoid X Receptors in Macrophage Biology. *Trends Endocrinol. Metab.* **2013**, *24*, 460–468. [CrossRef]
74. Kiss, M.; Czimmerer, Z.; Nagy, G.; Bieniasz-Krzywiec, P.; Ehling, M.; Pap, A.; Poliska, S.; Boto, P.; Tzerpos, P.; Horvath, A.; et al. Retinoid X Receptor Suppresses a Metastasis-Promoting Transcriptional Program in Myeloid Cells via a Ligand-Insensitive Mechanism. *Proc. Natl. Acad. Sci. USA* **2017**, *114*, 10725–10730. [CrossRef]
75. Ma, F.; Liu, S.-Y.; Razani, B.; Arora, N.; Li, B.; Kagechika, H.; Tontonoz, P.; Núñez, V.; Ricote, M.; Cheng, G. Retinoid X Receptor α Attenuates Host Antiviral Response by Suppressing Type I Interferon. *Nat. Commun.* **2014**, *5*, 5494. [CrossRef] [PubMed]
76. Standeven, A.M.; Thacher, S.M.; Yuan, Y.-D.; Escobar, M.; Vuligonda, V.; Beard, R.L.; Chandraratna, R.A.S. Retinoid X Receptor Agonist Elevation of Serum Triglycerides in Rats by Potentiation of Retinoic Acid Receptor Agonist Induction or by Action as Single Agents 2 2Abbreviations: RARs, Retinoic Acid Receptors; and RXRs, Retinoid X Receptors. *Biochem. Pharmacol.* **2001**, *62*, 1501–1509. [CrossRef] [PubMed]

cancers

MDPI

Article

Café-Au-Lait Macules in Neurofibromatosis Type 1: Birthmark or Biomarker?

Andrea Santangelo [1,2,†], Cristina Chelleri [1,†], Marco Tomasino [3,4], Mattia Pasquinucci [1], Francesca Cappozzo [1], Pasquale Striano [1,2], Maria Cristina Diana [2] and Marcello Scala [1,5,*]

1 Department of Neurosciences, Rehabilitation, Ophthalmology, Genetics, Maternal and Child Health, University of Genoa, 16132 Genoa, Italy; androsantangelo@gmail.com (A.S.); cristinachelleri@libero.it (C.C.); mattia.pasquinucci@aulss7.veneto.it (M.P.); s5283983@studenti.unige.it (F.C.); strianop@gmail.com (P.S.)
2 Pediatric Neurology and Muscular Diseases Unit, IRCCS Istituto Giannina Gaslini, 16147 Genova, Italy; mcristinadiana@gaslini.org
3 Cardiology Department, Vall d'Hebron University Hospital, 08035 Barcelona, Spain; marcotomasino21@gmail.com
4 Department of Medicine, Universitat Autònoma de Barcelona (UAB), 08193 Barcelona, Spain
5 Medical Genetics Unit, IRCCS Istituto Giannina Gaslini, 16147 Genoa, Italy
* Correspondence: mscala.md@gmail.com
† These authors contributed equally to this work.

Simple Summary: Neurofibromatosis type 1 (NF1) is a rare genetic disorder that affects multiple body systems and increases the risk of tumors. One of its earliest signs is café-au-lait macules (CALMs), pigmented skin spots that can help diagnose NF1 when six or more are present. This study investigated whether CALMs at birth could predict NF1 diagnosis and severity. We analyzed records of children with CALMs, aged four years or older, evaluated at our Institution. Among 208 patients, 147 had confirmed NF1. While some had no CALMs at birth, those with multiple spots were significantly more likely to develop NF1. The risk reached 95% in patients with at least five CALMs at birth. A higher number of CALMs also correlated with an increased risk of plexiform neurofibromas. These findings emphasize the importance of early monitoring for children with multiple CALMs, enabling timely diagnosis, better follow-up, and improved patient care.

Abstract: Background: Neurofibromatosis type 1 (NF1) is a rare multisystem disorder characterized by variable expressivity and increased tumor risk. Café-au-lait macules (CALMs) are a hallmark of the disease, often representing one of the earliest clinical manifestations and allowing a clinical NF1 diagnosis if six or more are present. In this study, we aimed to investigate the prognostic value of CALMs at birth in NF1 patients. Methods: We conducted a retrospective study in patients aged ≥ 4 years presenting with CALMs at our Institution between 2020 and 2021, with a minimum follow-up of four years. We retrospectively collected data on CALMs at birth and other clinical manifestations associated with NF1. Results: Among 208 patients evaluated, including 147 with a confirmed diagnosis of NF1, 110 did not show CALMs at birth, and 98 had at least one. The absence of CALMs at birth did not correlate with a lower likelihood of NF1. In contrast, the CALM number at birth directly correlated with the likelihood of NF1, up to 95% in patients with ≥ 5 macules. Additionally, a higher number of CALMs correlated with a greater prevalence of plexiform neurofibromas ($p < 0.001$). Conclusions: Our findings suggest that a higher number of CALMs may indicate a more severe form of NF1, with an increased risk of plexiform neurofibromas. These results emphasize the importance of a comprehensive evaluation of patients with CALMs, especially in case of multiple lesions, aiming at implementing early NF1 diagnosis, follow-up strategies, and overall patient management.

Cancers **2025**, *17*, 1490 https://doi.org/10.3390/cancers17091490

Keywords: neurofibromatosis; NF1; café-au-lait macules (CALMs); plexiform neurofibromas; early diagnosis; prognostic value

1. Introduction

Neurofibromatosis type 1 (NF1) is a rare cancer-predisposing syndrome with a wide range of clinical manifestations affecting the skin, nervous system, eyes, and bones [1]. It is an autosomal dominant disorder associated with mutations involving NF1, located on chromosome 17q11.2. Its diagnosis is based on the presence of at least two criteria, including six or more café-au-lait macules (CALMs), axillary or inguinal freckling, two or more neurofibromas or one plexiform neurofibroma (pNF), an optic pathway glioma, Lisch nodules or choroidal abnormalities, distinctive bone lesions, or a pathogenic variant in the *NF1* gene. Additionally, a child with a parent meeting these criteria is diagnosed if they exhibit one or more of these features [2].

NF1 significantly increases the risk of neoplasms. Patients experience a 2.7-fold higher cancer risk and a cumulative malignancy risk of 20% by the age of 50 [3]. Malignant peripheral nerve sheath tumors (MPNSTs) are the most common malignancy, accounting for 3–10% of all soft tissue sarcomas. Among these, 15–70% of cases occur in NF1 patients [4]. The lifetime cumulative risk of developing MPNSTs in NF1 is 8–13% compared with just 0.001% in the general population, making them a leading cause of death in this group [3,5]. Internal plexiform neurofibromas increase the risk of MPNSTs by 20-fold, and 10–50% of MPNSTs arise from malignant transformation of plexiform neurofibromas [6]. Notably, NF1-associated MPNSTs have a more severe prognosis compared to sporadic tumors, with a 5-year survival rate of 16–38% versus 42–57% for non-NF1 cases [3,7,8]. These tumors are highly aggressive and have the highest recurrence rate among sarcomas [9]. Optic pathway gliomas are other common NF1-associated neoplasms, occurring in up to 20% of pediatric cases [10]. These tumors often develop during early childhood and can significantly impact vision and quality of life.

The hallmark feature of NF1 is represented by multiple CALMs. These are flat hyperpigmented skin lesions typically appearing within the first few years of life. Although CALMs can appear in individuals without NF1, the presence of several lesions, especially in combination with other diagnostic features, strongly suggests a diagnosis of NF1 [11]. Given their frequent appearance in early childhood, CALMs are a critical marker for the early diagnosis and management of NF1 [11,12]. The number and size of CALMs can increase over time, especially in the early stages of the disorder. Their early onset represents a pivotal diagnostic tool, as they often appear before more severe NF1-related complications, such as neurofibromas or optic gliomas. While CALMs are a key diagnostic feature, they are not exclusive to NF1. In fact, up to 25% of the general population presents up to three CALMs [13]. Moreover, different disorders can also manifest with multiple CALMs. Legius syndrome is the most important phenocopy of NF1, manifesting with CALMs without the development of neurofibromas or other NF1-related tumors [14]. This phenotypic overlap complicates early diagnosis, particularly in young children. However, molecular testing of the *NF1* gene can differentiate NF1 from other conditions and help guide patient management.

In this study, we aimed at exploring the correlation between the presence of CALMs at birth and the subsequent risk of developing NF1. We also investigated the possible relevance of the presence of CALMs in relation to key prognostic factors of disease outcome, such as the likelihood of neurofibroma development, including plexiform neurofibromas, and other NF1-related complications.

2. Materials and Methods

2.1. Study Cohort

We retrospectively evaluated pediatric patients presenting with CALMs at birth to assess the risk of developing NF1 in these children. Data were collected from the medical records of subjects followed at the Specialized Center for NF1 Care in IRCCS G. Gaslini, Genoa, between 2020 and 2021. The inclusion criteria for the NF1 group were as follows: age of at least 4 years, the presence of at least one CALM at birth, fulfilling criteria for NF1 diagnosis according to NIH [2], and a minimum follow-up of 4 years at our Institution. Patients with pre-existing genetic diagnoses or conditions that could be confounding factors for a diagnosis of NF1 were excluded from this study. Inclusion criteria for the non-NF1 group included age of at least 4 years, the presence of at least one CALM at birth, clinical and genetic exclusion of NF1, and a follow-up of at least 4 years at our Institution.

2.2. Data Collection

Clinical and genetic data were retrospectively collected from electronic medical records. The following information was retrieved: number of CALMs at birth; development of clinical features associated with NF1 during follow-up (including neurofibromas, axillary or inguinal freckling, Lisch nodules, and optic pathway gliomas); family history of NF1 or other genetic disorders, or a genetic confirmation of a variant in *NF1*. Only typical CALMs (homogeneous pigmentation, regular borders) with a minimum diameter of 0.5 cm were considered, in accordance with NIH diagnostic criteria.

All individuals classified as non-NF1 underwent NF1 genetic testing. Conversely, patients with a clinical diagnosis based on $\geq$2 NIH criteria were included regardless of genetic confirmation.

2.3. Statistical Analysis

The CALM number, initially a continuous variable, was categorized into four groups (0, 1–2, 3–4, and 5 or more) based on clinical relevance and data distribution. Summary statistics for categorical variables, stratified by CALM group, were reported as frequencies and percentages. Group comparisons were conducted using the Pearson chi-square test or Fisher's exact test, as appropriate. Assumptions for the Pearson chi-square test, including the independence of observations and a minimum expected cell count of five in at least 80% of cells, were verified. For cases where these assumptions were not met, Fisher's exact test was used. Statistical significance was set at two-tailed p-values < 0.05. All analyses were performed using Stata software, version 17.0 (StataCorp, College Station, TX, USA).

3. Results

3.1. Cohort Description

We recruited 208 individuals, including 61 without NF1 and 147 with diagnosed NF1. Patients were categorized by the number of CALMs at birth: 110 with no CALMs, 38 with 1–2 CALMs, 20 with 3–4 CALMs, and 40 with 5 or more CALMs. The Fitzpatrick skin type distribution was recorded for all enrolled subjects. In both NF1 and non-NF1 groups, phototype III was the most frequent, observed in 88 out of 147 NF1 patients (59.9%) and 37 out of 61 non-NF1 patients (60.7%). Phototype II was present in 22 NF1 patients (15.0%) and 10 non-NF1 patients (16.4%), while phototype IV was found in 26 NF1 cases (17.7%) and 9 non-NF1 cases (14.8%). Less frequent were phototype I (four NF1 cases (2.7%), two non-NF1 cases (3.3%)), phototype V (four NF1 (2.7%), one non-NF1 (1.6%)), and phototype VI (three NF1 (2.0%), two non-NF1 (3.3%)). There was no significant difference in the distribution of skin types between the NF1 and non-NF1 groups ($p > 0.05$). The primary characteristics of the cohort are summarized in Table 1.

Table 1. Presence of CALMs at birth in NF1 and non-NF1 patients in our cohort.

Number of CALMs	0	1–2	3–4	5 or More
Non-NF1 patients	32 (29%)	19 (50%)	8 (40%)	2 (5%)
NF1 patients	78 (71%)	19 (50%)	12 (60%)	38 (95%)
Total	110	38	20	40

3.2. CALMs' Correlation with NF1 Diagnosis and pNF

The prevalence of NF1 increased with the number of CALMs. A prevalence of 71% (78 patients) was observed in subjects with no CALMs. The prevalence was 50% in subjects with 1–2 CALMs, 60% in those with 3–4 CALMs, and 95% in those with 5 or more CALMs ($p < 0.001$) (Table 1). Interestingly, a significant association was observed between CALM count and the prevalence of pNFs (Figure 1), with a higher prevalence in patients with five or more CALMs ($p = 0.001$) (Table 2).

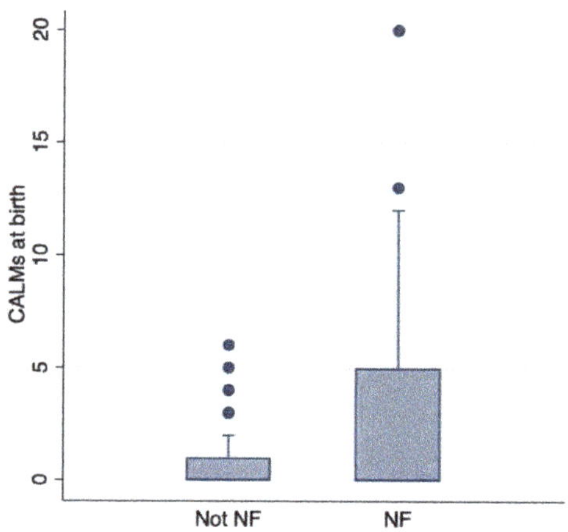

Figure 1. Association between CALMs at birth and NF1 diagnosis. Bar plot graph showing the prevalence of NF1 with an increasing number of CALMs at birth.

Table 2. Comorbidities found in our cohort and their association with CALMs at birth. OPG: optical pathway glioma, pNF: plexiform neurofibroma, ADHD: attention-deficit/hyperactivity disorder, ASD: autism spectrum disorder, CV: cardiovascular.

Comorbidities	CALMs at Birth				p-Value
	0 (78 Patients)	1–2 (19 Patients)	3–4 (12 Patients)	5 or More (38 Patients)	
OPG	21 (27%)	4 (21%)	5 (42%)	13 (34%)	0.320
Cutaneous/subcutaneous neurofibromas	31 (40%)	9 (47%)	7 (58%)	21 (55%)	0.084
pNFs	25 (32%)	6 (32%)	6 (50%)	24 (63%)	0.001
Other neoplasms	22 (28%)	3 (16%)	4 (33%)	14 (37%)	0.320
ADHD	9 (12%)	1 (5%)	0	3 (8%)	0.366
ASD	10 (13%)	0	1 (8%)	3 (8%)	0.374
Endocrinological manifestations	30 (38%)	9 (47%)	6 (50%)	20 (53%)	0.134
Allergic manifestations	27 (35%)	10 (53%)	6 (50%)	10 (26%)	0.536
CV manifestations	25 (32%)	5 (26%)	5 (42%)	15 (39%)	0.372

Additionally, a trend towards higher cutaneous neurofibroma prevalence was noted in the same group ($p = 0.084$) (Table 2).

4. Discussion

Beyond their diagnostic value, CALMs may have an important prognostic significance in NF1. In fact, research has already shown that the number and size of CALMs can correlate with disease severity [15], and larger CALMs or a higher number of lesions can occur in patients with more serious complications, such as MPNSTs and skeletal abnormalities [16]. Furthermore, CALMs occurring in patients with NF1 are often more intensely pigmented and larger than those found in individuals with other syndromes or isolated lesions [14,17]. Our findings revealed that children with five or more CALMs exhibited a 95% prevalence of NF1, compared to a 50% prevalence in those with 1–2 CALMs. This aligns with prior studies, such as a retrospective analysis by Ben-Schachar et al., which reported an 80.4% risk of being affected by NF1 in children younger than 29 months with more than six CALMs [18]. Overall, these observations support the relevance of the number and size of CALMs as predictors of disease severity in NF1 patients, highlighting the critical importance of early CALM count assessment as a potential screening tool for NF1.

The early identification of children with a high CALM burden may indeed allow clinicians to make a timely diagnosis, facilitating appropriate intervention in pediatric populations at elevated risk. Early diagnosis can enable tailored surveillance strategies, including genetic testing and regular imaging to monitor for complications such as optic gliomas, neurofibromas, or pNFs. However, not all patients with multiple CALMs will develop a full NF1 phenotype. A review of patients with isolated CALMs revealed that 19.5% to 57.1% of such cases did not meet the clinical criteria for NF1 upon follow-up [11]. This finding highlights the need for molecular confirmation of NF1 in cases where CALMs are the sole presenting feature, especially in the absence of other diagnostic signs.

Notably, none of the patients with negative *NF1* genetic testing developed additional clinical criteria for NF1 during the follow-up period, supporting the reliability of their classification as non-NF1.

Importantly, our findings raise a relevant clinical question regarding children presenting with two CALMs in early infancy, without other signs or genetic confirmation of NF1. While this presentation does not meet diagnostic criteria, we recommend close monitoring due to the potential for additional features to emerge over time. Specifically, we suggest scheduling a clinical re-evaluation at 12 months of age and a dedicated neurological/genetic assessment at 18 months, to ensure the early identification of any evolving NF1 phenotype.

The important impact that an early diagnosis may have on patient management in individuals affected with NF1 has led to the investigation of other possible early markers of disease. For instance, Parrozzani et al. demonstrated the diagnostic value of choroidal abnormalities detected through near-infrared imaging. These defects showed higher specificity than Lisch nodules for early NF1 detection in pediatric patients [19]. Similarly, Cnossen et al. identified minor features such as macrocephaly and thorax abnormalities as predictors of NF1 in children under six. Such markers may be very helpful in trying to enhance diagnostic accuracy when traditional criteria are insufficient [20].

Other early visible cutaneous signs may also support the clinical suspicion of NF1 in infancy. Among these, nevus anemicus and juvenile xanthogranulomas have been reported as additional early markers with diagnostic value in young children [21–23]. Notably, these features could be detectable on clinical examination and may aid early stratification, especially when combined with the CALM count.

The increased prevalence of neurofibromas and pNFs in patients with higher CALM counts further highlights the clinical significance of these tumors. Our analysis found that 40% of patients without CALMs exhibited subcutaneous or cutaneous neurofibromas, while this proportion increased to 58% in individuals with 3–4 CALMs. For pNFs, the prevalence increased dramatically from 32% in patients with no CALMs to 63% in those with five or more CALMs. These findings are supported by Nasi et al., who analyzed 63 Greek pediatric NF1 patients and observed that individuals with protein-truncating *NF1* variants presented not only a higher CALM count but also a greater incidence of pNFs [24]. Such genetic predispositions may lead to more severe disease manifestations in NF1 patients with high CALM counts. These observations support the potential utility of CALM assessment in the early clinical stratification and risk management of NF1 patients. The strong association between the number of CALMs and the prevalence of pNFs suggests that CALMs may serve not only as a diagnostic marker, but also as an early indicator of disease severity. As such, CALMs could also be an indicator of the likelihood of developing significant complications. The early identification of individuals with a high CALM burden could therefore enable targeted interventions, such as more frequent imaging studies for the early detection of pNFs or early administration of Selumetinib. The second point is particularly relevant since the side effects of Selumetinib can be age-related [25,26].

NF1 is a multisystem disorder with variable expressivity and elusive genotype–phenotype correlations [1,27–30]. This also applies to CALMs, where no significant evidence supporting an association between specific genetic variants and their presence or number was reported in the literature. The clinical manifestations of NF1 span diverse systems, including skeletal abnormalities, neurological features, and cardiovascular anomalies. Based on the results of our study, we cannot observe a significant correlation between CALM counts at birth and the presence of these diverse clinical manifestations. Additionally, our findings do not suggest the existence of genotype–phenotype correlations between specific variants in the *NF1* gene and the presence or number of CALMs. This observation highlights the well-known complexity of NF1 and suggests that CALMs alone may not fully capture the multifactorial nature of the disorder. Thus, the multifactorial nature of NF1 prompts the investigation of other potential diagnostic and prognostic markers that could be helpful for implementing clinical diagnosis and management in NF1 patients.

Our study presents some limitations. First, the retrospective design may have limited the availability of information regarding the presence of specific clinical manifestations in the enrolled NF1 patients, such as those that are more strictly age-related. Second, the inclusion in the study cohort of patients enrolled at a single Institution may have generated potential biases in the identification of specific clinical features in NF1 subjects, beyond CALMs, due to the preferential investigation and detection of some disease manifestations based on the expertise of the clinicians. Finally, although previous studies have suggested a possible correlation between CALM size and disease severity, our study did not analyze this parameter systematically. Further prospective investigations are warranted to explore the potential role of macule dimensions in predicting NF1 complications. While every effort has been made to limit the impact of these limitations, these aspects may still affect the generalizability of our findings. Therefore, we recognize the importance of prospective, multicenter studies with larger and more diverse populations to validate our observations and further refine our understanding of the prognostic significance of CALMs.

5. Conclusions

In conclusion, our study suggests that CALMs hold prognostic significance in NF1, beyond their diagnostic relevance. This is particularly evident when they are present at birth in higher numbers. Additionally, patients with higher CALM counts showed a significantly increased risk of developing pNFs, which are among the most severe complications associated with NF1. This observation highlights the need for closer surveillance and early intervention for these individuals. Integrating CALM assessment with genetic testing can be a very helpful tool to refine risk stratification in NF1 patients, potentially enabling personalized management and timely treatment. Overall, our findings support the utility of CALMs as a cost-effective tool for guiding early and proactive care strategies towards the improvement of long-term outcomes in NF1 patients.

Author Contributions: Conceptualization, M.S. and C.C.; methodology, M.S., C.C. and A.S.; software, M.T.; validation, M.T. and A.S.; formal analysis, A.S., C.C. and A.S.; investigation, M.P., F.C., P.S. and M.C.D.; resources, M.S.; data curation, A.S., C.C. and M.S.; writing—original draft preparation, A.S. and C.C.; writing—review and editing, M.S.; visualization, M.S.; supervision, M.S.; project administration, M.S. All authors have read and agreed to the published version of the manuscript.

Funding: This research was supported by PNRR-MUR-M4C2 PE0000006 Research Program "MNESYS"—A multiscale integrated approach to the study of the nervous system in health and disease.

Institutional Review Board Statement: This study was conducted in accordance with the Declaration of Helsinki and approved by the Institutional Review Board of Gaslini Institute (protocol code 163/2018, approved in August 2018).

Informed Consent Statement: Informed consent was obtained from all subjects involved in this study.

Data Availability Statement: The data generated by this study are available in the manuscript. Additional information is available from the authors upon reasonable request.

Acknowledgments: IRCCS 'G. Gaslini' is a member of ERN-Epicare.

Conflicts of Interest: The authors declare no conflicts of interest.

References

1. Scala, M.; Schiavetti, I.; Madia, F.; Chelleri, C.; Piccolo, G.; Accogli, A.; Riva, A.; Salpietro, V.; Bocciardi, R.; Morcaldi, G.; et al. Genotype-Phenotype Correlations in Neurofibromatosis Type 1: A Single-Center Cohort Study. *Cancers* **2021**, *13*, 1879. [CrossRef] [PubMed]
2. Legius, E.; Messiaen, L.; Wolkenstein, P.; Pancza, P.; Avery, R.A.; Berman, Y.; Blakeley, J.; Babovic-Vuksanovic, D.; Cunha, K.S.; Ferner, R.; et al. Revised diagnostic criteria for neurofibromatosis type 1 and Legius syndrome: An international consensus recommendation. *Genet. Med.* **2021**, *23*, 1506–1513. [CrossRef] [PubMed]
3. Patil, S.; Chamberlain, R.S. Neoplasms associated with germline and somatic NF1 gene mutations. *Oncologist* **2012**, *17*, 101–116. [CrossRef] [PubMed]
4. Bhattacharyya, A.K.; Perrin, R.; Guha, A. Peripheral nerve tumors: Management strategies and molecular insights. *J. Neurooncol.* **2004**, *69*, 335–349. [CrossRef]
5. Rasmussen, S.A.; Friedman, J.M. NF1 gene and neurofibromatosis 1. *Am. J. Epidemiol.* **2000**, *151*, 33–40. [CrossRef]
6. Tucker, T.; Wolkenstein, P.; Revuz, J.; Zeller, J.; Friedman, J.M. Association between benign and malignant peripheral nerve sheath tumors in NF1. *Neurology* **2005**, *65*, 205–211. [CrossRef]
7. Carli, M.; Ferrari, A.; Mattke, A.; Zanetti, I.; Casanova, M.; Bisogno, G.; Cecchetto, G.; Alaggio, R.; De Sio, L.; Koscielniak, E.; et al. Pediatric malignant peripheral nerve sheath tumor: The Italian and German soft tissue sarcoma cooperative group. *J. Clin. Oncol.* **2005**, *23*, 8422–8430. [CrossRef]
8. Cai, Z.; Tang, X.; Liang, H.; Yang, R.; Yan, T.; Guo, W. Prognosis and risk factors for malignant peripheral nerve sheath tumor: A systematic review and meta-analysis. *World J. Surg. Oncol.* **2020**, *18*, 257. [CrossRef]
9. Jansma, C.Y.M.N.; Acem, I.; Grünhagen, D.J.; Verhoef, C.; Martin, E.; MONACO Collaborators. Local recurrence in malignant peripheral nerve sheath tumours: Multicentre cohort study. *BJS Open* **2024**, *8*, zrae024. [CrossRef]
10. Chen, Y.; Yu, J.; Ge, S.; Jia, R.; Song, X.; Wang, Y.; Fan, X. An Overview of Optic Pathway Glioma With Neurofibromatosis Type 1: Pathogenesis, Risk Factors, and Therapeutic Strategies. *Investig. Ophthalmol. Vis. Sci.* **2024**, *65*, 8. [CrossRef]
11. Bernier, A.; Larbrisseau, A.; Perreault, S. Café-au-lait Macules and Neurofibromatosis Type 1: A Review of the Literature. *Pediatr. Neurol.* **2016**, *60*, 24–29.e1. [CrossRef]
12. Nunley, K.S.; Gao, F.; Albers, A.C.; Bayliss, S.J.; Gutmann, D.H. Predictive value of café au lait macules at initial consultation in the diagnosis of neurofibromatosis type 1. *Arch. Dermatol.* **2009**, *145*, 883–887. [CrossRef] [PubMed]
13. Jha, S.K.; Mendez, M.D. Cafe Au Lait Macules. [Updated 2023 Jul 31]. In *StatPearls [Internet]*; StatPearls Publishing: Treasure Island, FL, USA, 2024.

14. Messiaen, L.; Yao, S.; Brems, H.; Callens, T.; Sathienkijkanchai, A.; Denayer, E.; Spencer, E.; Arn, P.; Babovic-Vuksanovic, D.; Bay, C.; et al. Clinical and mutational spectrum of neurofibromatosis type 1-like syndrome. *JAMA* **2009**, *302*, 2111–2118; [published correction appears in *JAMA* **2010**, *303*, 2477]. [CrossRef] [PubMed]
15. Chelleri, C.; Brolatti, N.; De Marco, P.; Ognibene, M.; Diana, M.C.; Madia, F.; Duca, M.D.; Santangelo, A.; Capra, V.; Striano, P.; et al. Novel causative variants in Legius syndrome: SPRED1 Genotype spectrum expansion. *Am. J. Med. Genet. A.* **2024**, *194*, e63824. [CrossRef] [PubMed]
16. Sbidian, E.; Wolkenstein, P.; Valeyrie-Allanore, L.; Rodriguez, D.; Hadj-Rabia, S.; Ferkal, S.; Lacour, J.P.; Leonard, J.C.; Taillandier, L.; Sportich, S.; et al. NF-1Score: A prediction score for internal neurofibromas in neurofibromatosis-1. *J. Investig. Dermatol.* **2010**, *130*, 2173–2178. [CrossRef]
17. Tong, H.X.; Li, M.; Zhang, Y.; Zhu, J.; Lu, W.Q. A novel NF1 mutation in a Chinese patient with giant café-au-lait macule in neurofibromatosis type 1 associated with a malignant peripheral nerve sheath tumor and bone abnormality. *Genet. Mol. Res.* **2012**, *11*, 2972–2978. [CrossRef]
18. Boyd, K.P.; Gao, L.; Feng, R.; Beasley, M.; Messiaen, L.; Korf, B.R.; Theos, A. Phenotypic variability among café-au-lait macules in neurofibromatosis type 1. *J. Am. Acad. Dermatol.* **2010**, *63*, 440–447. [CrossRef]
19. Ben-Shachar, S.; Dubov, T.; Toledano-Alhadef, H.; Mashiah, J.; Sprecher, E.; Constantini, S.; Leshno, M.; Messiaen, L.M. Predicting neurofibromatosis type 1 risk among children with isolated café-au-lait macules. *J. Am. Acad. Dermatol.* **2017**, *76*, 1077–1083.e3. [CrossRef]
20. Parrozzani, R.; Clementi, M.; Frizziero, L.; Miglionico, G.; Perrini, P.; Cavarzeran, F.; Kotsafti, O.; Comacchio, F.; Trevisson, E.; Convento, E.; et al. In Vivo Detection of Choroidal Abnormalities Related to NF1: Feasibility and Comparison With Standard NIH Diagnostic Criteria in Pediatric Patients. *Investig. Ophthalmol. Vis. Sci.* **2015**, *56*, 6036–6042. [CrossRef]
21. DeBella, K.; Szudek, J.; Friedman, J.M. Use of the national institutes of health criteria for diagnosis of neurofibromatosis 1 in children. *Pediatrics* **2000**, *105 (Pt 1)*, 608–614. [CrossRef]
22. Marque, M.; Roubertie, A.; Jaussent, A.; Carneiro, M.; Meunier, L.; Guillot, B.; Pinson, L.; Pinson, S.; Bessis, D. Nevus anemicus in neurofibromatosis type 1: A potential new diagnostic criterion. *J. Am. Acad. Dermatol.* **2013**, *69*, 768–775. [CrossRef] [PubMed]
23. Cnossen, M.H.; Moons, K.G.; Garssen, M.P.; Pasmans, N.M.; de Goede-Bolder, A.; Niermeijer, M.F.; Grobbee, D.E. Minor disease features in neurofibromatosis type 1 (NF1) and their possible value in diagnosis of NF1 in children < or = 6 years and clinically suspected of having NF1. Neurofibromatosis team of Sophia Children's Hospital. *J. Med. Genet.* **1998**, *35*, 624–627. [PubMed]
24. Nasi, L.; Alexopoulos, A.; Kokkinou, E.; Roka, K.; Tzetis, M.; Tsipi, M.; Kakourou, T.; Kanaka-Gantenbein, C.; Chrousos, G.; Kattamis, A.; et al. Characteristics of Café-au-lait Macules and their Association with the Neurofibromatosis type I Genotype in a Cohort of Greek Children. *Acta Derm. Venereol.* **2023**, *103*, adv5758. [CrossRef] [PubMed]
25. Borgia, P.; Piccolo, G.; Santangelo, A.; Chelleri, C.; Viglizzo, G.; Occella, C.; Minetti, C.; Striano, P.; Diana, M.C. Dermatologic Effects of Selumetinib in Pediatric Patients with Neurofibromatosis Type 1: Clinical Challenges and Therapeutic Management. *J. Clin. Med.* **2024**, *13*, 1792. [CrossRef]
26. Morello, A.; Scala, M.; Schiavetti, I.; Diana, M.C.; Severino, M.; Tortora, D.; Piatelli, G.; Pavanello, M. Surgical revascularization as a procedure to prevent neurological complications in children with moyamoya syndrome associated with neurofibromatosis I: A single institution case series. *Childs Nerv. Syst.* **2024**, *40*, 1731–1741. [CrossRef]
27. Ognibene, M.; Scala, M.; Iacomino, M.; Schiavetti, I.; Madia, F.; Traverso, M.; Guerrisi, S.; Di Duca, M.; Caroli, F.; Baldassari, S.; et al. Moyamoya Vasculopathy in Neurofibromatosis Type 1 Pediatric Patients: The Role of Rare Variants of RNF213. *Cancers* **2023**, *15*, 1916. [CrossRef]
28. Tortora, D.; Scavetta, C.; Rebella, G.; Bertamino, M.; Scala, M.; Giacomini, T.; Morana, G.; Pavanello, M.; Rossi, A.; Severino, M. Spatial coefficient of variation applied to arterial spin labeling MRI may contribute to predict surgical revascularization outcomes in pediatric moyamoya vasculopathy. *Neuroradiology* **2020**, *62*, 1003–1015. [CrossRef]
29. Koczkowska, M.; Chen, Y.; Callens, T.; Gomes, A.; Sharp, A.; Johnson, S.; Hsiao, M.C.; Chen, Z.; Balasubramanian, M.; Barnett, C.P.; et al. Genotype-Phenotype Correlation in NF1: Evidence for a More Severe Phenotype Associated with Missense Mutations Affecting NF1 Codons 844-848. *Am. J. Hum. Genet.* **2018**, *102*, 69–87. [CrossRef]
30. Kehrer-Sawatzki, H.; Mautner, V.F.; Cooper, D.N. Emerging genotype-phenotype relationships in patients with large NF1 deletions. *Hum. Genet.* **2017**, *136*, 349–376. [CrossRef]

cancers

MDPI

Article

Identification of the Determinants of Plexiform Neurofibroma Morbidity in Pediatric and Young Adult Neurofibromatosis Type 1 Patients: A Pilot Multivariate Approach

Biagio de Brons [1], Britt Dhaenens [1], Rick van Minkelen [2] and Rianne Oostenbrink [1,3,*]

[1] Sophia, Department of General Pediatrics, Erasmus MC, 3015 GD Rotterdam, The Netherlands; 445070bb@student.eur.nl (B.d.B.)

[2] Department Genetics, Erasmus MC, 3015 GD Rotterdam, The Netherlands; r.vanminkelen@erasmusmc.nl

[3] The ENCORE Expertise Centre for Neurodevelopmental Disorders, Erasmus MC, 3015 GD Rotterdam, The Netherlands

* Correspondence: r.oostenbrink@erasmusmc.nl; Tel.: +31-6-1488-6807

Simple Summary: We studied a group of 90 patients with NF1-related plexiform neurofibromas (PNs) with an average age of 15.7 years and a follow-up period of 9.8 yrs. PNs in patients with older age and PNs located in the craniofacial region or trunk were most frequently associated with plexiform neurofibroma morbidity and most frequently underwent intervention (surgery or systemic treatment). These findings may contribute to decisions on whether or not to start what treatment in NF1 patients with PNs.

Abstract: Background: Plexiform neurofibromas (PNs) are histologically benign peripheral nerve sheath tumors associated with neurofibromatosis type 1 (NF1) and often lead to significant morbidity due to growth. Management includes watchful waiting, surgery for partial debulking, and, since recently, systemic treatment with MEK inhibitors. However, due to the scarcity of natural history studies, our understanding of the natural progression of PNs to guide clinicians in deciding in whom and when to intervene is scarce. This study aims to describe the characteristics of NF1 patients with PNs and compare those at high risk for PN progression or experiencing significant morbidity from PN (complex PN) with NF1 patients with PNs of lower complexity. Methods: In this retrospective cohort study using clinical data from hospital records of NF1 patients with PNs seen at the Sophia Children's Hospital in the Netherlands between 2012 and 2023, we assessed determinants of clinical phenotypes and PN characteristics predictive of outcomes, including PN complexity and the timing of intervention for PN. We assessed the outcomes using logistic regression analysis and Cox regression. Results: Ninety patients with a median age at last evaluation of 15.7 years and a median follow-up duration of 9.8 years were included. Out of 90 individuals with a benign PN, 37 developed plexiform neurofibroma morbidity during follow-up. Older age was (corrected for pathogenic NF1 variant and PN location) significantly associated with plexiform neurofibroma morbidity. Cox regression revealed that craniofacial and trunk PNs were associated with a higher intervention hazard compared to limb PNs. Conclusion: Our pilot multivariate approach identified older age and the location of the PN to be mostly associated with a higher chance of plexiform neurofibroma morbidity and higher intervention hazard. This may contribute to decisions regarding in whom and when to initiate treatment in NF1 patients with PNs.

Keywords: longitudinal history; plexiform neurofibroma; predictors; neurofibromatosis type 1

1. Introduction

Neurofibromatosis type 1 (NF1), although rare, with an incidence of approximately 1 in 2700, is one of the most frequent tumor-suppressor multisystem syndromes [1,2]. NF1 is characterized by a wide variability in manifestations and severity among patients. These include skin abnormalities (café au lait macules, axillary or inguinal freckling), eye abnormalities, musculoskeletal manifestations (scoliosis, pseudoarthrosis), nervous system tumors (neurofibromas, optic pathway gliomas (OPGs)), epilepsy, vascular complications, and cognitive problems [3,4]. NF1 is caused by a germline pathogenic variant in *NF1*, consisting of 57 exons (transcript NM_000267.3) that span over 350 kb of genomic DNA, located on chromosome 17q11.2 [5]. *NF1* encodes neurofibromin, a protein that serves as a negative regulator of the RAS/MAPK pathway [6]. This pathway plays a key role in cell growth, division, and differentiation. Therefore, the *NF1* gene functions as a tumor-suppressor gene 2.

A major complication in NF1 is plexiform neurofibroma (PN), occurring in 30% (visible) to 50% (on imaging) of NF1 patients [3,7]. PNs are present in principle from birth but may grow and develop into large benign tumors along large nerves in the body [8]. Due to their location or growth, they may cause neurological deficit, pain, or the obstruction of vital organs. A major risk of PN is the transformation into a malignant peripheral nerve sheath tumor (MPNST), with a 10% lifetime risk in patients with NF1, representing a major cause of mortality in NF1 patients [9,10]. Until the past decade, treatment was limited to surgery, which in many cases does not achieve complete tumor resection. Surgery also has a considerable risk of postoperative deficits due to the large size and the invasion of the surrounding structures of the PN [11]. Furthermore, long-term benefits of surgery are unlikely in patients under the age of 10 with craniofacial or trunk lesions, mainly because the resection is often incomplete. In 2020, selumetinib, an MEK inhibitor, was approved by the FDA (by EMA in 2021) for the treatment of children with inoperable symptomatic PNs [12,13].

Currently, it is unclear which NF1 patients with PNs are at risk for disease progression and need which therapy at which timepoint. The scientific community is trying to identify new outcomes to predict the course of PN using anatomical, radiological, and biological characteristics to identify PNs with a high risk for progression [14,15]. The scarcity of natural history studies on PNs limits our understanding of their natural progression. Natural history study data are imperative to uncover patient characteristics that can serve as predictors for the development of symptomatic or fast-growing PNs. Therefore, this study aims to outline the characteristics of NF1 patients with PN and compare those at high risk for PN progression or experiencing significant morbidity from PN with individuals who have lower morbidity or risk levels.

2. Materials and Methods

2.1. Study Design and Patients

This is a retrospective cohort study. We included patients currently alive with a diagnosis of PN and NF1, based on the revised diagnostic criteria for neurofibromatosis type 1 [16]. The patients were seen between 2012 and 2023 at the ENCORE-NF1 expertise center in the Erasmus MC-Sophia Children's Hospital in the Netherlands. Patients and/or their caregivers provided informed consent for the use of medical record data for research (local Institutional Review Board identifier MEC-2015-203).

2.2. Outcomes

The primary outcome of interest was the occurrence of a plexiform neurofibroma at risk of or causing morbidity, further referred to as 'plexiform neurofibroma morbidity', and was defined as a PN with progressive growth, a PN that causes morbidity (excluding disfigurement/cosmetic burden), or a PN that causes pain needing intervention (analgesics, or warranting systemic or surgical treatment). The secondary outcome measure was the age at first therapeutic intervention (surgery or MEK-inhibitor treatment) of the PN where therapy was targeted for the patient.

2.3. Data

We collected data from medical records, including biological sex, date of birth, age at NF1 diagnosis, date of first and last evaluation, inheritance (familial or de novo), type of NF1 pathogenic variant, and diagnostic criteria associated with NF1 [16]. At the PN level, we gathered data on location, date of diagnosis, and available imaging data. PN location was categorized as either trunk, craniofacial, or limb. At the patient level, we gathered data on the number of PNs and their morbidity and size measurement. Volumetric analysis was not performed routinely in our center. As bidimensional reported sizes do not correspond well to tumor volume [17], we did not include the (change in) size in further analyses. Comorbidities related to PNs were categorized as disfigurement and/or cosmetic burden, pain, neurological deficit, airway complications, vision impairment, bowel or bladder complications, and others. Details of interventions included the type of intervention (surgical or systemic) and its date.

2.4. Statistical Analyses

Descriptive statistics were computed for primary outcomes and determinants, including means and standard deviations for continuous variables and frequencies for categorical variables. Continuous variables were analyzed using Mann–Whitney U tests, while chi-squared or Fisher's exact tests were performed for categorical variables. Patients with MPNST were excluded from this analysis and described separately. Determinants for complex PN were assessed by multivariate logistic regression analysis. In addition, we assessed determinants for the timing of the intervention by Cox regression. To prevent overfitting for both logistic regression analyses, given the expected low number of cases, we pre-selected potential predictors from the literature and clinical experience in order to keep the number of variables used in both regression models about equal to one variable per ten events [18]. All calculations were performed using SPSS Predictive Analytics Software Version 29.0.2.0 (IBM Corp, Armonk, NY, USA). If not elsewhere specified, *p*-values were calculated at a 95% confidence interval.

3. Results

3.1. Demographics and Clinical Characteristics

Ninety patients were identified with a benign PN, of which 54.4% were male, with a median age at last evaluation of 15.7 years. The median age of NF1 diagnosis was 1.0 years (Table 1). The median follow-up time was 9.8 yrs. All patients fulfilled the NF1 criteria. The most frequent diagnostic criteria were six or more café-au-lait macules (100%), freckling in the axillary or inguinal regions (98%), and a detected pathogenic NF1 variant (89%). NF1-related bone deformities were present in nine patients (10%), all with sphenoid wing dysplasia, combined with pseudoarthrosis in two. Inheritance was mostly de novo (66%). Pathogenic variants were mostly nonsense/frameshift/splicing (81%), with a small proportion of our patients having NF1 microdeletion (4.8%). Twelve patients (13.3%) harbored an optic pathway glioma (OPG), which in four patients was combined with an orbital or periorbital plexiform neurofibroma (OPPN).

Table 1. Demographic and clinical characteristics of patients with benign PNs.

Characteristic	Study Population (*N* = 90)
Age at last evaluation, years, median (range)	15.7 (3.3–28.6)
Duration of follow-up, years, median (range)	9.8 (0–26.4)
	***N* = 76**
Age at NF1 diagnosis, years, median (range)	1.0 (0–14)
Sex, *N* (%)	***N* = 90**
Male	49 (54.4)
Inheritance, *N* (%)	***N* = 88**
Familial	31 (34.4)
De novo	57 (63.3)
Unknown	2 (2.2)
Variant type, *N* (%) *	***N* = 83**
Missense/in-frame deletion	11 (13.3)
Nonsense/frameshift/splicing	67 (80.7)
Intragenic deletion	1 (1.2)
Total NF1 deletion (microdeletion)	4 (4.8)

* Known pathogenic variants based on the LOVD classification in 83 patients (www.lovd.nl, access date 10 September 2024).

In addition to this cohort, we observed four patients who developed an MPNST in the same study period, occurring at a median age of 10 years (one child below 5 years and one child above 15 years). Genetic variant types were two nonsense/frameshift, one missense, and one microdeletion. The MPNSTs were in the cervical/thoracic region (n = 2), upper limb, and abdomen.

In the 90 patients with a benign PN present, the limbs were the predominant site (Table 2). Fourteen patients (15.5%) of the population had more than one PN. Forty-three patients experienced comorbidities associated with their PN, predominantly pain requiring intervention and disfigurement. Based on the earlier defined criteria, 37 patients had plexiform neurofibroma morbidity. Twenty-eight patients received an intervention: 19 underwent resection at a median age of 13.4 years; 3 were primarily treated with an MEK inhibitor (median age 16.4 yrs), which have been accessible in the Netherlands through a compassionate use program since 2021; and 6 were treated with MEK as an adjuvant therapy to previous surgery at a median age of 5.2 yrs.

Table 2. Characteristics of plexiform neurofibromas.

Characteristics of PNs	At the PN Level (*N* = 105)	At the Patient Level (*N* = 90)
Location, *N* (%)		
Craniofacial	36 (34.29)	
Trunk	26 (24.76)	NA
Limbs	43 (40.95)	NA
Number of PNs per person, *N* (%)		
1	NA	76 (84.4)
2	NA	13 (14.4)
3	NA	1 (1.1)
PN morbidity, *N* (%) *		*N* = 48
Pain requiring intervention	23 (21.7)	21 (43.8)
Disfigurement	16 (15.1)	16 (33.3)
Neurological deficit	6 (5.7)	6 (12.5)
Visual impairment **	9 (8.5)	9 (18.8)
ENT-related complaints	3 (2.8)	3 (6.2)
Ptosis	3 (2.8)	3 (6.2)
Skeletal complaints	3 (2.8)	3 (6.2)
Sensory complaints	2 (1.9)	2 (4.2)
Hemorrhage in the PN	1 (0.9)	1 (2.1)
Urogenital complaints	1 (0.9)	1 (2.1)

Table 2. *Cont.*

Characteristics of PNs	At the PN Level (N = 105)	At the Patient Level (N = 90)
Intervention, N (median age (yrs) of first intervention)		28 (11.4)
Surgery	x	19 (13.4)
MEK inhibitor	x	3 (16.4)
Both	x	6 (5.2)

NA not applicable; * more than one comorbidity can be related to one PN; ** in all cases caused by an OPPN.

3.2. Predictors of Complexity and Need for Intervention

At the patient level, we observed no differences in univariate analysis for age at last evaluation, follow-up duration, or distribution of sex for the development of plexiform neurofibroma morbidity (Table 3), nor in any diagnostic criteria or genetic mutation type. Trunk PNs had a higher plexiform neurofibroma morbidity in comparison to limb PNs, although not significant. Within the craniofacial PNs, we observed 11 OPPNs; 10 of them were related to plexiform neurofibroma morbidity (27%), versus only 1 (1.9%) in an individual without plexiform neurofibroma morbidity ($p < 0.001$).

Table 3. Univariate comparison of characteristics between patients with and without plexiform neurofibroma morbidity.

Characteristic	Plexiform Neurofibroma Without Morbidity (N = 53)	Plexiform Neurofibroma With Morbidity (N = 37)	p Value Category *	p Value *
Age at last evaluation, years, median (range)	15.7 (3.3–27.7)	15.9 (6.5–28.6)		0.36
Follow-up duration, years, median (range)	8.2 (0–23.8)	10.9 (0–3.4)		0.09
Sex, N (%)				
Male	30 (56.6)	19 (51.4)		0.63
Inheritance, N (%)	**N = 52**	**N = 36**		
Familial	19 (36.5)	12 (33.3)		
De novo	33 (63.5)	24 (66.6)		
Variant type, N (%) **	**N = 51**	**N = 32**	0.84	
Missense/in-frame deletion	6 (11.8)	4 (12.5)		
Nonsense/frameshift/splicing	42 (82.4)	26 (81.3)		
Total NF1 deletion (microdeletion)	2 (3.9)	2 (6.3)		
Intragenic deletion	1 (2.0)	0		
Location of target PN, N (%)	**N = 53**	**N = 37**	0.41	
Craniofacial	20 (37.7)	14 (37.8)		
Trunk	10 (18.9)	11 (29.7)		
Limbs	23 (43.4)	12 (32.4)		

* Statistical significance at $p < 0.0045$; ** missing in seven patients.

An analysis of independent predictors for PNs with morbidity could be performed in 83 cases (PN with morbidity $N = 32$) due to missing mutation type data for seven patients (Table 4). We considered clinically relevant variables, including age and gender (as general patient descriptors), variant type, and location [3,9,14,19]. As a first step, we modeled patient characteristics, and in the second step, we added PN location to the model. Older age was significantly related to the risk of plexiform neurofibroma morbidity, independent of variant type or location. This model accounted for 37.0% of the variance in the occurrence of complex PN. It demonstrated an overall predictive accuracy of 68.7%, correctly identifying 92.2% of PN cases without morbidity and 31.3% of PN cases with morbidity. The model's discriminative ability for PNs with morbidity was limited (area under the ROC curve (AUC) of 0.64 (95% CI, 0.52 to 0.76)). Regarding independently associated determinants for the need for PN intervention in 81 patients with complete data (patients with intervention $n = 25$), Cox regression identified the location of the PN, with craniofacial region as the strongest predictor (Table 5). The mutation type did not contribute further.

Table 4. Multivariate logistic regression model of determinants for plexiform neurofibroma morbidity, adjusted for age at last evaluation and biological sex.

	Model 1		Model 2	
Variable	**Odds Ratio (95% CI)**	***p* Value**	**Odds Ratio (95% CI)**	***p* Value**
Age at last evaluation	1.05 (0.98–1.13)	0.16	1.05 (0.98–1.13)	0.05
Biological sex *	0.75 (0.30–1.86)	0.53	0.65 (0.25–1.69)	0.38
Variant type **				0.96
Nonsense/frameshift/splicing	1.02 (0.26–4.03)	0.98	0.86 (0.21–3.53)	0.83
Total NF1 deletion (microdeletion)	1.85 (0.17–20.70)	0.62	1.47 (0.3–17.2)	0.76
Intragenic deletion	0.000(0–∞)	1.00	0.000 (0–∞)	1.000
Location of target PN ***				0.41
Trunk	x	x	2.32 (0.68–7.96)	0.18
Craniofacial	x	x	1.34 (0.45–3.97)	0.60
AUC (95% CI)	0.62 (0.49–0.74)		0.64 (0.52–0.76)	

* Reference category: female; ** reference category: missense/in-frame deletion; *** reference category: limb PN.

Table 5. Cox regression model of determinants for PN intervention (n = 81 patients with complete data, n = 25 patients with intervention).

	Coefficient (S.E.)	**Hazard Ratio (95% CI)**	***p* Value**
Biological sex *	0.51 (0.43)	1.67 (0.72–3.89)	0.24
Location of target PN **			0.08
Trunk	1.14 (0.65)	3.13 (0.88–11.17)	0.08
Craniofacial	1.42 (0.58)	4.15 (1.34–12.86)	0.01
Variant type ***			0.61
Nonsense/frameshift/splicing	−0.22 (0.64)	0.80 (0.23–2.81)	0.73
Total NF1 deletion (Microdeletion)	0.75(0.96)	2.13 (0.33–13.84)	0.43
Intragenic deletion	−11.70 (645.71)	0.00 (0.00–∞)	0.99

* Reference category: female; ** reference category: limb PN; *** reference category: missense/in-frame deletion.

4. Discussion

4.1. Main Findings

Among a pediatric population of 90 NF1 patients with PNs, 37 developed plexiform neurofibroma morbidity over a median follow-up duration of 10 years. Fifteen percent of the patients developed multiple PNs. Older age was related to plexiform neurofibroma complexity, independent of genetic variant type or location. In addition, craniofacial PNs were independently associated with the early need for intervention.

Comparing our outcomes with findings in the literature revealed that our population was mostly similar to the general NF1 population [20–22]. The age of diagnosis was based on retrospective reports and may be biased by the first moment of consultation, so it is difficult to compare with other cohorts. The low incidence of MPNST (5%) may be due to the relatively young patient population.

The higher need for intervention for plexiform neurofibroma morbidity in craniofacial and trunk PNs can be explained by their potential morbidity. The craniofacial location may yield more complaints due to its limited anatomical space, where vital structures are closely packed. This is supported by the fact that 73% of morbidity in our OPPN group was due to visual impairment. Studies report visual impairment to be caused by conditions such as congenital glaucoma and/or amblyopia, which may result from eyelid closure caused by severe ptosis due to a PN, often in combination with an associated OPG [23]. Notably, four of our cases involved both OPPN and OPG simultaneously. Early intervention may be applied to improve and/or preserve functional ability and cosmetic outcomes. Systemic treatment with an MEKi is positioned for the treatment of OPPN [13]. Trunk PNs (including spinal, thoracic, and abdominal PNs) may be considered to threaten vital structures and warrant earlier intervention before causing actual symptoms (this was included in our definition of plexiform neurofibroma morbidity). This explains their association with a higher probability of intervention compared to that for limb PNs. The limited number of cases did not allow us to assess functionally relevant sub-locations to the main anatomical sites, such as vision loss, hearing loss, spinal cord compression, airway compromise, bowel/bladder disfunction, or mobility. We were unable to identify a microdeletion of the NF1 gene as a determinant in the occurrence of plexiform neurofibroma morbidity, while current literature suggests an association between NF1 microdeletions and an increased incidence of high tumor burden in PNs [9,24]. However, this may be related to the small number of patients with microdeletions in our population, limiting the power of our comparison.

4.2. Strengths and Limitations

A strength of this study is that we were able to include a high number of children with NF1-PN, with a median follow-up of 10 years. The ENCORE-NF1 expertise center Erasmus MC is the only expertise center in the Netherlands and leads the national NF1 expertise network with 11 treatment centers. In this network, complex cases are referred to our center. In addition, the Erasmus MC provides integrated NF1 care for the southern and southwestern regions of the Netherlands, which accounts for a 25% country adherence area. So, we believe that our patients are representative of the general NF1 population in the Netherlands [25]. Next, we add to previous longitudinal studies on NF1-related PNs [8,19,20,26] regarding the potential roles of demographic and PN characteristics in NF1 patients in developing plexiform neurofibroma morbidity and a need for intervention. Our study also has several limitations. First, although we employed a substantially large cohort, we still had a small number of cases of plexiform neurofibroma morbidity and PN with intervention. This limited the number of variables included in our regression analyses, and the models may be subject to overfitting. To reduce overfitting, we applied an approach of preselecting potential determinants from the literature. This, however, limited the chance of new findings. Second, the study is based on routine care data, and thereby subjective to changes in clinical management over time. Not all data were available for all patients. Also, we do not include volumetry measurements from MRI in routine care, limiting the use of (change in) tumor volume as a predictor in this study. In addition, we did not have standardized MRI intervals but performed MRI on indication (patients showing symptoms or suspected growth that warranted potential intervention). Monitoring PN growth (in absence of symptoms) was not an indication for MRI in the period before MEK inhibitors became available. Next, intervention was decided by the discretion of the clinician but included the level of complaints (deficit, pain), potential threats to vital organ structure/function, growth, and patient preferences (despite the latter being rather subjective and potential variable). Treatment decisions, however, were made by the multidisciplinary team, including the neurology, ophthalmology, neurosurgery, and plastic surgery departments, the members of which have been quite stable in the past 10 years. The access to systemic treatment with MEK inhibitors since 2021 may have influenced the time to treatment for inoperable PNs. The retrospective nature forced us to use objective definitions of parameters. This caused us to decide to exclude disfigurement/cosmetic burden in our definition of plexiform neurofibroma morbidity, but these aspects can also have a significant impact on quality of life and may benefit from treatment. For future prospective longitudinal studies, we underline the importance of including functional and patient-reported outcomes, which are becoming increasingly available for NF1 specific manifestations [27–29].

4.3. Future Directions

Our study has provided valuable insights into NF1-related PN morbidity. Our results support initiating the treatment of PNs early in life, for craniofacial PNs in particular. The choice of surgery versus systemic MEK inhibitor treatment may depend on PN characteristics, accessibility, and experience and should be discussed in multidisciplinary teams. Of course, there remain several challenges for further research to enhance our understanding of PN natural progression. Some of our study limitations can be overcome by a prospective multicenter LNHS rather than selective patient populations from clinical trials or smaller observational cohorts from local institutions, as in the current study. This, however, is more financially and temporally demanding. Such a prospective approach also allows researchers to collect patient-derived material for new therapeutic targets and biomarkers for NF1-PN progression or transformation into MPNST [30–32]. There are some efforts to build networks for NF1, aiming to cover the general population of NF1 patients, e.g., the CTF clinical care network in the USA (https://www.ctf.org/nf-clinic-network/, accessed on 10 September 2024) and ERN-GENTURIS [33] in Europe, but not all NF1 patients have access to network centers. Next, a systematic data collection procedure with standardized protocols among network centers is needed, such that observational data can be harmonized and combined for studying rare outcomes in rare conditions. REiNS provide valuable recommendations for both imaging and functional or patient-reported outcome assessments [27], but these are not yet fully implemented in routine care. Integrating volumetric analysis holds promise for the more accurate and earlier detection of complex PNs, as well as the improved assessment of treatment response, but adopting this in routine practice requires (semi)automatic analyses [34]. Collaborators from REiNS and the EU-PEARL consortium have proposed content for longitudinal studies, but these are not broadly implemented yet [32,35].

5. Conclusions

Our pilot multivariate approach provides insights into the natural course of plexiform neurofibromas in neurofibromatosis type 1 patients and into potential factors independently influencing plexiform neurofibroma morbidity and the need for intervention. Our results support initiating the treatment of PNs early in life before complications become present. In addition, the location of the PN may contribute to the treatment decisions in NF1 patients. Harmonized approaches to follow-up on PNs among global NF centers are needed, as they will allow researchers to bundle longitudinal natural history cohorts. Such large multicenter cohorts may confirm our findings, identify additional prognostic determinants, accelerate our understanding of the PN course, and advance PN management strategies.

Author Contributions: Conceptualization, B.D. and R.O.; Data curation, B.d.B., B.D. and R.v.M.; Formal analysis, B.d.B. and R.O.; Investigation, R.v.M.; Methodology, B.d.B., B.D. and R.O.; Project administration, R.O.; Supervision, R.O.; Visualization, B.d.B.; Writing—original draft, B.d.B.; Writing—review & editing, B.D., R.v.M. and R.O. All authors have read and agreed to the published version of the manuscript.

Funding: This research received no external funding.

Institutional Review Board Statement: The study was conducted in accordance with the Declaration of Helsinki and approved by the Institutional Review Board (or Ethics Committee) of Erasmus MC (MEC-2015-203, 13 March 2015).

Informed Consent Statement: Informed consent was obtained from all subjects involved in the study.

Data Availability Statement: Data are available on request from the corresponding author. Data are available as .csv formats.

Conflicts of Interest: The authors declare no conflicts of interest.

References

1. Uusitalo, E.; Leppavirta, J.; Koffert, A.; Suominen, S.; Vahtera, J.; Vahlberg, T.; Poyhonen, M.; Peltonen, J.; Peltonen, S. Incidence and mortality of neurofibromatosis: A total population study in Finland. *J. Investig. Dermatol.* **2015**, *135*, 904–906. [CrossRef] [PubMed]
2. Evans, D.G.; Howard, E.; Giblin, C.; Clancy, T.; Spencer, H.; Huson, S.M.; Lalloo, F. Birth incidence and prevalence of tumor-prone syndromes: Estimates from a UK family genetic register service. *Am. J. Med. Genet.* **2010**, *152A*, 327–332. [CrossRef]
3. Peduto, C.; Zanobio, M.; Nigro, V.; Perrotta, S.; Piluso, G.; Santoro, C. Neurofibromatosis Type 1: Pediatric Aspects and Review of Genotype-Phenotype Correlations. *Cancers* **2023**, *15*, 1217. [CrossRef] [PubMed]
4. Carton, C.; Evans, D.G.; Blanco, I.; Friedrich, R.E.; Ferner, R.E.; Farschtschi, S.; Salvador, H.; Azizi, A.A.; Mautner, V.; Rohl, C.; et al. ERN GENTURIS tumour surveillance guidelines for individuals with neurofibromatosis type 1. *EClinicalMedicine* **2023**, *56*, 101818. [CrossRef] [PubMed]
5. van Minkelen, R.; van Bever, Y.; Kromosoeto, J.N.; Withagen-Hermans, C.J.; Nieuwlaat, A.; Halley, D.J.; van den Ouweland, A.M. A clinical and genetic overview of 18 years neurofibromatosis type 1 molecular diagnostics in the Netherlands. *Clin. Genet.* **2014**, *85*, 318–327. [CrossRef]
6. De Raedt, T.; Walton, Z.; Yecies, J.L.; Li, D.; Chen, Y.; Malone, C.F.; Maertens, O.; Jeong, S.M.; Bronson, R.T.; Lebleu, V.; et al. Exploiting cancer cell vulnerabilities to develop a combination therapy for ras-driven tumors. *Cancer Cell* **2011**, *20*, 400–413. [CrossRef] [PubMed]
7. Prada, C.E.; Rangwala, F.A.; Martin, L.J.; Lovell, A.M.; Saal, H.M.; Schorry, E.K.; Hopkin, R.J. Pediatric plexiform neurofibromas: Impact on morbidity and mortality in neurofibromatosis type 1. *J. Pediatr.* **2012**, *160*, 461–467. [CrossRef]
8. Nguyen, R.; Dombi, E.; Widemann, B.C.; Solomon, J.; Fuensterer, C.; Kluwe, L.; Friedman, J.M.; Mautner, V.F. Growth dynamics of plexiform neurofibromas: A retrospective cohort study of 201 patients with neurofibromatosis 1. *Orphanet J. Rare Dis.* **2012**, *7*, 75. [CrossRef] [PubMed]
9. De Raedt, T.; Brems, H.; Wolkenstein, P.; Vidaud, D.; Pilotti, S.; Perrone, F.; Mautner, V.; Frahm, S.; Sciot, R.; Legius, E. Elevated risk for MPNST in NF1 microdeletion patients. *Am. J. Hum. Genet.* **2003**, *72*, 1288–1292. [CrossRef]
10. Reilly, K.M.; Kim, A.; Blakely, J.; Ferner, R.E.; Gutmann, D.H.; Legius, E.; Miettinen, M.M.; Randall, R.L.; Ratner, N.; Jumbe, N.L.; et al. Neurofibromatosis Type 1-Associated MPNST State of the Science: Outlining a Research Agenda for the Future. *J. Natl. Cancer Inst.* **2017**, *109*, djx124. [CrossRef]
11. Nguyen, R.; Ibrahim, C.; Friedrich, R.E.; Westphal, M.; Schuhmann, M.; Mautner, V.F. Growth behavior of plexiform neurofibromas after surgery. *Genet. Med.* **2013**, *15*, 691–697. [CrossRef]
12. Gross, A.M.; Wolters, P.L.; Dombi, E.; Baldwin, A.; Whitcomb, P.; Fisher, M.J.; Weiss, B.; Kim, A.; Bornhorst, M.; Shah, A.C.; et al. Selumetinib in Children with Inoperable Plexiform Neurofibromas. *N. Engl. J. Med.* **2020**, *382*, 1430–1442. [CrossRef] [PubMed]
13. Fisher, M.J.; Blakeley, J.O.; Weiss, B.D.; Dombi, E.; Ahlawat, S.; Akshintala, S.; Belzberg, A.J.; Bornhorst, M.; Bredella, M.A.; Cai, W.; et al. Management of neurofibromatosis type 1-associated plexiform neurofibromas. *Neuro Oncol.* **2022**, *24*, 1827–1844. [CrossRef] [PubMed]
14. Lemberg, K.M.; Gross, A.M.; Sproule, L.M.; Liewehr, D.J.; Dombi, E.; Baldwin, A.; Steinberg, S.M.; Bornhorst, M.; Lodish, M.; Blakeley, J.O.; et al. Anthropometric measurements of children with neurofibromatosis type I: Impact of plexiform neurofibroma volume and treatment. *Pediatr. Res.* **2024**, 1–11. [CrossRef]
15. Schmalhofer, M.L.; Farschtschi, S.; Kluwe, L.; Mautner, V.F.; Adam, G.; Well, L.; Ristow, I. Whole-body MRI-based long-term evaluation of pediatric NF1 patients without initial tumor burden with evidence of newly developed peripheral nerve sheath tumors. *Orphanet J. Rare Dis.* **2024**, *19*, 412. [CrossRef]
16. Legius, E.; Messiaen, L.; Wolkenstein, P.; Pancza, P.; Avery, R.A.; Berman, Y.; Blakeley, J.; Babovic-Vuksanovic, D.; Cunha, K.S.; Ferner, R.; et al. Revised diagnostic criteria for neurofibromatosis type 1 and Legius syndrome: An international consensus recommendation. *Genet. Med.* **2021**, *23*, 1506–1513. [CrossRef]
17. Dombi, E.; Ardern-Holmes, S.L.; Babovic-Vuksanovic, D.; Barker, F.G.; Connor, S.; Evans, D.G.; Fisher, M.J.; Goutagny, S.; Harris, G.J.; Jaramillo, D.; et al. Recommendations for imaging tumor response in neurofibromatosis clinical trials. *Neurology* **2013**, *81*, S33–S40. [CrossRef] [PubMed]
18. Peduzzi, P.; Concato, J.; Kemper, E.; Holford, T.R.; Feinstein, A.R. A simulation study of the number of events per variable in logistic regression analysis. *J. Clin. Epidemiol.* **1996**, *49*, 1373–1379. [CrossRef]
19. Nguyen, R.; Kluwe, L.; Fuensterer, C.; Kentsch, M.; Friedrich, R.E.; Mautner, V.F. Plexiform neurofibromas in children with neurofibromatosis type 1: Frequency and associated clinical deficits. *J. Pediatr.* **2011**, *159*, 652–655 e652. [CrossRef]

20. Ejerskov, C.; Farholt, S.; Nielsen, F.S.K.; Berg, I.; Thomasen, S.B.; Udupi, A.; Ågesen, T.; de Fine Licht, S.; Handrup, M.M. Clinical Characteristics and Management of Children and Adults with Neurofibromatosis Type 1 and Plexiform Neurofibromas in Denmark: A Nationwide Study. *Oncol. Ther.* **2023**, *11*, 97–110. [CrossRef] [PubMed]
21. Tucker, T.; Friedman, J.M.; Friedrich, R.E.; Wenzel, R.; Funsterer, C.; Mautner, V.F. Longitudinal study of neurofibromatosis 1 associated plexiform neurofibromas. *J. Med. Genet.* **2009**, *46*, 81–85. [CrossRef]
22. Peltonen, S.; Kallionpaa, R.A.; Rantanen, M.; Uusitalo, E.; Lahteenmaki, P.M.; Poyhonen, M.; Pitkaniemi, J.; Peltonen, J. Pediatric malignancies in neurofibromatosis type 1: A population-based cohort study. *Int. J. Cancer* **2019**, *145*, 2926–2932. [CrossRef] [PubMed]
23. Oystreck, D.T.; Morales, J.; Chaudhry, I.; Alorainy, I.A.; Elkhamary, S.M.; Pasha, T.M.U.; Bosley, T.M. Visual Loss in Orbitofacial Neurofibromatosis Type 1. *Ophthalmology* **2012**, *119*, 2168–2173. [CrossRef] [PubMed]
24. Kluwe, L.; Nguyen, R.; Vogt, J.; Bengesser, K.; Mussotter, T.; Friedrich, R.E.; Jett, K.; Kehrer-Sawatzki, H.; Mautner, V.F. Internal tumor burden in neurofibromatosis Type I patients with large *NF1* deletions. *Genes Chromosomes Cancer* **2012**, *51*, 447–451. [CrossRef] [PubMed]
25. Rietman, A.B.; Oostenbrink, R.; van Noort, K.; Franken, M.J.P.; Catsman-Berrevoets, C.E.; Aarsen, F.K.; Hendriksen, J.G.; de Nijs, P.F.A. Development of emotional and behavioral problems in neurofibromatosis type 1 during young childhood. *Am. J. Med. Genet.* **2017**, *173*, 2373–2380. [CrossRef]
26. Akshintala, S.; Baldwin, A.; Liewehr, D.J.; Goodwin, A.; Blakeley, J.O.; Gross, A.M.; Steinberg, S.M.; Dombi, E.; Widemann, B.C. Longitudinal evaluation of peripheral nerve sheath tumors in neurofibromatosis type 1: Growth analysis of plexiform neurofibromas and distinct nodular lesions. *Neuro Oncol.* **2020**, *22*, 1368–1378. [CrossRef]
27. Plotkin, S.R.; Blakeley, J.O.; Dombi, E.; Fisher, M.J.; Hanemann, C.O.; Walsh, K.S.; Wolters, P.L.; Widemann, B.C. Achieving consensus for clinical trials: The REiNS International Collaboration. *Neurology* **2013**, *81*, S1–S5. [CrossRef] [PubMed]
28. Merker, V.L.; Thompson, H.L.; Wolters, P.L.; Buono, F.D.; Hingtgen, C.M.; Rosser, T.; Barton, B.; Barnett, C.; Smith, T.; Haberkamp, D.; et al. Recommendations for assessing appearance concerns related to plexiform and cutaneous neurofibromas in neurofibromatosis 1 clinical trials. *Clin. Trials* **2024**, *21*, 6–17. [CrossRef]
29. Dhaenens, B.A.E.; van Dijk, S.A.; Taal, W.; Noordhoek, D.C.; Coffey, A.; McKenna, S.P.; Oostenbrink, R. The PlexiQoL, a patient-reported outcome measure on quality of life in neurofibromatosis type 1-associated plexiform neurofibroma: Translation, cultural adaptation and validation into the Dutch language for the Netherlands. *J. Patient Rep. Outcomes* **2024**, *8*, 33. [CrossRef] [PubMed]
30. Szymanski, J.J.; Sundby, R.T.; Jones, P.A.; Srihari, D.; Earland, N.; Harris, P.K.; Feng, W.; Qaium, F.; Lei, H.; Roberts, D.; et al. Cell-free DNA ultra-low-pass whole genome sequencing to distinguish malignant peripheral nerve sheath tumor (MPNST) from its benign precursor lesion: A cross-sectional study. *PLoS Med.* **2021**, *18*, e1003734. [CrossRef] [PubMed]
31. Masliah-Planchon, J.; Pasmant, E.; Luscan, A.; Laurendeau, I.; Ortonne, N.; Hivelin, M.; Varin, J.; Valeyrie-Allanore, L.; Dumaine, V.; Lantieri, L.; et al. MicroRNAome profiling in benign and malignant neurofibromatosis type 1-associated nerve sheath tumors: Evidences of PTEN pathway alterations in early NF1 tumorigenesis. *BMC Genom.* **2013**, *14*, 473. [CrossRef]
32. Hanemann, C.O.; Blakeley, J.O.; Nunes, F.P.; Robertson, K.; Stemmer-Rachamimov, A.; Mautner, V.; Kurtz, A.; Ferguson, M.; Widemann, B.C.; Evans, D.G.; et al. Current status and recommendations for biomarkers and biobanking in neurofibromatosis. *Neurology* **2016**, *87*, S40–S48. [CrossRef]
33. Vos, J.R.; Giepmans, L.; Rohl, C.; Geverink, N.; Hoogerbrugge, N.; Ern, G. Boosting care and knowledge about hereditary cancer: European Reference Network on Genetic Tumour Risk Syndromes. *Fam. Cancer* **2019**, *18*, 281–284. [CrossRef]
34. Cai, W.; Steinberg, S.M.; Bredella, M.A.; Basinsky, G.; Somarouthu, B.; Plotkin, S.R.; Solomon, J.; Widemann, B.C.; Harris, G.J.; Dombi, E. Volumetric MRI Analysis of Plexiform Neurofibromas in Neurofibromatosis Type 1: Comparison of Two Methods. *Acad. Radiol.* **2018**, *25*, 144–152. [CrossRef] [PubMed]
35. Leubner, J.; Legius, E.; Carton, C.; Dhaenens, B.; Oostenbrink, R.; Bakker, A.; Nievo, M.; Heimann, G. Protocol for a Longitudinal Natural History Study in NF. 2023. Available online: https://eu-pearl.eu/wp-content/uploads/2023/06/D7.3-Protocol-for-a-Longitudinal-Natural-History-Study-LNHS-in-NF.pdf (accessed on 10 September 2024).

cancers

MDPI

Article

Close Follow-Up of Patients with Neurofibromatosis Type 1 Reduces the Incidence of Malignant Peripheral Nerve Sheath Tumour

Maria Pia Iasella [1,†], Dries Ruttens [2,3,†], Daphne Hompes [4], Vincent Vandecaveye [5], Raf Sciot [6], Christophe Deroose [7], Thomas Douchy [4], Thomas Decramer [8], Sandra Jacobs [2], Ellen Denayer [1], Frank Van Calenbergh [8], Eric Legius [1] and Hilde Brems [1,*]

1 Centre for Human Genetics, University Hospitals Leuven, KU Leuven, 3000 Leuven, Belgium
2 Department of Paediatric Oncology, University Hospitals Leuven, 3000 Leuven, Belgium
3 Department of Paediatric Oncology, Princess Máxima Centre for Pediatric Oncology, 3584 CS Utrecht, The Netherlands
4 Department of Surgical Oncology, University Hospitals Leuven, 3000 Leuven, Belgium
5 Radiology Department, University Hospitals Leuven, 3000 Leuven, Belgium
6 Department of Pathology, University Hospitals Leuven, KU Leuven, 3000 Leuven, Belgium
7 Nuclear Medicine, University Hospitals Leuven, and Nuclear Medicine and Molecular Imaging, Department of Imaging and Pathology, KU Leuven, 3000 Leuven, Belgium
8 Department of Neurosurgery, University Hospitals Leuven, 3000 Leuven, Belgium
* Correspondence: hilde.brems@kuleuven.be
† These authors contributed equally to this work.

Simple Summary: Neurofibromatosis type 1 is one of the most common cancer predisposition syndromes, with affected individuals facing an increased risk of various benign and malignant tumours. Among these, malignant peripheral nerve sheath tumours are the leading cause of cancer-related mortality in NF1 patients. Complete surgical removal is necessary for a cure, but this is often unfeasible due to the tumour's extensive growth and challenging anatomical location. Malignant peripheral nerve sheath tumours frequently arise from pre-existing plexiform neurofibromas, often progressing through a premalignant stage known as atypical neurofibromatous neoplasm of uncertain biologic potential. Unlike malignant peripheral nerve sheet tumours, these lesions can be effectively treated with surgical excision using minimal resection margins, preventing malignant transformation. Our retrospective study provides evidence supporting the benefits of strict surveillance through whole-body imaging. By enabling early detection and timely surgical intervention for premalignant lesions, this approach can significantly reduce progression to malignancy, ultimately improving both morbidity and mortality in these patients.

Abstract: Background/Objectives: Neurofibromatosis type 1 (NF1) patients have an increased risk for benign and malignant neoplasms, leading to increased morbidity and mortality. Of these, malignant peripheral nerve sheath tumours (MPNSTs) are the most common malignant neoplasms causing death in NF1 patients. MPNSTs mostly originate from pre-existing plexiform neurofibromas (PNs). Many MPNSTs first pass through the premalignant stage of atypical neurofibromatous neoplasm with uncertain biologic potential (ANNUBP). With this study, we aimed to test whether active surveillance in adults with NF1 changes the natural history of MPNST development. More specifically, we wanted to evaluate the hypothesis that early detection of peripheral nerve sheath tumours (PNSTs) suspected of ANNUBP can lead to timely surgical removal of ANNUBPs, which in turn might reduce the incidence of MPNST in NF1 individuals. **Methods:** We retrospectively collected data on NF1 patients who were under surveillance with whole-body diffusion-weighted magnetic resonance imaging (WB-DW/MRI or DWI) and clinical exams at University Hospitals Leuven (UZL) or in one of the UZL network hospitals between 2012 and 2022 and who were 16 years or older at the time of their first WB-DW/MRI. The expected number of MPNST cases was calculated based on prior population-based studies, with statistical comparison using Poisson and Binomial distributions. **Results:** We included 276 patients with a total observation period of 1329.2 person-years. In total, 65 surgical interventions were performed in 58 individuals (21% of the cohort). WB-DW/MRI was followed by surgical intervention in 15.5% of the cases. We diagnosed 15 ANNUBPs in 14 patients. No cases of MPNST were observed against the expected 3.96 cases ($p = 0.019$). **Conclusions:** Active surveillance, incorporating WB-DW/MRI and timely surgical interventions for ANNUBP, significantly reduced the incidence of MPNST in this cohort.

Keywords: neurofibromatosis type 1; WB-DW/MRI; ANNUBP; MPNST

1. Introduction

Neurofibromatosis type 1 (NF1) is an autosomal dominant genetic condition with a birth incidence of one in 2000 to one in 3000 [1–3]. The disease is caused by germline loss-of-function variants in the *NF1* tumour suppressor gene at 17q11.2 [4]. *NF1* encodes the protein neurofibromin, a negative regulator of the RAS proto-oncogene, which is a key signalling molecule in the control of cell growth [5]. The disease is characterised by café-au-lait macules (CALMs), lentiginous macules in the axillary and inguinal region, iris Lisch nodules, multiple benign and malignant neoplasms and other features [6].

Malignancies associated with NF1 are high-grade intracranial glioma, malignant peripheral nerve sheath tumour (MPNST), breast cancer, gastrointestinal stromal tumour (GIST), and pheochromocytoma/paraganglioma (PPGL), with malignant glioma and MPNST having the highest malignant potential [7]. The incidence of cancer (including brain glioma) is higher in NF1 patients, and several cancers occur at a younger age compared to the general population. This is demonstrated in a Finnish cohort study showing a standardized incidence ratio (SIR) of 5.03 in NF1 patients, with the highest SIR values in children (including benign brain glioma: SIR 62.9 in children aged 0–14 years). In this cohort, the cumulative risk was 38.8% at 50 years of age, with a lifetime cancer risk of 59.6% (compared to 3.9% and 30.8%, respectively, in the general population) [8]. Furthermore, survival in NF1 patients with cancer is lower compared to matched controls [8]. This holds especially true for MPNST [7,8].

MPNSTs often originate from plexiform neurofibromas (PNs), which are a type of benign peripheral nerve sheath tumour (PNST) arising from single or multiple branches of nerves or nerve plexuses [9]. Some MPNSTs develop from plexiform neurofibromas through a premalignant stage of atypical neurofibromatous neoplasm with uncertain biologic potential (ANNUBP) [10]. Clinically, these tumours often show continuous growth over time and may cause pain. Further, they present an increased glucose uptake on fluorine-18-labeled fluorodeoxy-glucose (^{18}FDG)-PET scan [11]. On MRI, an ANNUBP might present as a distinct nodular lesion (DNL) [12]. Histologically, these lesions are characterised by at least two of the following features: cytologic atypia, loss of neurofibroma architecture, hypercellularity, and a mitotic index >1/50 high-power fields (HPF) and <3/10 HPF [10]. Genetically, these tumours frequently show loss of the *CDKN2A/B* gene locus [13,14]. According to the 2024 proposed integrated consensus criteria for ANNUBP *CDKN2A/B* homozygous inactivation alone or heterozygous inactivation with at least one of the aforementioned histological features is sufficient for a diagnosis of ANNUBP [15]. MPNSTs histologically have features of ANNUBP but with a mitotic index of ≥10/10

HPF or 3–9/10 HPF combined with necrosis. Molecularly, the presence of *SUZ12/EED* inactivating mutation, *TP53* inactivating mutation, or significant aneuploidy (segmental gain or loss of at least eight different chromosome arms) is sufficient for diagnosis of MPNST [15]. The lifetime risk for developing an MPNST is 8–15.8% (compared to 0.003% in the general population), with a median age at diagnosis between 20 and 40 years [7,8,16,17]. The 5-year disease-specific survival remains poor, ranging from 31.6 to 60% [7,18]. Overall, MPNST is the most common malignant neoplasm causing death in NF1 patients [7,8].

PPGL and GIST are also more frequent in NF1 patients compared to the general population. Concerning PPGL, the lifetime risk is 1–5% with the highest prevalence during the fourth and fifth decade. Current guidelines do not recommend routine screening for PPGL [19]. GIST presents in NF1 patients most frequently during the fourth to seventh decade. It is estimated that a little over half of these tumours are asymptomatic, and the remaining half present with gastrointestinal bleeding, obstruction, abdominal pain, palpable mass, nausea, or weight loss [20–22]. A Japanese prospective cohort study showed a prevalence of 6.3% in NF1 individuals who are 30 years or older [23].

Taken together, NF1 patients are at risk of developing multiple neoplasms, leading to increased morbidity and mortality in these patients. In order to improve the clinical outcome of these patients, a surveillance program to detect NF1-associated neoplasms in adults is highly relevant. Early detection of tumours is recommended to minimize tumour-related morbidity and mortality. With this study, we aimed to test whether active surveillance in adults with NF1 influences the incidence of MPNST. Early detection of PNSTs suspected of ANNUBP can lead to further investigation, resulting in timely surgical removal of ANNUBPs, which, in turn, can reduce the incidence of MPNST in NF1 individuals.

2. Materials and Methods

2.1. Patients

Basic surveillance of adult NF1 patients at our centre consists of a clinical visit with history taking and physical exam every two to three years, whole-body diffusion-weighted magnetic resonance imaging (WB-DW/MRI) at the age of 16–18 years (or later if not yet performed) and an annual breast MRI for women between 30 and 50 years. If WB-DW/MRI shows a tumour suspected of ANNUBP, an FDG-PET scan is performed. A tumour suspected of being ANNUBP based on clinical, radiological, and PET findings is removed surgically, if safely possible, using nerve-sparing surgery.

We retrospectively collected data on patients with a clinical or genetic diagnosis of NF1 who were under surveillance with WB-DW/MRI and clinical exams at University Hospitals Leuven (UZL) or in one of the UZL network hospitals between 2012 and 2022. The clinical diagnosis of NF1 was established in accordance with the revised diagnostic criteria [6]. All patients 16 years or older at the time of their first WB-DW/MRI were included. The follow-up time was calculated starting from the date of the first WB-DW/MRI that took place after 1 January 2012. We considered the last follow-up before 31 December 2022 or death as follow-up endpoints. The data collection regarding the information on demographics, medical events (occurrence of PN, ANNUBP, MPNST, PPGL, and GIST), and interventions was performed by a single person to ensure reliability under the supervision of two MDs. The date of a medical event or intervention was noted when available. If only the month was known, we used the first day of that month. If only the year was known, we used the first day of that year. Data collection was conducted in compliance with the declaration of Helsinki. Approval for this study was given by the ethics committee of UZ Leuven (MP021514 and S69071). Data were encrypted, and access to the data was restricted to individuals directly involved in the study. Informed consent was not required since the study concerns retrospective data collection. All data were treated confidentially by the investigators.

2.2. Whole-Body MRI

Three Tesla WB-DW/MRI (Ingenia, Philips Healthcare, Best, The Netherlands) was performed with parallel radiofrequency transmission and phased-surface coils. Free-breathing WB-DWI was acquired in the transverse plane at b0 and b1000 s/mm^2 in 4 stacks from head to pelvis. The scanner software created apparent diffusion coefficient (ADC) maps from the DWI data. All DWI image sets were reformatted to coronal and transverse WB images. Correlative anatomic imaging consisted of free breathing coronal WB short tau inversion recovery fat-suppressed T2-weighted turbo spin-echo sequence acquired in 3 stacks and free breathing/dual breath-hold single-shot turbo spin-echo T2-weighted sequences acquired in 4 transverse stacks (Table S1). Anatomical images were also reformatted to WB images. No intravenous contrast material was administered.

WB-DW/MRI images were assessed by radiologists experienced in abdominal and oncologic imaging (V.V.). Characterization of PNSTs was based on T2-weighted (tumour size, margin, perilesional oedema, presence of split fat, fascicular and target sign) and DWI characteristics (b1000 signal intensity and ADC with mean threshold of 1.15×10^{-3} mm^2) [24]. Adrenal gland tumours and GIST were similarly identified and characterized using T2-weighted and DWI characteristics.

2.3. [^{18}F]FDG-PET/CT Scanning and Quantitative Analysis

[^{18}F]FDG-PET/CT scans were performed with Siemens Biograph 16 HiRez, Siemens Truepoint 40 (Siemens Healthcare, Erlangen, Germany), or GE Healthcare Discovery MI4 (GE Healthcare, Chicago, IL, USA). Patients fasted for a minimum of 6 h before intravenous administration of 3–4.25 MBq [^{18}F]FDG/kg body weight. Three hours after [^{18}F]FDG administration, a high dose CT scan (85 mAs for Siemens and 50–450 for GE (modulated); 120 kV) with intravenous and oral iodinated contrast was performed, immediately followed by a PET scan (vertex to mid-thigh, or until feet if clinically indicated). The CT data were used for attenuation correction of the PET images. Scan acquisition was performed according to The European Association of Nuclear Medicine (EANM) procedure guidelines for tumour imaging and reconstruction parameters compliant with EANM Research (EARL 1.0) recommendations [25].

Image analysis of [^{18}F]FDG-PET/CT was performed using hybrid orthogonal viewer (Hermes Hybrid Viewer (Hermes Medical Solutions, Stockholm, Sweden) or MIM Software (MIM Software Inc., Cleveland, OH). Maximum Standardized uptake values (SUV_{max}) were calculated within each lesion. SUV_{max} values > 5.0 were considered of concern for (pre-)malignant transformation, and SUV_{max} values > 10 were considered highly suspicious for MPNST [26–28].

2.4. Pathological Definitions and Genetic Analysis

The diagnosis of PN, MPNST, PPGL, GIST, and glioma was based on the criteria defined by WHO panels [29–31]. Diagnosis of ANNUBP was based on the latest consensus criteria [15]. If clinically necessary, PNs, ANNUBPs, and MPNSTs were further analysed by array CGH, next-generation sequencing on an Illumina platform using Sanger sequencing and MLPA (MRC Holland).

2.5. Statistical Methods

The expected number of MPNST cases per year was calculated using the data from Uusitalo et al. (2016) [8]. p-values for both Poisson and Binomial distributions were calculated.

3. Results

3.1. Demographics

We included 276 individuals, of which 158 were women (57.2%) and 118 were men (42.8%), with at least one WB-DW/MRI and subsequent clinical and/or radiological follow-up. The total observation period was 1329.2 person-years with, respectively, 760.6 and 568.6 person-years in women and men. Age at last observation ranged from 16 to 77 years (mean 37 years, median 34 years).

3.2. Whole-Body MRI

In total, 419 WB-DW/MRI scans were performed, with an average of 1.5 scans per individual. Of the total cohort, 88 patients (31.9%) had more than one WB-DW/MRI.

3.3. Interventions

In total, 65 surgical interventions were performed in 58 individuals, 21% of the cohort. WB-DW/MRI was followed by surgical intervention in 15.5% of the cases. The surgical intervention and subsequent histopathological examination led to the identification of 15 ANNUBPs in 14 people (age range 16.2–60.7 years; mean age 30.4 years, median age 26.4), 14 secretory pheochromocytomas (age range 23.0–56.5 years; mean age 39.0 years, median 38.2), 5 GISTs (age range 35.2–68.8 years; mean age 53.5 years, median 53.9 years), 1 brain tumour (age 18.4 years) and 28 benign neurofibromas of different types. One desmoid tumour of the small intestine and one lymph node consistent with Castleman disease were removed surgically.

3.4. Tumours Detected During the Study Period

Table 1 shows the numbers of the tumours detected by WB-DW/MRI (ANNUBP, MPNST, PPGL, GIST, and brain tumour), specifying whether the tumour was diagnosed as a result of the surveillance program or not. Recurrences of tumours initially detected and treated before the surveillance period were excluded from this table.

Table 1. Tumours observed.

Tumour Type	Male	Female	Total
GIST			
Interval tumours [a]	0	2	2
Cases detected through surveillance [b]	0	5	5
Total	0	7	7
PPGL			
Interval tumours [a]	0	0	0
Cases detected through surveillance [b]	7	7	14
Total	7	7	14
ANNUBP			
Interval tumours [a]	0	0	0
Cases detected through surveillance [b]	3	12	15
Total	3	12	15
MPNST			
Interval tumours [a]	0	0	0
Cases detected through surveillance [b]	0	0	0
Total	0	0	0
BRAIN TUMOUR			
Interval tumours [a]	4	1	5
Cases detected through surveillance [b]	0	1	1
Total	4	2	6

[a], [b]: Tumours were considered detected as a consequence of the surveillance program if diagnosis was made through physical exam/imaging performed at one of the regular clinical visits. If the tumour was diagnosed during the surveillance period but not on a scheduled visit, it was considered an interval tumour.

During surveillance, a total of 321 PNs were visualized on WB-DW/MRI. This corresponds to a total of 152 people (55%) of the cohort, with an average of 2.11 lesions per person (average in complete cohort: 1.16 lesions; range 0–9). Of these lesions, 220 were previously known, and 101 were newly discovered. Table 2 shows the number of PNs, either previously known or detected through active surveillance, according to the anatomic site.

Table 2. Number of PNs.

Location	Cases in Previous Medical History	Cases Detected Through WB-DW/MRI	Total
Head and neck	50	16	66
Arms	39	10	49
Thorax	39	12	51
Abdomen	27	15	42
Pelvis	13	16	29
Legs	52	32	84
Total	220	101	321

In total, 15 ANNUBPs were removed (age range 16.2–60.7 years, mean age 30.4 years, median age 26.4 years) as a consequence of active surveillance. In all but one, there was a suspicion of ANNUBP based on pain, clinical or radiographic appearance/growth, and/or PET scan. Eight lesions met the criteria for ANNUBP as per the 2017 consensus histologic criteria. Through molecular analysis, we could detect *CDKN2A/B* deletion in another seven lesions. As per the 2024 proposed integrated consensus criteria, the total number of ANNUBP cases is 15 [15]. Molecular analysis was not systematically performed for all lesions as this was performed on clinical indication. An FDG-PET scan was performed prior to surgery in all but three patients, and every pictured ANNUBP showed increased FDG uptake. We observed no MPNST and expected 3.96 cases of MPNST when accounting for age using the Finnish population data ($p = 0.019$, Poisson, $p = 0.019$, Binomial distribution) [8]. Table 3 shows the person-years follow-up with the expected and observed number of MPNSTs per age group.

Table 3. Cumulative incidence of MPNSTs in different age groups.

Age Group (Years)	Person-Years Follow-up	C.I. °	Expected MPNST per Year/Group	MPNST = 0 *p*-Value Poisson/Binomial
$10 < x \leq 30$	627.6	0.085	0.0043/2.67	
$31 < x \leq 50$	487.4	0.123	0.0021/1.01	
$51 < x \leq 80$	214.2	0.158	0.0013/0.29	
Total	1329.2	-	0.0030/3.96	0.019/0.019

° C.I.: cumulative incidence till 30, 50, and 80 years.

In total, 5 GISTs (age range 35.2–68.8 years; mean age 53.5 years, median 53.9 years) were discovered through active surveillance. Two more GISTs were discovered outside routine clinical visits because of new symptoms (abdominal pain/diarrhoea and melena, respectively; last MRI 44 months and 9 months before diagnosis, respectively).

Fourteen secretory pheochromocytomas (age range 23.0–56.6 years; mean age 39.1 years) were diagnosed through active surveillance. There were no interval pheochromocytomas.

3.5. Follow-Up

At the last follow-up, 72 individuals were considered tumour-free, 199 had one or more tumours, and 5 were deceased (all of them males). Of the 199 persons with a tumour, 1 had a potential pheochromocytoma, and 4 had a lesion suspected to be ANNUBP. These people did not undergo surgery either because the operation was planned after the moment of data collection because of the high risk of postoperative neurological deficit or because caregivers and patients opted for a "watchful waiting" approach. The deceased individuals died of the following causes: cholangiocarcinoma (age 45 years), progressive brain stem tumour (age 39 years), oral carcinoma (smoking-related, age 60 years), sudden death (age 46 years) and unknown cause but unrelated to oncological problems (age 35 years).

4. Discussion

In this retrospective study, we show that one-fifth of the patients underwent surgery as a direct result of active surveillance. WB-DW/MRI was followed by an intervention in 15.5% of the cases, leading to the diagnosis of a (pre)malignant lesion in over half of these cases.

In the retrospective cohort, we were able to demonstrate a significant decrease in the incidence of MPNST when compared to the expected incidence based on population data from Finland, supporting the hypothesis that the detection and timely removal of PNSTs suspected of being ANNUBP can prevent further transformation to MPNST. We calculated the expected number of MPNST cases in our cohort using data from Uusitalo et al., 2016 [8], which, to our knowledge, represents the most reliable population-based data currently available. In contrast, our cohort comprises a university hospital-based population, potentially introducing a bias towards more severely affected patients.

In our cohort, a PN was present in 55% of the patients, corresponding to the upper end of the reported prevalences in the literature [32]. A total of 15 ANNUBPs were removed. Eight lesions met the criteria for ANNUBP as per the 2017 consensus histologic criteria. As per the proposed 2024 integrated consensus criteria, we could classify an additional seven lesions as ANNUBP because of *CDKN2A/B* deletion in combination with one histological criterion. We do not have an explanation for the high proportion of females with ANNUBP in our cohort (12/15; 80%). In a previous study of 63 patients with atypical neurofibromas, 31 females were reported (49%) [33]. The five cases of GIST were also females. A cohort study of 95 adult NF1 individuals in Japan showed GIST in 2 females and 4 males [23].

Currently, a combination of clinical information (growth in adulthood, pain), MRI-scan findings (growth in adulthood, nodular lesion), and PET-scan findings (FDG-avidity) are used to aid in the differentiation between ANNUBP and PN [10,34]. Further research is needed in order to expand the knowledge of existing biomarkers to predict the potential of ANNUBPs to transform into MPNST. An important first step in this direction would be to improve the definition of MRI imaging modalities and to identify the difference in FDG-PET characteristics between PN, ANNUBP, and MPNST in order to more effectively distinguish these conditions through imaging. Tissue biopsy can give valuable information but presents some important limitations, such as the often difficult accessibility of the lesions and heterogeneity within the tumour. The latter issue can be partly remedied by PET-guided biopsy [35]. The addition of *CDKN2A/B* deletion to the diagnostic criteria will improve the accuracy of the classification of ANNUBP. In our study, the incorporation of these molecular features led to the classification of seven additional tumours as ANNUBPs, which would not have met the criteria otherwise [10]. Likewise, pathological discrimination of ANNUBP from MPNST can be difficult. Also, here, molecular features of early MPNST can help discriminate these lesions from ANNUBP [15]. Regarding biomarkers, liquid biopsy would be an interesting approach, but this is currently poorly explored in the setting of ANNUBP and looking for copy number alterations might have little additive value to discriminate ANNUBP from early MPNST. The possibility of fragmentomics on cell-free DNA seems more promising [36]. A recent study demonstrated the biological role of ENG (endoglin) in MPNSTs and its potential role as a liquid biopsy biomarker and therapeutic target [37]. A similar approach for ANNUBP would be of great interest.

It is known that PNs have heterogenous growth behaviour, with frequently the central part of the lesion showing malignant degeneration. It has also been shown that some lesions might show spontaneous regression [38,39]. Also, some MPNSTs originate from PNs without going through an observable ANNUBP stage [33]. Currently, there are no good predictors for this tumoral behaviour [40]. Determining the appropriate frequency of clinical visits and imaging, as well as identifying the age range with the highest risk for malignant transformation, remains a key research priority. Most centres will remove ANNUBPs when feasible, provided there is no significant risk of serious surgical complications. However, the ability to accurately distinguish between ANNUBPs with a high versus low risk of malignant transformation would help avoid unnecessary interventions. This is particularly important given the potential burden of over-treatment, which can lead to financial strain on both patients and healthcare systems, as well as unnecessary treatment-related adverse effects from interventions that may not have been essential. Developing predictive markers for malignant transformation would enable a more personalized surveillance and treatment approach, ensuring that only those at the highest risk undergo surgical intervention while minimizing unnecessary procedures and associated burdens.

Since 2020, Selumetinib, a MEK1/2-inhibitor, has been FDA-approved for the treatment of symptomatic, inoperable PN in children with NF1 [41]. The drug negatively affects cell proliferation in NF1-deficient cells, reducing tumour burden and proving particularly effective in decreasing the size of PNs [42]. A recent study shows promising results on symptomatic PNs in NF1 adults and a broader-scale clinical trial has recently been published showing promising results also in adults [43]. Researchers have also begun exploring the potential of MEK inhibitors in the treatment of MPNST, though results have been mixed [44,45]. Future research should explore whether patients undergoing or having completed Selumetinib treatment develop ANNUBP and MPNST at the same rate as those who have not received the treatment. Additionally, it would be valuable to assess whether administering this drug (alone or in combination with drugs targeted towards other pathways) in cases of ANNUBP could prevent or delay the development of MPNST, potentially widening the therapeutic window for intervention.

Through this screening strategy, we diagnosed and treated 14 cases of secretory pheochromocytoma detected by WB-DW/MRI, followed by urinary catecholamine and metanephrine excretion analysis in cases with abnormal adrenal glands. There were no interval tumours reported. These findings demonstrate that WB-DW/MRI is also effective for the detection of PPGL, possibly decreasing the rates of morbidity and potential mortality associated with the condition. Two GIST cases were not discovered through the screening program. Although the number of patients is low, this finding suggests that follow-up through WB-DW/MRI does not allow for the detection all cases of GIST.

A limitation of this study is its retrospective nature, and prospective studies are needed to confirm the potential benefits of close surveillance on tumour management in adolescents and adults with NF1. Prospective studies are also needed to improve the diagnosis of the different types of PNSTs and their malignant potential using imaging modalities, including MRI with ADC, DWI, chemical exchange saturation transfer imaging [46], and FDG-PET. We also need to further study the added value of cell-free DNA fragmentomics, single-cell RNA sequencing, and spatial transcriptomics of tumour biopsies. The ultimate goal would be to identify those individuals that would benefit from nerve-sparing surgery or targeted drug therapy to prevent imminent malignant transformation using an individualised surveillance programme for adolescents and adults with NF1.

5. Conclusions

This study demonstrates that a surveillance program consisting of regular clinical examination and WB-DW/MRI followed by further investigations, if necessary, results in the detection of premalignant PNSTs, preventing further malignant transformation of these tumours. Most importantly, we could demonstrate a significant reduction in the number of MPNSTs in our retrospective cohort. This supports the approach for surgical removal of ANNUBPs to prevent evolution towards MPNST. Further prospective studies to optimize existing biomarkers and to develop new biomarkers are needed to help clinicians select the patients for nerve-sparing surgery at the optimal time point. The role of MEK-inhibition and other targeted treatments on natural tumour progression needs to be explored, as surgery for PN/ANNUBP can be associated with high morbidity.

Supplementary Materials: The following supporting information can be downloaded at: https://www.mdpi.com/article/10.3390/cancers17081306/s1. Table S1: Acquisition protocol.

Author Contributions: Conceptualization, H.B. and E.L.; methodology, H.B. and E.L.; formal analysis, M.P.I., D.R. and E.L.; investigation, M.P.I. and D.R.; resources, D.H., V.V., R.S., C.D., E.D., F.V.C., T.D. (Thomas Douchy), T.D. (Thomas Decramer), S.J., E.L. and H.B.; writing—original draft preparation, M.P.I. and D.R.; writing—review and editing, D.H., V.V., R.S., C.D., E.D., F.V.C., T.D. (Thomas Douchy), T.D. (Thomas Decramer), S.J., H.B. and E.L.; supervision, H.B. and E.L. All authors have read and agreed to the published version of the manuscript.

Funding: This research is supported by the fund Inès Costa.

Institutional Review Board Statement: Data collection, processing, and analysis were approved by the institutional review board in compliance with the principles of the Declaration of Helsinki.

Informed Consent Statement: Not applicable.

Data Availability Statement: The data that support the findings of this study are included in the article. Further inquiries can be directed at the corresponding author.

Acknowledgments: We thank the individuals with NF1 who collaborated in this study. The authors particularly thank the Inès Costa Fund of KU Leuven for financial support.

Conflicts of Interest: E.L. receives occasional consultancy fees from Alexion and Springworks Therapeutics. The other authors declare no conflicts of interest.

References

1. Huson, S.M.; Harper, P.S.; Compston, D.A. Von Recklinghausen neurofibromatosis. A clinical and population study in south-east Wales. *Brain A J. Neurol.* **1988**, *111 Pt 6*, 1355–1381. [CrossRef]
2. Lammert, M.; Friedman, J.M.; Kluwe, L.; Mautner, V.F. Prevalence of neurofibromatosis 1 in German children at elementary school enrollment. *Arch. Dermatol.* **2005**, *141*, 71–74. [CrossRef]
3. Kallionpää, R.A.; Uusitalo, E.; Leppävirta, J.; Pöyhönen, M.; Peltonen, S.; Peltonen, J. Prevalence of neurofibromatosis type 1 in the Finnish population. *Genet. Med. Off. J. Am. Coll. Med. Genet.* **2018**, *20*, 1082–1086. [CrossRef]
4. Gutmann, D.H.; Wood, D.L.; Collins, F.S. Identification of the neurofibromatosis type 1 gene product. *Proc. Natl. Acad. Sci. USA* **1991**, *88*, 9658–9662. [CrossRef]
5. Cichowski, K.; Jacks, T. NF_1 Tumor Suppressor Gene Function: Narrowing the GAP. *Cell* **2001**, *104*, 593–604. [CrossRef]
6. Legius, E.; Messiaen, L.; Wolkenstein, P.; Pancza, P.; Avery, R.A.; Berman, Y.; Blakeley, J.; Babovic-Vuksanovic, D.; Cunha, K.S.; Ferner, R.; et al. Revised diagnostic criteria for neurofibromatosis type 1 and Legius syndrome: An international consensus recommendation. *Genet. Med. Off. J. Am. Coll. Med. Genet.* **2021**, *23*, 1506–1513. [CrossRef]

7. Landry, J.P.; Schertz, K.L.; Chiang, Y.J.; Bhalla, A.D.; Yi, M.; Keung, E.Z.; Scally, C.P.; Feig, B.W.; Hunt, K.K.; Roland, C.L.; et al. Comparison of Cancer Prevalence in Patients with Neurofibromatosis Type 1 at an Academic Cancer Center vs in the General Population from 1985 to 2020. *JAMA Netw. Open* **2021**, *4*, e210945. [CrossRef]
8. Uusitalo, E.; Rantanen, M.; Kallionpää, R.A.; Pöyhönen, M.; Leppävirta, J.; Ylä-Outinen, H.; Riccardi, V.M.; Pukkala, E.; Pitkäniemi, J.; Peltonen, S.; et al. Distinctive Cancer Associations in Patients With Neurofibromatosis Type 1. *J. Clin. Oncol. Off. J. Am. Soc. Clin. Oncol.* **2016**, *34*, 1978–1986. [CrossRef]
9. Farid, M.; Demicco, E.G.; Garcia, R.; Ahn, L.; Merola, P.R.; Cioffi, A.; Maki, R.G. Malignant peripheral nerve sheath tumors. *Oncologist* **2014**, *19*, 193–201. [CrossRef]
10. Miettinen, M.M.; Antonescu, C.R.; Fletcher CD, M.; Kim, A.; Lazar, A.J.; Quezado, M.M.; Reilly, K.M.; Stemmer-Rachamimov, A.; Stewart, D.R.; Viskochil, D.; et al. Histopathologic evaluation of atypical neurofibromatous tumors and their transformation into malignant peripheral nerve sheath tumor in patients with neurofibromatosis 1-a consensus overview. *Hum. Pathol.* **2017**, *67*, 1–10. [CrossRef]
11. Meany, H.; Dombi, E.; Reynolds, J.; Whatley, M.; Kurwa, A.; Tsokos, M.; Salzer, W.; Gillespie, A.; Baldwin, A.; Derdak, J.; et al. 18-fluorodeoxyglucose-positron emission tomography (FDG-PET) evaluation of nodular lesions in patients with Neurofibromatosis type 1 and plexiform neurofibromas (PN) or malignant peripheral nerve sheath tumors (MPNST). *Pediatr. Blood Cancer* **2013**, *60*, 59–64. [CrossRef]
12. Akshintala, S.; Baldwin, A.; Liewehr, D.J.; Goodwin, A.; Blakeley, J.O.; Gross, A.M.; Steinberg, S.M.; Dombi, E.; Widemann, B.C. Longitudinal evaluation of peripheral nerve sheath tumors in neurofibromatosis type 1: Growth analysis of plexiform neurofibromas and distinct nodular lesions. *Neuro-Oncology* **2020**, *22*, 1368–1378. [CrossRef]
13. Beert, E.; Brems, H.; Daniëls, B.; De Wever, I.; Van Calenbergh, F.; Schoenaers, J.; Debiec-Rychter, M.; Gevaert, O.; De Raedt, T.; Van Den Bruel, A.; et al. Atypical neurofibromas in neurofibromatosis type 1 are premalignant tumors. *Genes Chromosomes Cancer* **2011**, *50*, 1021–1032. [CrossRef]
14. Pemov, A.; Hansen, N.F.; Sindiri, S.; Patidar, R.; Higham, C.S.; Dombi, E.; Miettinen, M.M.; Fetsch, P.; Brems, H.; Chandrasekharappa, S.C.; et al. Low mutation burden and frequent loss of CDKN2A/B and SMARCA2, but not PRC2, define premalignant neurofibromatosis type 1-associated atypical neurofibromas. *Neuro-Oncology* **2019**, *21*, 981–992. [CrossRef]
15. Lucas, C.G.; Gross, A.M.; Romo, C.G.; Dehner, C.A.; Lazar, A.J.; Miettinen, M.; Pekmezci, M.; Quezado, M.; Rodriguez, F.J.; Stemmer-Rachamimov, A.; et al. Symposium on Atypical Neurofibroma: State of the Science Members Consensus recommendations for an integrated diagnostic approach to peripheral nerve sheath tumors arising in the setting of Neurofibromatosis type 1 (NF1). *Neuro-Oncology* **2024**, *27*, noae235. [CrossRef]
16. Evans, D.G.; Baser, M.E.; McGaughran, J.; Sharif, S.; Howard, E.; Moran, A. Malignant peripheral nerve sheath tumours in neurofibromatosis. *J. Med. Genet.* **2002**, *39*, 311–314. [CrossRef]
17. Widemann, B.C. Current status of sporadic and neurofibromatosis type 1-associated malignant peripheral nerve sheath tumors. *Curr. Oncol. Rep.* **2009**, *11*, 322–328. [CrossRef]
18. Watson, K.L.; Al Sannaa, G.A.; Kivlin, C.M.; Ingram, D.R.; Landers, S.M.; Roland, C.L.; Cormier, J.N.; Hunt, K.K.; Feig, B.W.; Ashleigh Guadagnolo, B.; et al. Patterns of recurrence and survival in sporadic, neurofibromatosis Type 1-associated, and radiation-associated malignant peripheral nerve sheath tumors. *J. Neurosurg.* **2017**, *126*, 319–329. [CrossRef]
19. Carton, C.; Evans, D.G.; Blanco, I.; Friedrich, R.E.; Ferner, R.E.; Farschtschi, S.; Salvador, H.; Azizi, A.A.; Mautner, V.; Röhl, C.; et al. ERN GENTURIS NF1 Tumour Management Guideline Group ERN GENTURIS tumour surveillance guidelines for individuals with neurofibromatosis type 1. *eClinicalMedicine* **2023**, *56*, 101818. [CrossRef]
20. Miettinen, M.; Fetsch, J.F.; Sobin, L.H.; Lasota, J. Gastrointestinal stromal tumors in patients with neurofibromatosis 1: A clinicopathologic and molecular genetic study of 45 cases. *Am. J. Surg. Pathol.* **2006**, *30*, 90–96. [CrossRef]
21. Salvi, P.F.; Lorenzon, L.; Caterino, S.; Antolino, L.; Antonelli, M.S.; Balducci, G. Gastrointestinal stromal tumors associated with neurofibromatosis 1: A single centre experience and systematic review of the literature including 252 cases. *Int. J. Surg. Oncol.* **2013**, *2013*, 398570. [CrossRef]
22. Ylä-Outinen, H.; Loponen, N.; Kallionpää, R.A.; Peltonen, S.; Peltonen, J. Intestinal tumors in neurofibromatosis 1 with special reference to fatal gastrointestinal stromal tumors (GIST). *Mol. Genet. Genom. Med.* **2019**, *7*, e927. [CrossRef]
23. Nishida, T.; Tsujimoto, M.; Takahashi, T.; Hirota, S.; Blay, J.Y.; Wataya-Kaneda, M. Gastrointestinal stromal tumors in Japanese patients with neurofibromatosis type I. *J. Gastroenterol.* **2016**, *51*, 571–578. [CrossRef]
24. Yun, J.S.; Lee, M.H.; Lee, S.M.; Lee, J.S.; Kim, H.J.; Lee, S.J.; Chung, H.W.; Lee, S.H.; Shin, M.J. Peripheral nerve sheath tumor: Differentiation of malignant from benign tumors with conventional and diffusion-weighted MRI. *Eur. Radiol.* **2021**, *31*, 1548–1557. [CrossRef]
25. Boellaard, R.; Delgado-Bolton, R.; Oyen, W.J.; Giammarile, F.; Tatsch, K.; Eschner, W.; Verzijlbergen, F.J.; Barrington, S.F.; Pike, L.C.; Weber, W.A.; et al. FDG PET/CT: EANM procedure guidelines for tumour imaging: Version 2.0. *Eur. J. Nucl. Med. Mol. Imaging* **2015**, *42*, 328–354. [CrossRef]

26. Moharir, M.; London, K.; Howman-Giles, R.; North, K. Utility of positron emission tomography for tumour surveillance in children with neurofibromatosis type 1. *Eur. J. Nucl. Med. Mol. Imaging* **2010**, *37*, 1309–1317. [CrossRef]
27. Benz, M.R.; Czernin, J.; Dry, S.M.; Tap, W.D.; Allen-Auerbach, M.S.; Elashoff, D.; Phelps, M.E.; Weber, W.A.; Eilber, F.C. Quantitative F18-fluorodeoxyglucose positron emission tomography accurately characterizes peripheral nerve sheath tumors as malignant or benign. *Cancer* **2010**, *116*, 451–458. [CrossRef]
28. Warbey, V.S.; Ferner, R.E.; Dunn, J.T.; Calonje, E.; O'Doherty, M.J. [18F]FDG PET/CT in the diagnosis of malignant peripheral nerve sheath tumours in neurofibromatosis type-1. *Eur. J. Nucl. Med. Mol. Imaging* **2009**, *36*, 751–757. [CrossRef]
29. Who Classification of Tumours Editorial Board. *Soft Tissue and Bone Tumours*, 5th ed.; WHO Classification of Tumours: Geneva, Switzerland, 2020.
30. Who Classification of Tumours Editorial Board. *Central Nervous System Tumours*, 5th ed.; WHO Classification of Tumours: Geneva, Switzerland, 2022.
31. Mete, O. Special Issue On the 2022 WHO Classification of Endocrine and Neuroendocrine Tumors: A New Primer for Endocrine Pathology Practice. *Endocr. Pathol.* **2022**, *33*, 1–2. [CrossRef]
32. Perreault, S.; Larouche, V.; Tabori, U.; Hawkin, C.; Lippé, S.; Ellezam, B.; Décarie, J.C.; Théoret, Y.; Métras, M.É.; Sultan, S.; et al. A phase 2 study of trametinib for patients with pediatric glioma or plexiform neurofibroma with refractory tumor and activation of the MAPK/ERK pathway: TRAM-01. *BMC Cancer* **2019**, *19*, 1250. [CrossRef]
33. Higham, C.S.; Dombi, E.; Rogiers, A.; Bhaumik, S.; Pans, S.; Connor SE, J.; Miettinen, M.; Sciot, R.; Tirabosco, R.; Brems, H.; et al. The characteristics of 76 atypical neurofibromas as precursors to neurofibromatosis 1 associated malignant peripheral nerve sheath tumors. *Neuro-Oncology* **2018**, *20*, 818–825. [CrossRef]
34. Ferner, R.E.; Golding, J.F.; Smith, M.; Calonje, E.; Jan, W.; Sanjayanathan, V.; O'Doherty, M. [18F]2-fluoro-2-deoxy-D-glucose positron emission tomography (FDG PET) as a diagnostic tool for neurofibromatosis 1 (NF1) associated malignant peripheral nerve sheath tumours (MPNSTs): A long-term clinical study. *Ann. Oncol. Off. J. Eur. Soc. Med. Oncol.* **2008**, *19*, 390–394. [CrossRef]
35. Yao, C.; Zhou, H.; Dong, Y.; Alhaskawi, A.; Hasan Abdullah Ezzi, S.; Wang, Z.; Lai, J.; Goutham Kota, V.; Hasan Abdulla Hasan Abdulla, M.; Lu, H. Malignant Peripheral Nerve Sheath Tumors: Latest Concepts in Disease Pathogenesis and Clinical Management. *Cancers* **2023**, *15*, 1077. [CrossRef]
36. Sundby, T.R.; Szymanski, J.J.; Pan, A.; Jones, P.A.; Mahmood, S.Z.; Reid, O.H.; Srihari, D.; Armstrong, A.E.; Chamberlain, S.; Burgic, S.; et al. Early detection of malignant and pre-malignant peripheral nerve tumors using cell-free DNA fragmentomics. *medRxiv* **2024**. [CrossRef]
37. González-Muñoz, T.; Di Giannatale, A.; García-Silva, S.; Santos, V.; Sánchez-Redondo, S.; Savini, C.; Graña-Castro, O.; Blanco-Aparicio, C.; Fischer, S.; De Wever, O.; et al. Endoglin, a Novel Biomarker and Therapeutical Target to Prevent Malignant Peripheral Nerve Sheath Tumor Growth and Metastasis. *Clin. Cancer Res. Off. J. Am. Assoc. Cancer Res.* **2023**, *29*, 3744–3758. [CrossRef]
38. Moon, C.I.; Tompkins, W.; Wang, Y.; Godec, A.; Zhang, X.; Pipkorn, P.; Miller, C.A.; Dehner, C.; Dahiya, S.; Hirbe, A.C. Unmasking Intra-tumoral Heterogeneity and Clonal Evolution in NF1-MPNST. *Genes* **2020**, *11*, 499. [CrossRef]
39. Carrió, M.; Gel, B.; Terribas, E.; Zucchiatti, A.C.; Moliné, T.; Rosas, I.; Teulé, Á.; Ramón YCajal, S.; López-Gutiérrez, J.C.; Blanco, I.; et al. Analysis of intratumor heterogeneity in Neurofibromatosis type 1 plexiform neurofibromas and neurofibromas with atypical features: Correlating histological and genomic findings. *Human mutation* **2018**, *39*, 1112–1125. [CrossRef]
40. Ly, K.I.; Merker, V.L.; Cai, W.; Bredella, M.A.; Muzikansky, A.; Thalheimer, R.D.; Da, J.L.; Orr, C.C.; Herr, H.P.; Morris, M.E.; et al. Ten-Year Follow-up of Internal Neurofibroma Growth Behavior in Adult Patients with Neurofibromatosis Type 1 Using Whole-Body MRI. *Neurology* **2023**, *100*, e661–e670. [CrossRef]
41. Casey, D.; Demko, S.; Sinha, A.; Mishra-Kalyani, P.S.; Shen, Y.L.; Khasar, S.; Goheer, M.A.; Helms, W.S.; Pan, L.; Xu, Y.; et al. FDA Approval Summary: Selumetinib for Plexiform Neurofibroma. *Clin. Cancer Res. Off. J. Am. Assoc. Cancer Res.* **2021**, *27*, 4142–4146. [CrossRef]
42. Campagne, O.; Yeo, K.K.; Fangusaro, J.; Stewart, C.F. Clinical Pharmacokinetics and Pharmacodynamics of Selumetinib. *Clin. Pharmacokinet.* **2021**, *60*, 283–303. [CrossRef]
43. Gross, A.M.; O'Sullivan Coyne, G.; Dombi, E.; Tibery, C.; Herrick, W.G.; Martin, S.; Angus, S.P.; Shern, J.F.; Rhodes, S.D.; Foster, J.C.; et al. Selumetinib in adults with NF1 and inoperable plexiform neurofibroma: A phase 2 trial. *Nat. Med.* **2025**, *31*, 105–115. [CrossRef] [PubMed]
44. Borcherding, D.C.; Amin, N.V.; He, K.; Zhang, X.; Lyu, Y.; Dehner, C.; Bhatia, H.; Gothra, A.; Daud, L.; Ruminski, P.; et al. MEK Inhibition Synergizes with TYK2 Inhibitors in NF1-Associated Malignant Peripheral Nerve Sheath Tumors. *Clin. Cancer Res. Off. J. Am. Assoc. Cancer Res.* **2023**, *29*, 1592–1604. [CrossRef] [PubMed]

45. Kohlmeyer, J.L.; Lingo, J.J.; Kaemmer, C.A.; Scherer, A.; Warrier, A.; Voigt, E.; Raygoza Garay, J.A.; McGivney, G.R.; Brockman, Q.R.; Tang, A.; et al. CDK4/6-MEK Inhibition in MPNSTs Causes Plasma Cell Infiltration, Sensitization to PD-L1 Blockade, and Tumor Regression. *Clin. Cancer Res. Off. J. Am. Assoc. Cancer Res.* **2023**, *29*, 3484–3497. [CrossRef] [PubMed]
46. Hu, L.S.; Smits, M.; Kaufmann, T.J.; Knutsson, L.; Rapalino, O.; Galldiks, N.; Sundgren, P.C.; Cha, S. Advanced Imaging in the Diagnosis Response Assessment of High-Grade Glioma: AJR Expert Panel Narrative Review. *Am. J. Roentgenol.* **2025**, *224*, e2330612. [CrossRef]

cancers

MDPI

Article

Recent Developments in Surgical Treatment of Spinal Deformity in Pediatric Patients: Experience from a Single-Center Series of 42 Neurofibromatosis Type 1 Patients

Kiril V. Mladenov [1,2,*] and Ralf Stücker [1,2]

[1] Pediatric Orthopedic Department, Altona Children's Hospital, Bleickenallee 38, D-22763 Hamburg, Germany; ralf.stuecker@kinderkrankenhaus.net

[2] Department of Orthopedics, University Medical Center Hamburg-Eppendorf, D-20246 Hamburg, Germany

* Correspondence: kiril.mladenov@kinderkrankenhaus.net

Simple Summary: Approximately 60% of the patients with neurofibromatosis type 1 (NF-1) demonstrate involvement of the skeletal system, with the spine being the most commonly affected element. In the vast majority of the cases with an NF-1-associated spinal deformity, the natural history is unfavorable and worsening is observed in cases that proceed without treatment. Non-operative management is rarely successful and surgery is necessary in most of the cases, especially in the presence of the characteristic osseous dystrophic changes. Since the disease is rare and features a heterogeneous presentation, evidence-based treatment protocols are not available. The aim of this retrospective study is to share the experience and to report the outcomes after treatment of spinal deformities in pediatric patients with NF-1. The results show that good and sustainable correction of spinal deformities can be achieved by means of early surgical treatment even in immature patients. However, surgery remains challenging, and the complication rate is higher than in patients with spinal deformities of other etiologies.

Abstract: Background: The management of spinal deformities in patients with NF-1 is challenging. The study aimed to assess the outcomes of the surgical treatment of spine deformities in children with neurofibromatosis type 1 with our treatment approach. Methods: A retrospective single-center study on pediatric patients with spinal deformities associated with NF-1 who received surgical treatment between 2006 and 2024. Results: The study group comprised 42 patients with a mean age at surgery of 9.8 years. Twenty-five patients (60%) were treated by means of growth-preserving techniques and 17 patients (40%) by means of definitive fusion. Preoperative halo-gravity traction was used in 14 (33%) cases. In the group treated with a growth-preserving technique, a 54.1% mean curve correction was observed at the latest follow-up, and growth of the thoracic spine was maintained at a physiological rate; however, 25 unplanned revision surgeries (mostly due to mechanical complications) were necessary. In the group treated by definitive fusion, a 66% curve correction was achieved at initial surgery, which remained unchanged at latest follow-up, and revision surgery was performed in three cases for augmentation of the fusion mass. There was one neurological complication (2%). Another patient developed a deep wound infection (2%). Conclusions: Good and sustainable surgical correction of spinal deformities can be achieved in pediatric patients with NF-1. Due to the bony dystrophic changes, surgical treatment is challenging and the complication rate is higher than in spinal deformities of other etiologies.

Keywords: spinal deformity; neurofibromatosis type 1

1. Introduction

Neurofibromatosis type 1 (NF-1) is one of the most common genetic disorders in human beings, affecting 1/3000–4000 individuals. An estimated 1,000,000 persons are affected worldwide without gender or racial predisposition [1–3]. Spinal deformities in patients with NF-1 are considered the most common skeletal manifestation in NF-1 patients and have been reported in up to 60% of the affected individuals [1,4]. Typically, spinal deformities are very severe and rigid and are accompanied by characteristic NF-1 dystrophic osseous changes with involvement of the vertebrae and/or the ribs [5,6], which make treatment very challenging [7]. Non-operative approaches, such as observation and bracing, can be applied only for a very small number of patients with mild non-dystrophic "idiopathic like" curves [5,6]. In opposition to this, surgical treatment is advocated in most of the patients presenting with dystrophic spinal deformity due to the history of such cases featuring constant worsening [8,9]. Despite the development of modern surgical techniques for stable spinal instrumentation, the complication rate after surgical correction of spine deformities remains relatively high due to biological and mechanical factors. Spinal instrumentation may be very challenging due to dystrophic vertebral body and lamina, as well as absent or tiny pedicles, dura ectasia and soft bony structures. The most common complications are delayed union, pseudarthrosis, curve progression, implant failure and perioperative bleeding, which have been reported at a rate of up to 64% [10,11]. Current treatment strategies have been proposed by some authors [12,13]; however, well-established evidence-based treatment protocols, especially for the pediatric population, are still lacking. The current study aimed at evaluation of the results after treatment of spinal deformities in children with NF-1 with our treatment protocol, highlighting pitfalls and presenting different approaches depending on curve morphology and patient-specific factors.

2. General Knowledge on NF-1

2.1. Genetics, Pathogenesis and Diagnosis

Neurofibromatosis type 1 is caused by a defect in the tumor suppressor gene located on the long arm of chromosome 17, which encodes production of the ubiquitously present protein neurofibromin, its major function being the downregulation of the RAS protein [14–16]. NF-1 is classified as a "RAS-opathy", which is a group of clinically related disorders that includes Costello syndrome, Noonan syndrome and gingival fibromatosis. Lack of neurofibromin results in increased RAS signaling and the development of NF-1-associated neoplasms such as peripheral nerve sheath tumors, pheochromocytoma, myeloid dysplasia and neurofibromas [17,18]. Since downregulation of the RAS follows the protein kinase pathway, protein kinase inhibitors such as Trametinib underwent clinical trials, with promising results [19–21]. Data on the positive effects of medical treatment on the development of spinal deformities are currently not available.

Inheritance is autosomal dominant; however, 50% of the cases are "de novo" mutations, and genetic identification of mutation can be achieved in 95% of the affected patients [22]. Since the gene is very large and affection is heterogeneous, clinical expressivity between patients is highly variable and no clear genotype–phenotype correlation exists, which makes the predictive value of the genetic testing concerning clinical presentation unreliable.

2.2. Clinical Presentation of NF-1

NF-1 is a multisystem disorder affecting the skin, the peripheral nerve sheaths and the cardio vascular system. Cognitive disabilities are present in 60–80% of the children [23], and skeletal manifestations, such as scoliosis, kyphosis and tibia dysplasia (congenital tibia pseudarthrosis), have been documented in up to 60% of the affected individuals. Although the disease is mostly fully present by the age of 5 years, phenotypic appearance and presentation may be highly variable between individuals and even between relatives. Typical skin manifestations are the "café-au-lait" hyperpigmented macules, the axillary and inguinal freckling, the cutaneous neurofibromas and the plexiform neurofibromas. About 10% of the patients develop malignant peripheral nerve sheath tumors (MPNSTs) with a median time of diagnosis of between 20 and 40 years; MPNSTs have a poor prognosis and may be lethal [24,25]. Ocular manifestations, such as the pathognomonic iris "Lisch" nodules (iris hamartoma), are present in children above 6 years of age and may be seen in most adult patients by slit lamp examination. Optic glioma (a pilocytic astrocytoma) is seen in 15–20% of children with NF-1, with median age of 4.9 years at presentation. It remains often asymptomatic and may cause visual abnormalities which may progress to optic nerve atrophy and blindness in certain cases [26–28]. The diagnosis of NF-1 is based on clinical criteria defined by the Consensus Development Conference of the National Institutes of Health from 1987 [29]. The diagnostic criteria were recently revised in order to add the importance of genetic testing as a diagnostic tool supporting the diagnosis of NF-1 and differentiating it from similar conditions with overlapping clinical presentation [30].

2.3. *Spinal Deformity in NF-1 Patients*

Spinal deformity (scoliosis, kyphosis) is the most common musculo-skeletal manifestation in NF-1 patients. The high incidence was described more than a century ago [31], and the real prevalence in NF-1 patients is unknown. However, current observations report that over 60% of the NF-1 patients may present with spinal deformities [1,4]. The exact etiology is unknown, and current hypotheses include mesodermal dysplasia, erosion and infiltration of the bone by local neurofibromas, osteomalacia and endocrine factors [4]. Curves are mostly localized in the thoracic spine, but the cervical and the lumbar spine may be involved as well [32,33]. Depending on curve appearance and radiologic bone morphology, curves can be differentiated in terms of being "non-dystrophic" and "dystrophic" deformities [4,6]. The differentiation between those two presentations is very important since deformity behavior, prognosis and management are largely different.

2.3.1. Non Dystrophic Spinal Deformity

Non-dystrophic coronal curves (scoliosis) are also called "idiopathic like"; they typically present without morphological changes in the single vertebral elements (absent signs of osseous dysplasia) and behave similarly to idiopathic scoliosis. The prognosis is favorable, and the mainstays of treatment are observation for curves <20° and brace treatment for curves 20–40°, usually with a Cheneaux-type brace [6]. Particular attention should be paid to these patients, and regular clinical and radiologic curve monitoring in 6–12 month intervals is mandatory since dystrophic features may occur over time and may be followed by transformation into dystrophic deformities—a process called "modulation" [34].

2.3.2. Dystrophic Spinal Deformity

Dystrophic osseous changes are best seen on upright plain whole-spine radiographs, and meticulous evaluation for dystrophic features should be performed since management and prognosis of spinal deformity are highly dependent on the presence of dystrophic signs. Characteristic dystrophic features are listed in Table 1 and extensively described in Figure 1.

Table 1. Radiographic features of dystrophic changes in NF-1 patients.

Feature	Location	Definition
Scalloping	Vertebral body	scalloping of the posterior, anterior or lateral wall *
Rotation	Vertebra	rotational deformity as compared to adjacent vertebra
Penciling	Rib	narrowing of the medial portion of the rib **
Wedging	Vertebral body	wedge shaped vertebral body ***
Spindling	Transverse process	transverse process thinned like a spindle
Widening	Spinal canal	enlarged interpedicular distance ****
Enlargement	Neuroforamen	enlarged neuroforamen *****
Soft tissue mass	Paravertebral	seen mostly on MRI

* >3 mm thoracic spine, >4 mm lumbar spine. ** Width of the rib is smaller than that of the narrowest portion of the second rib. *** Similar to congenital hemivertebra. **** Seen in the ap projection compared to the adjacent vertebra. ***** Seen in the lateral view compared to the adjacent vertebra.

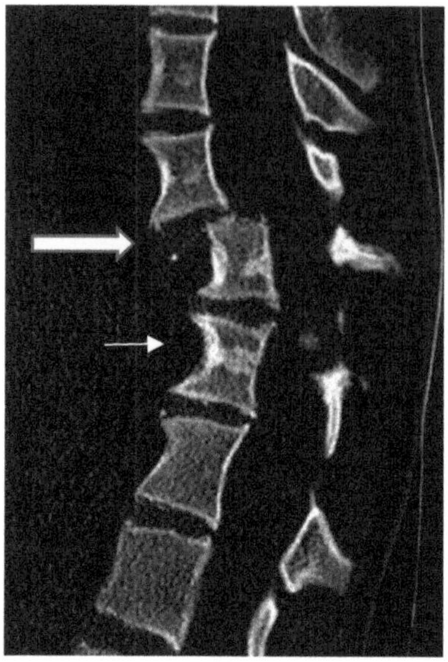

(a)

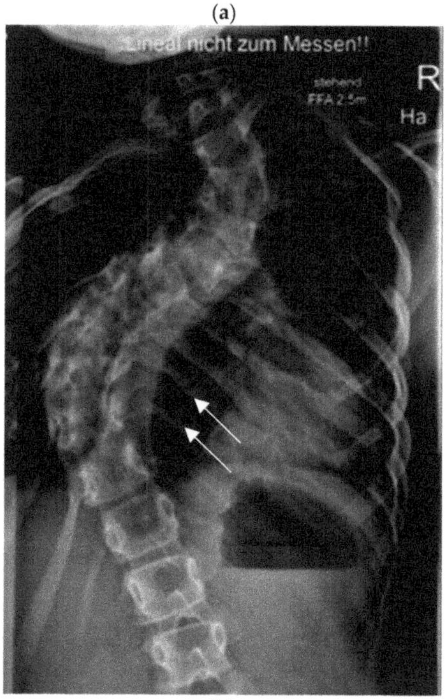

(b)

Figure 1. *Cont.*

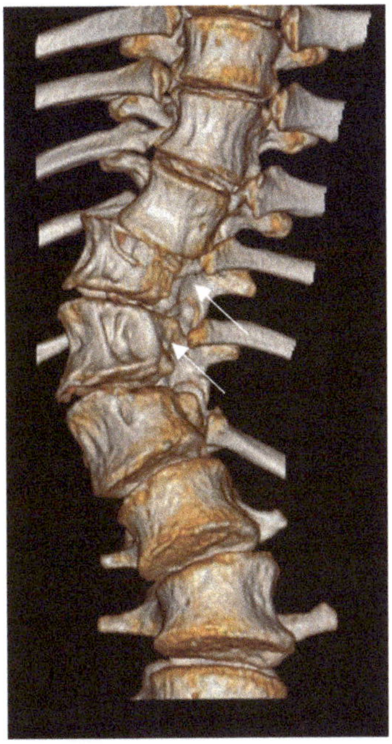

(c)

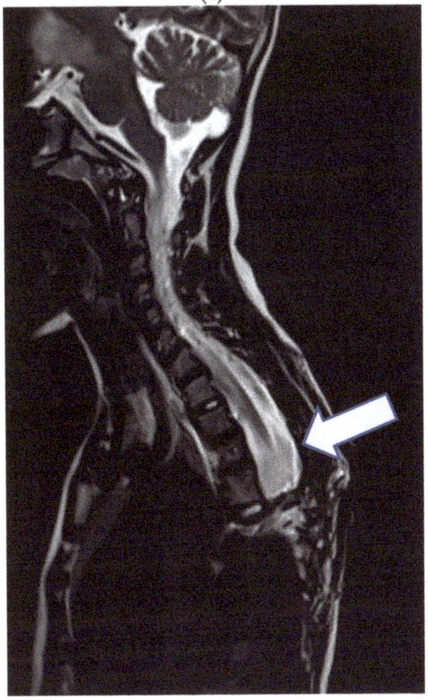

(d)

Figure 1. Dystrophic osseous features: (**a**) scalloping (thin arrow), rotation and dislocation with pathologic kyphosis (thick arrow), (**b**) rib penciling (white arrows), (**c**) wedging and rotatory dislocation (arrows) in a 3-D CT reconstruction, (**d**) widening of the spinal canal and dural ectasia (thick white arrow).

Dystrophic curves are typically short, extending over 3–5 spinal segments with poorly visible vertebral structures and a significant spinal rotation which occasionally leads to rotatory subluxation or complete dislocation, frequently accompanied by pathologic kyphosis (Figure 1a). It has been hypothesized that dystrophic changes are either intrinsic (due to primary bone deformation) or appear secondary to increased pressure from dural ectasia or nerve root enlargement, leading to scalloping or neuroforaminal enlargement [35]. The presence of dystrophic changes is of very important prognostic value. As a general rule, the more pronounced the dystrophic changes, the more unfavorable the prognosis. The presence of three or more dystrophic features has been related to worsening of the spinal deformity in over 85% of the cases [34].

2.3.3. Imaging Modalities of Spinal Deformity in NF-1

Upright whole-spine antero-posterior and lateral plain radiographs are the gold standard for the evaluation of spinal deformity in NF-1 patients. These allow for exact measurements of the severity of the coronal and the sagittal deformity by means of the Cobb angle and the evaluation of dystrophic changes. Whole-spine MRIs are considered essential in the evaluation of spinal deformities in NF-1 patients and have become mandatory in the preoperative assessment of all patients in order to detect intraspinal and paravertebral pathologies in recent years. A combined incidence of paraspinal and intraspinal tumor pathologies has been reported in 37% of the patients with non-dystrophic and dystrophic curves [13].

Bone morphology can be best evaluated by means of a CT scan. Despite concerns of x-ray exposure, a thin-slice CT scan with coronal, sagittal and 3-D reconstructions is very valuable for the preoperative planning and for the evaluation of the fusion mass. The scan surface should be restricted to the area of interest, which mostly corresponds to the dystrophic portion of the spine in order to reduce the negative effects of radiation exposure.

3. Materials and Methods

3.1. Data Collection, Measurements

A retrospective study with prospective data collection of all patients who received surgical treatment for spinal deformities associated with NF-1 in a single institution between 2006 and 2024. Patient charts, available medical records, spinal radiographs, and other imaging studies (MRI, CT) were used for data collection.

Initial upright spine radiographs were used for the analysis of location and type of spinal deformity (scoliosis, kyphosis) as well as the presence of osseous dystrophic changes already listed in Table 2. The amount of coronal and sagittal spinal deformity were evaluated by means of standardized measurement of the Cobb angle on upright radiographs performed before surgery on the first erect postoperative radiography and at the latest follow-up. Patients were divided into groups according to the location of deformity (cervical vs. thoracic and/or lumbar), type of procedure (growth-preserving vs. definitive Fusion), and type of surgical approach (anterior, posterior or combined). In the patient cohort treated by means of a growth-preserving technique, the T1-12 height was measured on the first postoperative index image and ultimate AP radiographs in order to evaluate spinal growth. Based on the cumulative height gain during the observation period, the T1-12 growth ratio was calculated and presented as millimeter per year. Achieved correction at final follow-up was calculated as percent from the initial amount of spinal deformity. Presence of spinal fusion in the group treated by means of definitive spondylodesis was estimated on the latest available imaging study (x-ray, MRI, CT).

Information about the number of surgical procedures, the necessity for planned or unplanned revision surgery as well as perioperative and late complications was collected from patients' records.

Demographics are reported in mean and SD values; a paired students *t*-test was used for evaluation of achieved curve correction using SPSS software, (Version 29.0.0.0) and the statistical significance was set at 0.05.

Table 2. Results according to type of initial surgical procedure.

Type of Index Surgical Procedure	Age at Surgery *	Duration of Follow-Up *	Curve ° Pre-Op	Curve ° Last Follow-Up	% Curve Correction	T1-12 Postoperative †	T1-12 Last Follow-Up †	Growth T1-12 ‡
Growth-preserving	7.7 (±2.3)	6.7 (±3.6)	77 (±11.4)	33.1 (±10.6)	54.1 (±14.7)	19.6 (±3)	22.8 (±2.9)	0.73 (±0.17)
Fusion	13.4 (±2.3)	3.1 (±1.7)	66 (±13.6)	26 (±11.3)	66 (±23.7)			

Legend: *—years; °—Cobb angle; T1-12—thoracic spine height; †—in centimeters; ‡—in centimeters per year.

3.2. Treatment Protocol

Our treatment protocol is based on patient-specific and deformity-specific factors such as bone age, skeletal maturity curve location, magnitude and flexibility, as well as the presence of dystrophic osseous changes. The currently widely accepted bone age of <10 years was chosen as a treshold to define "early onset" spinal deformity as proposed by the SRS. [36]. The Sanders classification was used for the definition of bone age, with Sanders stage 7b defining end of spinal growth [37].

With respect to location, spinal deformity was divided into cervical, thoracic, thoraco-lumbar, lumbar and lumbo-sacral. According to the magnitude of coronal deformity (scoliosis), curves were divided into mild (20–40°), moderate (40–60°) and severe (>60°). With respect to osseous dystrophic changes, we divided spinal deformity into "non-dystrophic" and "dystrophic". The treatment strategy is presented through the following case scenarios:

3.2.1. Non Dystrophic Spinal Deformity

Spinal deformity in the absence of osseous dysrtophic changes in patients with NF-1 behave like idiopathic spinal deformities, and spinal curves are called "idiopathic like" [13]. Management follows the guidelines for idiopathic scoliosis treatment. Simple observation is sufficient in soliosis <20° independent of patient maturity, and the prognosis is generally good, especially after completion of skeletal growth. Immature patients with curves of 20–40° are treated with a brace until the end of growth. Curves above 50° Cobb usually need surgical treatment since worsening is observed in most of the untreated cases. The method of choice depends on skeletal maturity, with growth-preserving techniques being adequate for immature patients and definitive fusion being the recommended method after the completion of growth. Particular attention should be paid in these patients, and follow-up radiographs should be performed once a year and meticulously evaluated for dystrophic osseous signs since those may develop with time in initially non-dystrophic vertebral bodies.

3.2.2. Dystrophic Spinal Deformity

The risk of deterioration of spinal deformity in the presence of dystrophic osseous changes is high and increases proportionally with the severity of bone dystrophy. Brace treatment is not efficient to stop deformity progression and is not recommended in these cases. Our approach in immature patients is to perform an anterior fusion at the apex of the deformity, which usually extends over 2–4 segments, and then perform a spine-based growth-preserving instrumentation through a posterior approach in order to correct and control the global spinal deformity. After the end of growth, instrumentation is converted to the final spinal fusion. Skeletally mature patients with scoliosis 40–60° Cobb at initial presentation underwent posterior spinal fusion (PSF) with segmental instrumentation. Patients with very severe dystrophic curves (>60° Cobb) at index presentation were treated by means of combined anterior and posterior spinal fusion.

3.3. Surgical Treatment Methods

3.3.1. Anterior Spinal Fusion

The rationale of anterior spinal fusion in dystrophic curves is to control the deformity at the apex of the curve through achievement of a solid fusion and preservation of the stability of the spinal column, thus avoiding the risk of neurological damage of the spinal cord.

This is especially important in cases with pathologic kyphosis or rotational dislocation. Depending on the levels to be addressed, we performed the anterior part of the procedure through an open transthoracic, a retroperitoneal or a combined approach from the convex side. In the thoracic spine, anterior fusion was performed through a convex-sided thoracotomy using the intercostal space 2 levels above the apex of the curve. A partial resection of the corresponding rib was performed and the rib was preserved as a bone graft. The apical intervertebral disks (usually 2–4 segments) were meticulously removed, generously exposing the subchondral vertebral end plates. Violation of the cancellous bone of the vertebral end plates was avoided in order to avoid severe uncontrolled bleeding. A part of the rib graft was morselized and filled in the intervertebral disk spaces. An anterior screw–rod instrumentation was used, as shown in Figure 2.

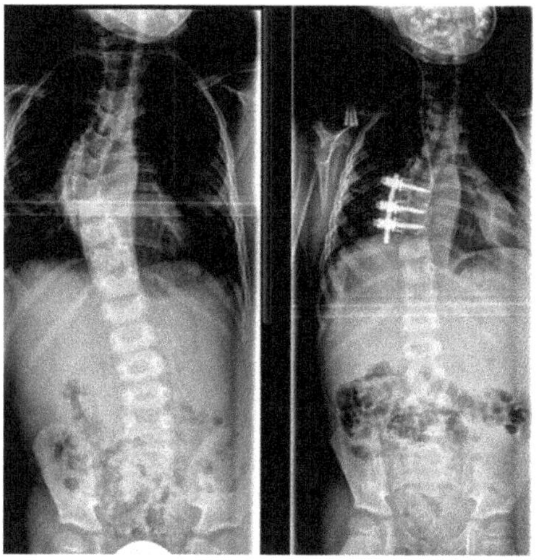

(a) (b)

Figure 2. (**a**) Six-year old patient with dystrophic scoliosis of the thoracic spine. (**b**) After anterior spinal fusion Th 7–9 with instrumentation.

In patients with severe dystrophic changes and insufficient bony substance of the vertebral bodies, the remaining portion of the rib was anchored as a strut bone graft in a gap created with a rongeur in the antero-lateral portion on the convex side of the apical and the juxta apical vertebral bodies, as shown in Figure 3.

In the lumbar spine, the fusion was achieved through a retroperitoneal approach, and titanium mesh cages filled with autologous cancellous bone graft from the iliac crest were used for anterior support in order to maintain physiologic lordosis. If the apex was located in the thoraco-lumbar junction, a combined transthoracic–retroperitoneal approach with diaphragmatic release was used.

3.3.2. Posterior Growth-Preserving Instrumentation

Preservation of the thoracic spine growth in immature patients has been shown to play an essential role in the physiologic development of the lung tissue and is of vital importance in terms of preserving normal lung function and avoiding the development of iatrogenic thoracic insufficiency syndrome [38]. We used the following spinal growth-preserving techniques, all of which are based on active distraction:

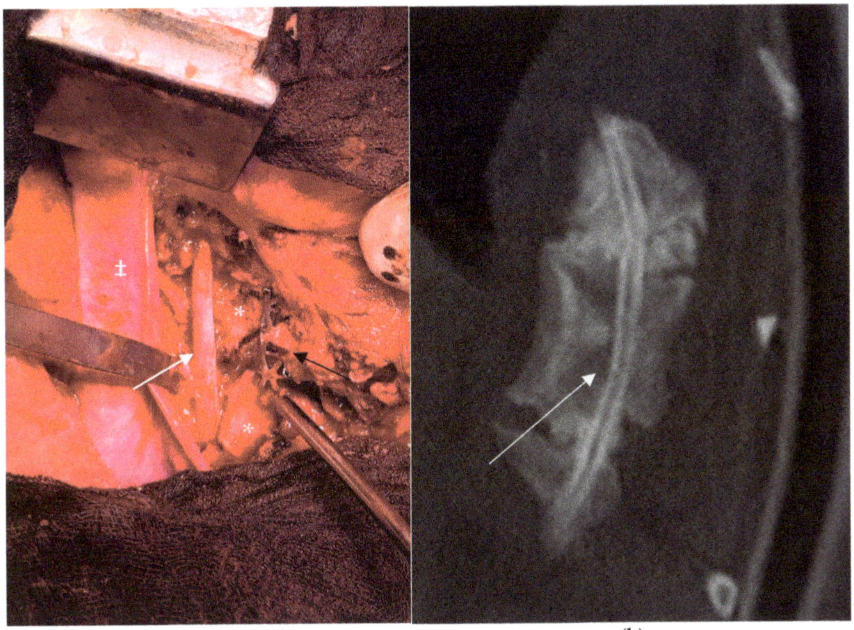

(a) (b)

Figure 3. Transthoracic approach to the thoracic spine in a 15-year-old patient with dystrophic scoliosis and kyphotic deformity (**a**). Anterior strut rib graft (white arrow), anterior vertebral body support with an intercorporal mesh cage (black arrow), vertebral bodies (*), aorta (‡); (**b**) The rib graft (white arrow) in place with a bony fusion confirmed by a thin-slice CT scan.

VEPTR

The vertical expandable prosthetic titanium rib (VEPTR®, De Puy Synthes, Raynham, MA, USA) was initially designed for the treatment of congenital scoliosis associated with rib anomalies and chest-wall deformities. Later, the device was approved for clinical use in immature patients with scoliosis of a non-idiopathic origin. The technique consists of proximal and distal anchors connected with a telescoping device which can be lengthened surgically, usually every 6 months, by a minimally invasive approach. The proximal anchors are attached to the ribs, and the distal may be attached to the ribs, directly to the spine by means of a laminar hook or to the pelvis by means of an ilium "S" shaped hook. We used this technique upon performing index surgery in an early series of immature patients; however, due to the high number of mechanical complications due mostly to aseptic loosening of the anchors which migrated through dystrophic bone its use was abandoned Figure 4.

Traditional Growing Rods (TGRs)

The surgical technique consists of cranial and caudal anchors (laminar hooks or pedicle screws) attached directly to the spine which are placed through a less-invasive posterior surgical approach. Each anchor is connected with a rod. The cranial and the caudal rods connected to the anchors are coupled to each other with a longitudinal or a parallel connector in such a manner that instrumentation extends from the upper to the lower end vertebra of the curve. The rods are left overlapping each other for 3–5 cm, allowing repetitive lengthening of the construct between the cranial and the caudal anchor (Figure 5). In that way, control of the curve may be achieved, and further growth of the spine is possible by repetitive lengthening of the rods by means of a small surgical procedure, thus avoiding growth disturbance, which is one of the main drawbacks of definitive fusion.

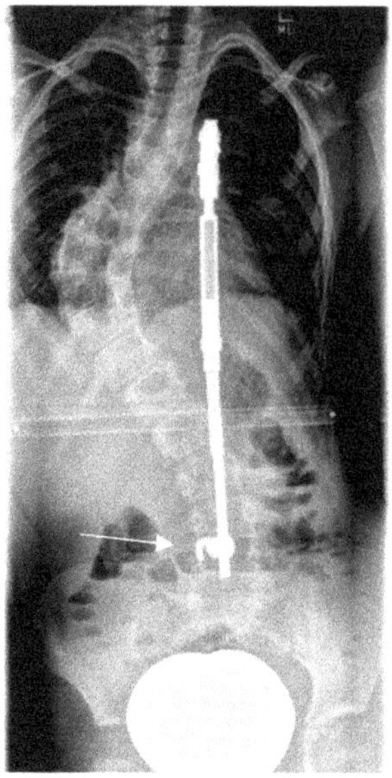

Figure 4. Rib-to-ilium VEPTR construct in a 9-year-old patient with a dystrophic curve. Distal migration of the laminar caudal anchor (white arrow) with loss of correction.

Lengthening is marked with double arrow.

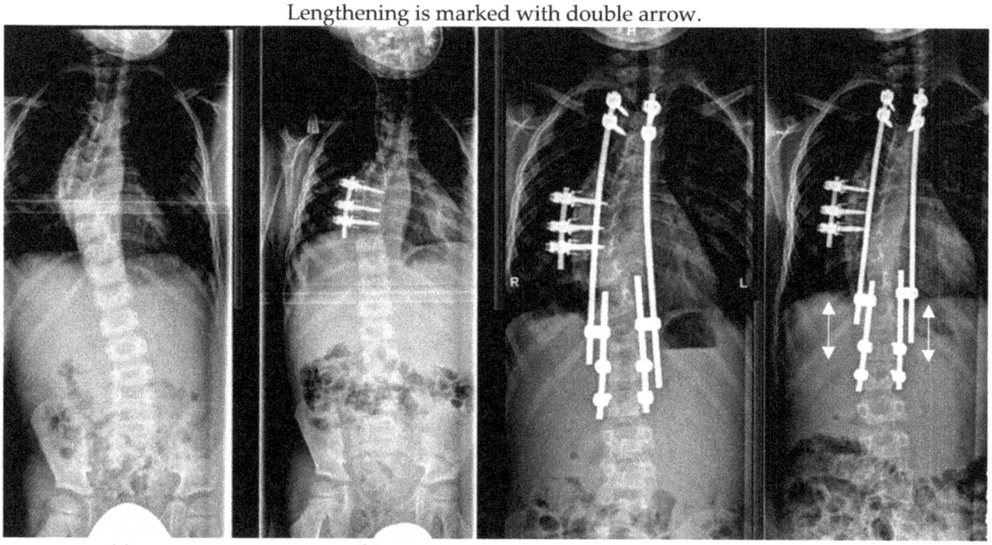

(a) (b) (c) (d)

Figure 5. Six-year-old patient with dystrophic scoliosis (**a**). After a short-segment anterior fusion T7-9 (**b**). After TGR application T3-L2 (**c**), and after 3 years of follow-up and 5 TGR lengthenings (**d**).

Magnetically Controlled Growing Rods (MCGRs)

To avoid the necessity of multiple surgeries for rod lengthening, growing rods which can be lengthened without surgical intervention were introduced (Figure 6). The principles of anchor placement are similar to those of TGRs, but the magnetically controlled growing rod incorporates a magnet unit ("motor") which is coupled with a threaded rod. The "motor" is activated by means of transcutaneous magnetic waves produced by an external device (called a controller) which is placed directly on the skin. In this way, non invasive lengthening of the rod can be achieved without skin incisions and without the need for anesthesia. Our lengthening protocol comprises rod lengthenings of 5 mm every 4 to 6 months, which are performed in the outpatient department. Despite the benefits of MCGRs in terms of avoiding multiple surgeries for lengthening of the device, their application is limited and practically impossible in cases which need MRI follow-ups since the magnetic unit produces a strong magnetic artifact extending 20 cm in diameter around the magnet unit, making MRI assessment of the structures located in this field impossible. Another limitation are patients with severe kyphotic deformities, since the lengthening unit of the MCGR rod should remain straight and cannot be contoured in order to match spinal deformities.

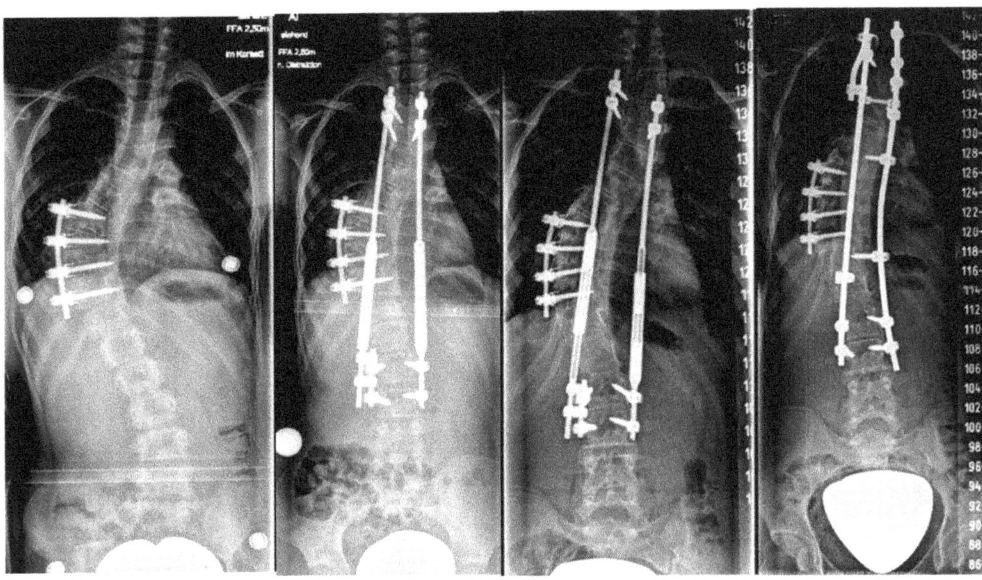

(a) (b) (c) (d)

Figure 6. Nine-year-old patient with a dystrophic thoracic curve after short-segment anterior spinal fusion Th8-11 (**a**). After MCGR application Th3-L3 (**b**). After 5 years of follow-up and a 4.5 cm lengthening (**c**). After definitive fusion at maturity (**d**).

3.3.3. Posterior Spinal Fusion

In this classical technique, the posterior vertebral elements are subperiosteally exposed through a posterior surgical approach. Segmental instrumentation of the vertebral column is performed using transpedicular screws or sublaminar fixation by means of hooks or bands. Spinal deformity is corrected by means of forces applied to the fixation points, which are then connected to longitudinal rods and locked in the corrected position. The facet joints are removed and the posterior vertebral elements are meticulously exposed and decorticated in order to assure good bone graft–recipient contact. Subperiosteal exposure is performed very cautiously using electrocautery in order to control bleeding and to avoid inadvertent penetration and violation of the spinal canal, especially if bone erosion is present and significant dural ectasia was seen in a preoperative MRI. This is followed by a generous bone graft application by abundant autologous iliac crest cancellous bone in order to achieve fusion.

Levels of posterior fusion extended from the cranial to the caudal end vertebra. Vertebra-based dual rod segmental instrumentation was used with transpedicular screws.

In the presence of bone erosion and pedicle dystrophy, hooks or sublaminar bands are used, and care was taken to prevent violation of the dura (Figure 7).

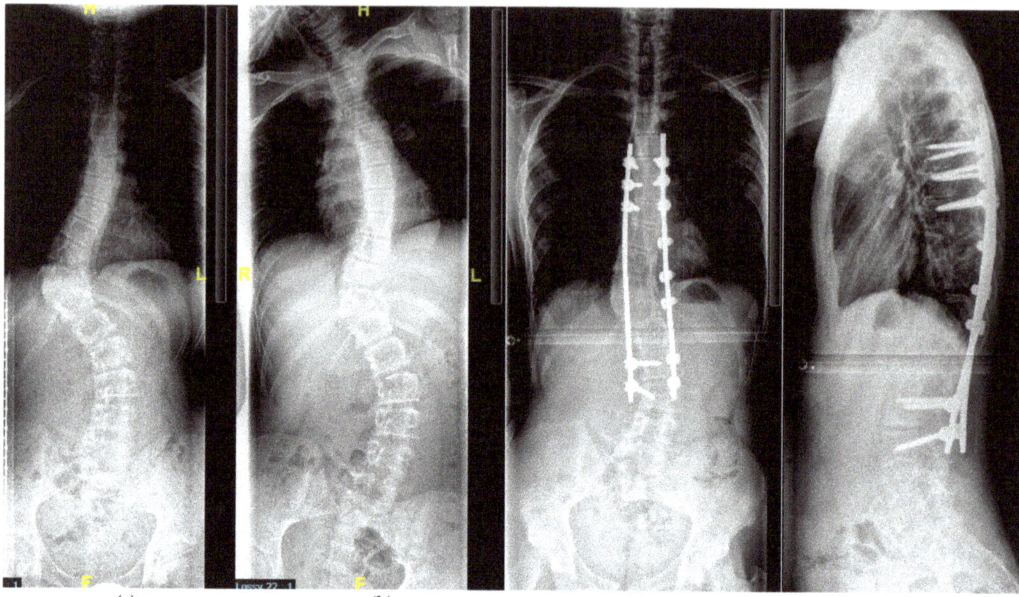

(a) (b) (c) (d)

Figure 7. Sixteen-year-old patient with severe scoliosis of 65° Cobb (**a**). Good curve flexibility on the lateral bending film (**b**). AP (**c**) and lateral (**d**) radiographs after posterior-only spinal fusion T7-L3. Fixation in the upper thoracic and the lumbar spine with transpedicular screws, fixation in the apical dystrophic area with sublaminar wires.

3.3.4. Combined Anterior and Posterior Spinal Fusion

This is a combination of anterior and posterior fusion techniques. If a combined anterior–posterior spinal fusion was indicated, critical assessment of the stability of the vertebral column was performed. If the spine was stable, an anterior approach was performed as an initial procedure in order to achieve better correction through removal of the disks. In the presence of a proven or questionable instability, a posterior approach was performed first in order to achieve stability and prevent neurological injury (Figure 8).

3.3.5. Halo-Gravity Traction

The method is used for temporary preoperative correction in severe, rigid, dystrophic curves independent of the age of the patient. The rationale of HGT is a slow deformity correction by means of continuous longitudinal distraction, allowing for adjustment of neurological structures and avoiding perfusion compromise of the spinal cord. Furthermore, a significant amount of the spinal deformity is reduced before surgery; in that way, no strong corrective forces need to be applied. At our institution, the patient is treated with a short general anesthesia and a Halo ring is applied to the head and fixed to the skull with 4–8 pins. Each pin penetrates just the outer skull lamina and is tightened with a torque of 3–8 Pound/Inch^2 depending on the age of the patient. The patient is admitted to the hospital and a continuous longitudinal traction (24/24 h) is applied, beginning with 10% of the body weight and increasing up to 60% of the body weight of the patient. The patient is provided with an individually fitted wheelchair and posterior walker; additionally, they are placed in bed traction for a duration of 4 weeks before spine surgery. Vital-sign monitoring and neurologic examination (cranial nerves included) are performed every 8 h. Oxygen saturation is continuously recorded during sleep. Curve correction is monitored clinically on a daily basis and by means of serial radiographs every 7 days during the traction period. (Figure 9).

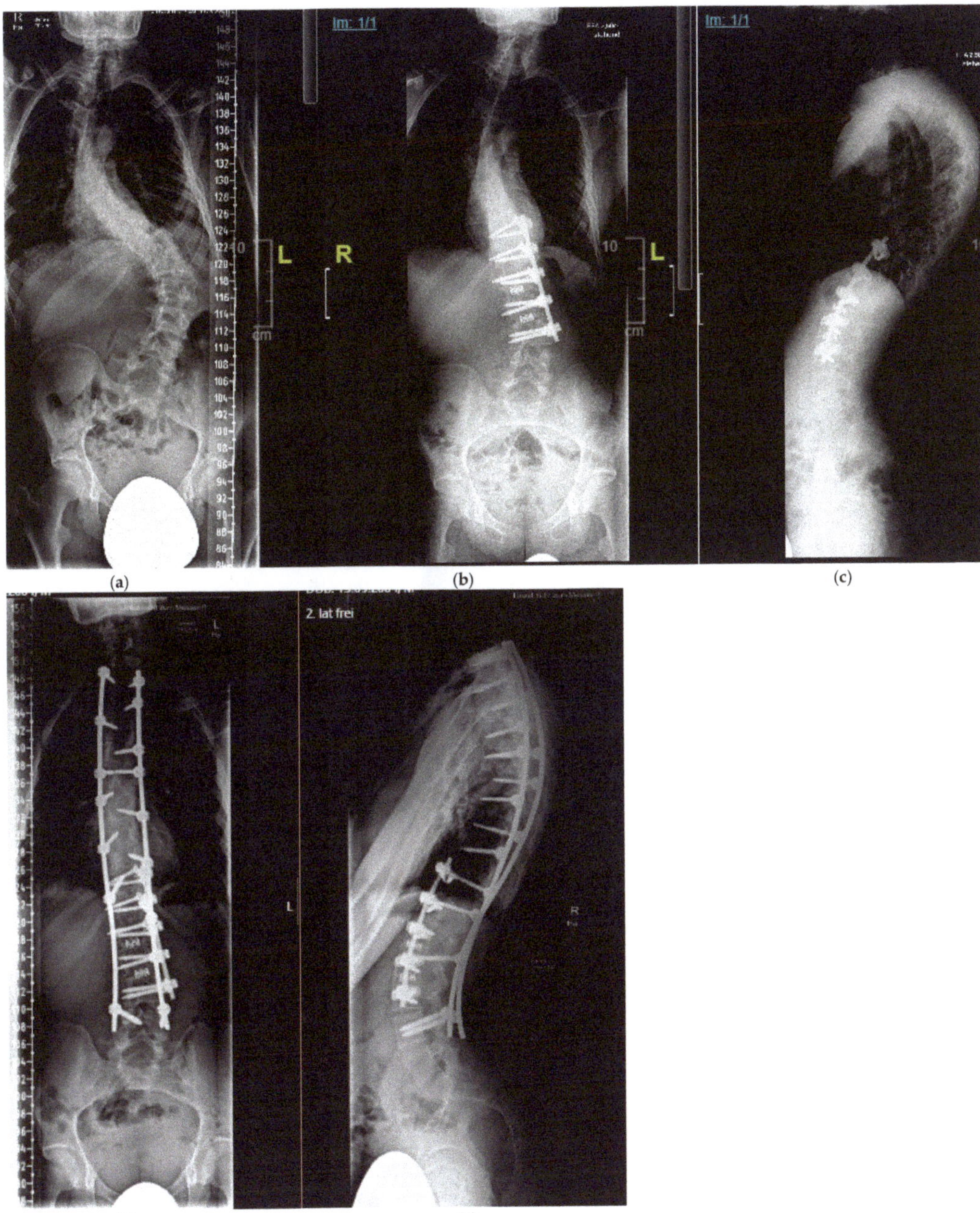

(a) (b) (c)

(d) (e)

Figure 8. Sixteen-year-old patient with severe, rigid dystrophic scoliosis (**a**). After anterior instrumented spinal fusion T11-L3 with intervertebral mesh cages for restoration of physiologic lumbar lordosis (**b**,**c**). After combined anterior and posterior Fusion T2-L4 (**d**,**e**).

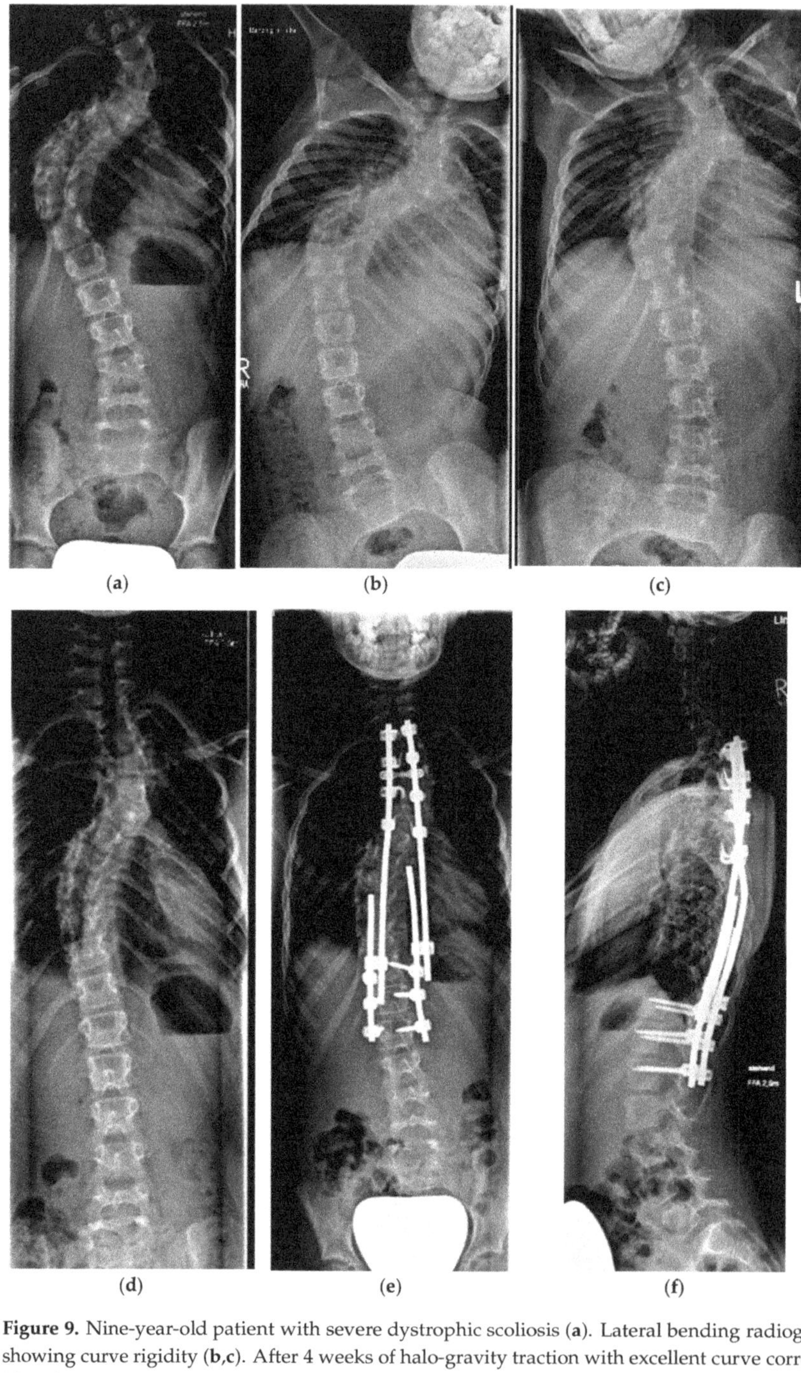

Figure 9. Nine-year-old patient with severe dystrophic scoliosis (a). Lateral bending radiographs showing curve rigidity (b,c). After 4 weeks of halo-gravity traction with excellent curve correction (d). After TGR application (e,f).

We set the following indications for preoperative HGT *:
Severe coronal curve (scoliosis) of >90 °Cobb angle

Rigid curve which does not improve <50° Cobb angle on bending film, especially in association with dystrophic osseous changes.
Severe kyphotic deformity (>45° Cobb in the cervical spine or >90° Cobb in the thoracic spine)
* Presence of at least one criterium.

3.3.6. Bone Grafting

At our institution, a combination of autologous bone graft obtained from the resected facet joints and cancellous bone obtained from the posterior iliac crest combined with heterologous stripes of beta tricalcium phosphate is routinely used for cases receiving posterior fusion.

A morselized autologous rib graft is used in instrumented anterior fusion and a rib strut graft is used in non instrumented cases, as previously described.

A human recombinant bone morphogenic protein (Rh-BMP-2) is used "off-label" in cases with severe osseous dystrophy with menacing vertebral column instability and risk of spinal cord compromise in order to achieve rapid fusion and stability. Critical assessment of local morphology is performed on MRI images before application in order to avoid proximity of application to areas affected by neurofibromatosis tumor tissue. Informed consent is obtained from the official patient guardian(s) before rh-BMP-2 application.

4. Results

Between 2006 and 2024, a total of 42 NF-1 pediatric and adolescent patients received surgical treatment for spinal deformities at our institution. The mean age at initial surgery for the complete cohort was 9.87 years (range 4.3–17.5) and the mean follow-up was 5.28 years (range 2 months–15.1 years). At index surgery, 17 patients (40%) had definitive fusion (mean age 13.4 years; mean follow-up 3.1 years) and 25 (60%) were treated with growth-preserving instrumentation. A total of 14 patients (33%) received preoperative halo-gravity traction (HGT) based on our indication criteria. Preoperative HGT allowed for achieving very good curve correction even in the presence of severe, rigid deformity, averaging at 61%, which was similar to the correction in the non-HGT group (59,6%). Recombinant human bone morphogenic protein type 2 (rhBMP-2) was used "off label" in seven patients (at the time of the index procedure n = 3 and at time of revision or last procedure n = 4). No adverse effects related to rhBMP-2 application were encountered during the observation period. Unplanned revision surgery was needed in 18 patients (42%); in six of these patients, more than one revision surgery was indicated. In all cases, the curve was corrected and progression of deformity could be stopped. Results according to type of initial surgery are summarized in Table 2. Data are reported as a mean and (±1 SD).

4.1. Cervical Spine

The cervical spine was affected in three patients (7%), all of them presented with severe dystrophic kyphosis and were treated with preoperative halo-gravity traction followed by combined anterior and posterior spinal fusion. Initial cervical kyphosis measured preoperatively 97° (range 70–125°) and was corrected to 25° (range 10–52°) at latest follow-up, corresponding to a mean correction of 77% (range 59–87%).

4.2. Thoracic and Lumbar Spine

The patients treated for deformity below the cervical spine were divided depending on the age at which the index surgery was performed.

4.2.1. "Early Onset Spinal Deformity"

Growth-preserving instrumentation was used in 25 cases representing 60% of the whole study group. The mean age at index surgery was 7.7 years (range 4.3–11.1), and the mean follow-up was 6.7 years (range 0.2–15.1). The initial growth-preserving surgical method was VEPTR in 10; MCGRs in 9 and TGRs in 6 patients. In a total of 10 cases from this group, growth-preserving instrumentation was combined with short apical anterior fusion. The Cobb angle of the major coronal curve (scoliosis) was measured immediately before surgery 77° (range 50–88°) and was corrected to 33.1° on latest follow-up, representing a 54.1% deformity correction. Immediate postoperative height of the thoracic spine (T1-12) averaged 19.6 cm (range 13.6–23.4 cm) and increased during the treatment period to 22.8 cm (range 16.8–28.1 cm) at latest follow-up, corresponding to a T1-12 growth rate of 0.73cm/year. Lengthening procedures were routinely performed at 6–9 month intervals, averaging 1.7 lengthening per patient and per year follow-up. A total of 25 unplanned revision surgeries were performed, averaging one revision surgery per patient. The most frequent reasons for revision surgery were anchor dislocation or implant failure (n = 16), as well as exhaustion of the lengthening reserve of the implant (n = 8). A deep late infection was encountered in one patient. Neurologic symptoms in association with spinal deformity in one patient who developed incomplete, flaccid lower paraparesis 10 years after index intervention for deformity correction. In this patient, kyphotic deformity worsened during the observation period due to progressive dystrophic osseous changes representing the characteristic NF-1-related "modulation process". The patient was treated by removal of the growth-preserving instrumentation and the intermittent application of HGT for slow correction of kyphosis over 4 weeks, followed by anterior and posterior spinal fusion and anterior strut grafting in the same surgical setting. Flaccid lower paraparesis improved partially during the 6 months following the revision surgery, and the patient was able to ambulate short distances with a posterior walker at the most recent follow-up 5 years after the revision procedure. During the observation period, seven of the patients from this group reached skeletal maturity and growth-preserving instrumentation was converted to definitive spinal fusion.

4.2.2. Adolescent Spinal Deformity

We performed definitive spinal fusion at index surgery in 17 patients. In nine of them, posterior fusion was performed as a "stand alone" procedure. Seven patients underwent combined anterior and posterior fusion either during the same anesthesia session or as staged procedures. The preoperative Cobb angle of the major coronal curve measured 66° and was corrected to 21° on latest follow-up, corresponding to a 66% average curve correction. No early neurologic or inflammatory complications were observed. Revision surgeries with simultaneous augmentation of fusion mass were necessary in three patients (loss of correction due to "modulation process"—1 patient; implant failure due to pseudarthrosis—2 patients).

5. Discussion

Involvement of the skeletal system has been reported in up to 60% of the patients with NF-1 [1,4], with the spine and the tibia being mostly involved. The management of the spinal deformities in those patients requires particular attention since most of the cases need surgical treatment, which is very challenging due to the severity of the curves, the presence of dystrophic changes and the high risk of complications, such as pseudarthrosis, bleeding and infection [12]. It is obvious that, due to the very heterogenic presentation of NF-1-associated spinal deformities, it is very difficult to create categorical divisions of the patients in clearly defined subgroups based on the morphological aspect of the deformity or on other criteria. We focused on the treatment approach depending on the skeletal maturity and the expected spinal growth of the patients studying the outcomes after growth-preserving surgery and definitive fusion methods. Since the treatment rationale of different "growth preserving" techniques is identical, our purpose was not to compare those techniques nor to compare the results in immature patients with older patients who received final fusion. Instead, we aimed at evaluation of the outcomes with our treatment protocol, focusing on spinal deformity correction, spinal growth preservation and complication rate. Since presentation and management of spinal deformities in NF-1 patients differ in relation to the affected segment of the spine, those entities will be discussed separately.

5.1. Cervical Spine

The cervical spine is affected in up to 30% of the NF-1 patients presenting with spinal deformities [39]. Characteristic diagnosis can easily be overlooked since patients are asymptomatic and more attention is paid to the more pronounced thoracic or lumbar deformities. The most common subjective complaint is usually neck pain. On clinical observation, a tumor mass or kyphosis may be present. The patient evaluation includes a questioning for neck symptoms and a thorough examination of the C-spine, including proof of range of motion and a complete neurologic exam. In the presence of clinical abnormalities, AP and lateral radiographs should be obtained, especially before endotracheal anesthesia or a halo-gravity traction in order to exclude instability. Evaluation of standard flexion/extension radiographs is difficult due to the complexity of the deformity, and the presence of dystrophic changes and advanced imaging MRIs or a thin-slice CT scan is recommended in most of the cases. C-spine deformities are mostly dystrophic and need surgical treatment since there is underlying or impending instability with a high risk of neurologic compromise due to spinal cord compression. The purpose of treatment is to correct deformity and to obtain solid fusion in order to preserve neurologic function. Anterior-only, posterior-only or combined fusion are discussed in the literature [40]. In our institution, a combined anterior and posterior fusion with instrumentation is the method of choice. All patients in our cohort presented with severe dystrophic kyphosis and were treated with preoperative halo-gravity traction followed by combined anterior and posterior fusion. A structural anterior support is necessary in order to restore the height of the anterior column in cases with significant dystrophic alterations of the vertebral bodies. We used a mesh titanium cage filled with autologous cancellous bone. In all our cases, a posterior fusion using autologous ilium bone graft with segmental fixation and double rod instrumentation was additionally performed. A halo vest was applied to protect instrumentation until solid union was confirmed by means of a CT scan performed 3 months after surgery. In two patients, solid fusion was achieved after the index procedure, and one of the patients showed delayed union and needed an augmentation procedure that included an autologous cancellous bone graft and "off-label" rhBMP-2 application.

5.2. Thoracic and Lumbar Spine

Deformities located in the thoracic and the lumbar spine are treated identically.

The natural history of spinal deformities in the presence of dystrophic osseous changes is unfavorable, with inevitable deterioration occurring in untreated cases [9,10]. Brace treatment has been shown to be ineffective in those patients, and surgical treatment is generally recommended in order to correct deformity and achieve a well-balanced, stable spine and preserve neurological function [6,41].

"Curve-specific" and "patient-specific" factors play an important role in decision-making and establishment in regard to surgical strategy.

The curve-specific factors include:

- Severity and rigidity of the deformity;
- Extent of dystrophic bone changes;
- Presence of paraspinal or intraspinal abnormalities (neurofibroma, dural ectasia, meningocele, etc.).

The patient-specific factors include:

- Expected residual growth of the spine (in particular the thoracic portion);
- Patient's general condition and nutritional status;
- Co-morbidities such as hypertension, pulmonary insufficiency etc.;
- Accompanying malignant transformation of neurofibromas.

5.2.1. Growth-Preserving Techniques

The historically well-established gold standard of treatment for dystrophic spinal deformities in NF-1 patients in order to achieve corrections and to stop deformity progression is instrumented spinal fusion. However, the negative effects of early spinal fusion in very immature patients in terms of producing growth inhibition of the thoracic spine, resulting in an iatrogenic extrinsic respiratory restrictive disease known as "thoracic insufficiency syndrome" (TIS), have been well recognized [42]. The severity of growth inhibition is directly related to the number of the fused thoracic spine segments [38]. Accordingly, as few segments as possible should be fused in an immature patient in order to preserve thoracic and lung growth. Despite this observation, consensus about the best type of procedure in early onset scoliosis NF-1 patients is still lacking. Tauchi et al. [43] reported their results after circumferential anterior and posterior spinal fusion in 11 immature patients with NF-1. Patient age at surgery averaged at 8.4 years and 67% initial correction was achieved and remained unchanged at the latest follow-up at 14 years. Solid fusion was documented in all cases. Despite observed acceptable values for lung function averaging 75.0% of the predicted amount, the observed spinal growth inhibition (T1-S1) in this study was significant and averaged only 0.39 cm/year, representing 32% of the expected amount.

Jain et al. recommended the traditional growing rods technique as a stand-alone method for the treatment of early onset spine deformity in NF-1 patients and reported an average curve correction of 51% of the initial curve [43]. In the same study, successful preservation of spinal growth (T1-S1) was observed and was measured at 1.12 cm/year. In our study, a 54.1% correction of the major curve was observed at an average follow-up of 6.7 years. We focused our evaluation on preservation of thoracic spine growth, since this is much more important for pulmonary function, and observed an average T1-12 growth of 0.73 cm/year, which does not significantly deviate from normal thoracic growth, which is reported as 0.84 cm/year (range 0.7–1.2 cm/year). Even in the patient cohort (10 out of 26 patients in our series) who received short anterior fusion in combination with growth-preserving posterior instrumentation, thoracic spinal growth was well preserved and was comparable with the subgroup without short apical fusion. Despite good deformity control, the literature-reported rate of implant-related complications with growth-preserving techniques remains very high at 57% [43]. The most common complication is proximal anchor failure, occurring in 35% of the cases [43]. Our observations are in accordance with previous reports. Of the 25 patients in our cohort treated with growth-preserving techniques, mechanical complications due to implant failure were observed in 16 patients, representing 64% of the cases. In eight patients, revision surgery was needed due to the exhausted lengthening possibility of the implant, which is an expected event and does not represent a complication in treatment. Only one patient in our series (4%) needed revision surgery due to deep infection.

It is evident that growth-preserving surgical techniques are associated with lower correction rates and higher incidence of implant-related complications for scoliosis associated with NF-1 patients as compared to definitive fusion [44]. However, thorax and lung growth preservation plays a key role in the treatment of early onset scoliosis.

Our favorite treatment approach to an immature NF-1 patient with a dystrophic curve is to perform a posterior growth-preserving instrumentation (preferably vertebra based traditional growing rods) extending from the upper to the lower end vertebrae of the major spinal curve combined with short anterior instrumented (preferred) or uninstrumented fusion extending only to the dystrophic segments. Due to the dystrophic osseous changes, a normal growth in the affected segments is not to be expected and a fusion of 3–5 levels would not lead to significant growth disturbances. Our results confirm the advantages of this approach, comprising growth preservation, achievement of stability in the dystrophic portion of the spine through solid fusion and restoration of spinal balance by straightening the spine with a concurrent restoration of thorax symmetry, which is important for the chest wall breathing excursions.

5.2.2. Definitive Spinal Fusion

The treatment strategy in NF-1-associated spinal deformity after skeletal maturity aims at deformity correction and the achievement of solid spinal fusion through anterior, posterior or combined approaches.

Moderate curves (45–60° Cobb) or severe curves (>60°) can be treated by a single posterior fusion provided that the deformity is flexible and straightens to <25° upon side bending.

Severe, rigid, dystrophic curves (>60° Cobb) are best treated by a combined anterior and posterior fusion [8,12,45–48] which can be performed in the same or in two separate surgical settings. Due to the poor bone quality, the dystrophic osseous changes and the severity of the deformity, surgery is very challenging and meticulous preoperative evaluation of the osseous vertebral morphology, the paravertebral structures as well as the spinal canal are mandatory and of utmost importance. Besides upright native whole-spine radiographs and bending films, a whole-spine MRI should be performed in order to define critical space-occupying lesions, spinal cord compression, dural ectasia or vertebral erosion. Additionally, a thin-slice CT scan with sagittal, coronal and 3-D reconstructions is needed in order to assess the vertebral morphology and rotational deformity, as well as for the choice of instrumentation (transpedicular screws vs. sublaminar fixation). Particular attention is paid to the dystrophic apical region where osseous changes are the most pronounced. Meticulous analysis of the morphology, especially in severe cases, is mandatory. The presence of rib-head protrusion into the spinal canal through a neuroforamen, which is a typical finding on the convex side of the apical vertebra, should be ruled out since it may migrate more medially into the spinal canal during curve correction and exposes the spinal cord to high risk of compression and neurological damage (Figure 10).

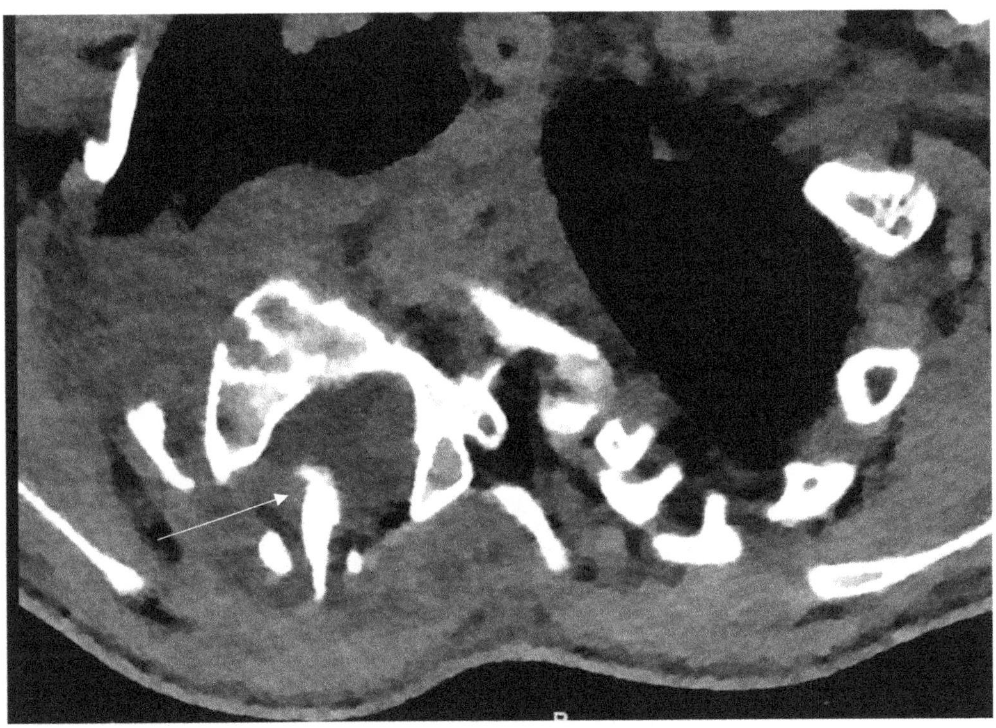

Figure 10. Concave rib-head protrusion into the spinal canal (arrow).

Koptan et al. [12] reported on their experience with spinal fusion and dystrophic NF-1-associated spinal deformities. The authors achieved 61% deformity correction with two-staged anterior and posterior fusion using a segmental spinal instrumentation augmented with sublaminar wires. Our approach comprised a preoperative evaluation of curve characteristics in order to define the needs of the combined anterior and posterior approach. Moderate (45–60° Cobb angle) and severe (>60° Cobb angle) curves which were flexible in preoperative bending films were treated by posterior-only fusion. In contrast to this, patients with severe, rigid (unflexible) dystrophic curves received anterior and posterior fusion. In our series, definitive fusion was performed as the initial surgery in 17 patients. In nine of them, a posterior-only fusion was performed as a "stand alone" procedure. Achieved correction averaged a 66° Cobb angle, corresponding to a 66% deformity correction upon follow-up at 3.4 years. A pseudarthrosis rate after an attempted spinal fusion of up to 31% has been reported in NF-1 patients [5]. We did not observe pseudarthrosis development in our series; however, deformity progression after performed fusion associated with osseous modulation changes occurred in three cases (17%). These cases needed revision surgery for augmentation of the fusion mass.

Based on observations of delayed bone healing and pseudarthrosis after attempted fusion procedures in NF-1 patients, some authors suggested the use of biologic osteoinductive substances such as rhBMP-2 in order to promote bone union [49]. However, rhBMP-2 application is controversially discussed, and its routine use, especially in immature patients, is not recommended due to the unknown systemic effects in pediatric patients and the hypothetic risk of malignant transformation. In our series, rhBMP-2 was used on an "off-label" basis during the index procedure in the presence of severe dystrophic osseous changes and bone erosions with an insufficient contact bone surface and anticipated delayed bone union 6 months after surgery. We empirically defined "bone contact surface insufficiency" as anterior intervertebral contact of less than 1 cm^2 and/or a bone gap between the posterior elements of more than one segment.

In the presence of severe, rigid spinal deformity, a preoperative halo-gravity traction should be considered in order to achieve sufficient correction. Our observations showed that a similar deformity correction can be achieved by means of preoperative HGT even in the presence of a severe, rigid deformity. Curve correction in the HGT group averaged 61% and was comparable to the non-HGT group (59.6%). We used rhBMP-2 in eight patients. Complications related to BMP application were not encountered in any of the patients. Despite solid fusion, which was observed in all these cases, no representative statistical data in support of the rhBMP-2 effect in promoting bone union can be presented due to the small number of patients. It should be emphasized that BMP application in the pediatric population is "off-label". Its use should be discussed individually and the decision remains at the discretion of the surgeon. BMP application should be avoided in the proximity of existing tumor masses due to the potential risk of malignant transformation.

Since NF-1 patients present with many comorbidities, such as hypertension, intraabdominal and intrathoracic tumors, optic glioma, nutritional issues, Vitamin D deficiency [50], cognitive disabilities, etc., a multidisciplinary approach was recommended [51]. We can strongly support this recommendation and perform a preoperative multisystemic interdisciplinary evaluation of all NF-1 patients on a routine basis, which, besides orthopedic surgical assessment, also includes cardio-pulmonary, anesthesiologic, neurologic and psychological assessments in order to minimize peri- and postoperative complication risks.

The study has several limitations. Data collection was prospective, but this was not a randomized controlled study. Not all of the patients reached skeletal maturity at the latest follow-up, and some of the patients with growth-preserving instrumentation are still under treatment. However, heterogeneity of presentation and variability of surgical approaches make the feasibility of a randomized controlled study (with a random selection of either treatment or simple observation or comparison of different surgical approaches) not feasible in the current state since such a study design would face severe ethical issues, making randomization impossible. Collection of observational data on rare conditions is first needed. A strong side of the study is the uniform treatment protocol and the single-center study design.

6. Conclusions

Surgical correction is the mainstay of treatment for dystrophic NF-1-associated spinal deformities. This differs significantly from idiopathic scoliosis, where less than 10% of the patients need surgery.

The treatment of choice for immature patients is posterior growth-preserving spinal instrumentation from the upper to the lower end vertebra combined with short apical fusion of the dystrophic segments.

In immature NF-1 patients, spinal growth can be preserved by means of "growth preserving surgical methods" at a near physiological rate; however, the rate of revision surgery due to mechanical complications is high, with 64% of the patients needing unplanned surgery when treated with the "growth preserving" technique.

Preoperative halo-gravity traction should be considered in cases of severe rigid NF-1-associated spinal deformity. A satisfactory curve correction averaging 60% of the initial curve can be achieved, which is comparable to patients with milder and flexible deformities.

Definitive spinal fusion is recommended for patients older than 10 years. In the presence of dystrophic bone changes, the method of choice is combined anterior and posterior spinal fusion with segmental instrumentation.

As opposed to idiopathic spinal deformity, which is usually treated by instrumented posterior-only fusion, more than 50% of the patients with NF-1-associated spinal deformities need combined anterior and posterior spinal surgery in order to achieve solid fusion and avoid pseudarthrosis.

Treatment of NF-1-associated spinal deformities is very complex and challenging due to bone dystrophic changes and poor bone stock, making instrumentation very difficult. A meticulous preoperative evaluation and perioperative interdisciplinary approach is mandatory since co-morbidities are very frequent.

Author Contributions: Conceptualization, K.V.M. and R.S.; methodology, K.V.M. and R.S.; formal statistical analysis, K.V.M.; data curation, K.V.M.; writing—original draft preparation, K.V.M.; writing—review and editing, R.S. All authors have read and agreed to the published version of the manuscript.

Funding: The patient cohort treated with growth preserving instrumentation is part of the "Early onset scoliosis" Registry funded by the "Vereinigung für Kinderorthopädie–Nuvasive Grant ID 459".

Institutional Review Board Statement: The study was conducted in accordance with the Declaration of Helsinki. Approval by the Ethics Committee of Medical Board Hamburg, Germany: PV5886 from 8 October 2018 was granted for the patient cohort with growth-preserving instrumentation, and patient observation is ongoing prospectively.

Informed Consent Statement: Patient consent was waived due to the retrospective nature of this study.

Data Availability Statement: All medical data are available on request and will be provided if needed by the corresponding author.

Conflicts of Interest: The authors declare no conflicts of interest.

References

1. Akbarnia, B.A.; Gabriel, K.R.; Beckman, E.; Chalk, D. Prevalence of scoliosis in neurofibromatosis. *Spine* **1992**, *17*, S244–S248. [CrossRef]
2. Cnossen, M.H.; de Goede-Bolder, A.; van den Broek, K.M.; Waasdorp, C.M.; Oranje, A.P.; Stroink, H.; Simonsz, H.J.; van den Ouweland, A.M.; Halley, D.J.; Niermeijer, M.F. A prospec tive 10 year follow up study of patients with neurofibromatosis type 1. *Arch. Dis. Child.* **1998**, *78*, 408–412. [CrossRef]
3. Huson, S.M.; Harper, P.S.; Compston, D.A. Von Recklinghausen neurofi bromatosis: A clinical and population study in south-east Wales. *Brain* **1988**, *111*, 1355–1381. [CrossRef] [PubMed]
4. Funasaki, H.; Winter, R.B.; Lonstein, J.B.; Denis, F. Pathophysiology of spinal deformities in neurofibromatosis. *J. Bone Jt. Surg.* **1994**, *76*, 692–700. [CrossRef] [PubMed]
5. Sirois, J.L.; Drennan, J.C. Dystrophic spinal deformity in neurofibromatosis. *J. Pediatr. Orthop.* **1990**, *10*, 522–526. [CrossRef] [PubMed]

6. Winter, R.B.; Moe, J.H.; Bradford, D.S.; Lonstein, J.E.; Pedras, C.V.; Weber, A.H. Spine deformity in neurofibromatosis. A review of one hundred and two patients. *J. Bone Jt. Surg.* **1979**, *61*, 677–694. [CrossRef]
7. Vitale, M.G.; Guha, A.; Skaggs, D.L. Orthopaedic manifestations of neurofibromatosis in children: An update. *Clin. Orthop.* **2002**, *401*, 107–118. [CrossRef]
8. Betz, R.R.; Iorio, R.; Lombardi, A.V.; Clancy, M.; Steel, H.H. Scoliosis surgery in neurofibromatosis. *Clin. Orthop. Relat. Res.* **1989**, *245*, 53–56. [CrossRef]
9. Calvert, P.T.; Edgar, M.A.; Webb, P.J. Scoliosis in neurofibromatosis. Natural history without operation. *J. Bone Jt. Surg.* **1989**, *71*, 246–251. [CrossRef]
10. Winter, R.B.; Lonstein, J.E.; Anderson, M. Neurofibromatosis hyperkyphosis: A review of 33 patients with kyphosis of 80 degrees or greater. *J. Spinal Disord.* **1988**, *1*, 39–49. [CrossRef]
11. Li, M.; Fang, X.; Li, Y.; Ni, J.; Gu, S.; Zhu, X. Successful use of posterior instrumented spinal fusion alone for scoliosis in 19 patients with NF-1 followed up for at least 25 months. *Arch. Orthop. Trauma. Surg.* **2009**, *129*, 915–921. [CrossRef] [PubMed]
12. Koptan, W.; ElMiligui, Y. Surgical correction of severe dystrophic neurofibromatosis scoliosis: An experience of 32 cases. *Eur. Spine J.* **2010**, *19*, 1569–1575. [CrossRef]
13. Tsirikos, A.I.; Saifuddin, A.; Noordeen, M.H. Spinal deformity in neurofibromatosis type-1: Diagnosis and treatment. *Eur. Spine J.* **2005**, *14*, 427–439. [CrossRef] [PubMed]
14. Guha, A.; Lau, N.; Huvar, I.; Gutmann, P.; Provias, J.; Pawson, T.; Boss, G. Ras GTP levels are elevated in human NF1 peripheral nerve tumors. *Oncogene* **1996**, *12*, 507–513. [CrossRef]
15. Gutmann, D.H.; Wood, D.L.; Collins, F.S. Identification of the neurofibromatosis type 1 gene product. *Proc. Natl. Acad. Sci. USA* **1991**, *88*, 9658–9662. [CrossRef]
16. Gutmann, D.H.; Geist, R.T.; Wright, D.E.; Snider, W.D. Expression of the neurofibromatosis 1 (NF1) isoforms in developing and adult rat tissues. *Cell Growth Differ.* **1995**, *6*, 315–323. [PubMed]
17. Legius, E.; Marchuk, D.A.; Collins, F.S.; Glover, T.W. Somatic deletion of the neurofibromatosis type 1 gene in a neurofibrosarcoma supports a tumour suppressor gene hypothesis. *Nat. Genet.* **1993**, *3*, 122–126. [CrossRef]
18. Walker, J.A.; Upadhyaya, M. Emerging therapeutic targets for neurofibromatosis type 1. *Expert. Opin. Ther. Targets* **2018**, *22*, 419–437. [CrossRef] [PubMed] [PubMed Central]
19. Armstrong, A.E.; Belzberg, A.J.; Crawford, J.R.; Hirbe, A.C.; Wang, Z.J. Treatment decisions and the use of MEK inhibitors for children with neurofibromatosis type 1-related plexiform neurofibromas. *BMC Cancer* **2023**, *23*, 553. [CrossRef]
20. Ronsley, R.; Hounjet, C.D.; Cheng, S.; Rassekh, S.R.; Duncan, W.J.; Dunham, C.; Gardiner, J.; Ghag, A.; Ludemann, J.P.; Wensley, D.; et al. Trametinib therapy for children with neurofibromatosis type 1 and life-threatening plexiform neurofibroma or treatment-refractory low-grade glioma. *Cancer Med.* **2021**, *10*, 3556–3564. [CrossRef]
21. Gross, A.M.; Wolters, P.L.; Dombi, E.; Baldwin, A.; Whitcomb, P.; Fisher, M.J.; Weiss, B.; Kim, A.; Bornhorst, M.; Shah, A.C.; et al. Selumetinib in Children with Inoperable Plexiform Neurofibromas. *N. Engl. J. Med.* **2020**, *382*, 1430–1442. [CrossRef] [PubMed]
22. Messiaen, L.M.; Callens, T.; Mortier, G.; Beysen, D.; Vandenbroucke, I.; Van Roy, N.; Speleman, F.; Paepe, A.D. Exhaustive mutation analysis of the NF1 gene allows identification of 95% of mutations and reveals a high frequency of unusual splicing defects. *Hum. Mutat.* **2000**, *15*, 541–555. [CrossRef] [PubMed]
23. Acosta, M.T.; Gioia, G.A.; Silva, A.J. Neurofibromatosis type 1: New insights into neurocognitive issues. *Curr. Neurol. Neurosci. Rep.* **2006**, *6*, 136–143. [CrossRef] [PubMed]
24. Evans, D.G.R.; E Baser, M.; McGaughran, J.; Sharif, S.; Howard, E.; Moran, A. Malignant peripheral nerve sheath tumours in neurofibromatosis 1. *J. Med. Genet.* **2002**, *39*, 311–314. [CrossRef]
25. Farid, M.; Demicco, E.G.; Garcia, R.; Ahn, L.; Merola, P.R.; Cioffi, A.; Maki, R.G. Malignant peripheral nerve sheath tumors. *Oncologist* **2014**, *19*, 193–201. [CrossRef]
26. Listernick, R.; Darling, C.; Greenwald, M.; Strauss, L.; Charrow, J. Optic pathway tumors in children: The effect of neurofibromatosis type 1 on clinical manifestations and natural history. *J. Pediatr.* **1995**, *127*, 718–722. [CrossRef]
27. Guillamo, J.; Créange, A.; Kalifa, C.; Grill, J.; Rodriguez, D.; Doz, F.; Barbarot, S.; Zerah, M.; Sanson, M.; Bastuji-Garin, S.; et al. Prognostic factors of CNS tumours in Neurofibromatosis 1 (NF1): A retrospective study of 104 patients. *Brain* **2003**, *126*, 152–160. [CrossRef]
28. Balcer, L.J.; Liu, G.T.; Heller, G.; Bilaniuk, L.; Volpe, N.J.; Galetta, S.L.; Molloy, P.T.; Phillips, P.C.; Janss, A.J.; Vaughn, S.; et al. Visual loss in children with neurofibromatosis type 1 and optic pathway gliomas: Relation to tumor location by magnetic resonance imaging. *Am. J. Ophthalmol.* **2001**, *131*, 442–445. [CrossRef]
29. Neurofibromatosis. Conference statement. National Institute of Health Consensus Develpment Conference. *Arch. Neurol.* **1987**, *45*, 575–578.
30. Legius, E.; Messiaen, L.; Wolkenstein, P.; Pancza, P.; Avery, R.A.; Berman, Y.; Blakeley, J.; Babovic-Vuksanovic, D.; Cunha, K.S.; Ferner, R.; et al. Revised diagnostic criteria for neurofibromatosis type 1 and Legius syndrome: An international consensus recommendation. *Genet. Med.* **2021**, *23*, 1506–1513. [CrossRef]
31. Gould, E.P. The bone changes occurring in Von Recklinghausen's disease. *Q. J. Med.* **1918**, *11*, 221–228. [CrossRef]
32. Crawford, A.H. Neurofi bromatosis. In *The Pediatric Spine: Principles and Practice*, 2nd ed.; Weinstein, S.L., Ed.; Lippincott Williams & Wilkins: Philadelphia, PA, USA, 2001; pp. 471–490.
33. Rezaian, S.M. The incidence of scoliosis due to neurofibromatosis. *Acta Orthop. Scand.* **1976**, *147*, 534–539. [CrossRef] [PubMed]

34. Durrani, A.; Crawford, A.H.; Choudhry, S.N.; Saifuddin, A.; Morley, T.R. Modulation of spinal deformities in patients with neurofibromatosis type 1. *Spine* **2000**, *25*, 69–75. [CrossRef] [PubMed]
35. Kim, H.W.; Weinstein, S.L. Spine update: The management of scoliosis in neurofibromatosis. *Spine* **1997**, *22*, 2770–2776. [CrossRef] [PubMed]
36. El-Hawary, R.; Akbarnia, B.A. Letter to the editor, early onset scoliosis: Time for consensus. *Spine Deform.* **2015**, *3*, 105–106. [CrossRef]
37. Sanders, J.O.; Khoury, J.G.; Kishan, S.; Browne, R.H.; Mooney, J.F., 3rd; Arnold, K.D.; McConnell, S.J.; Bauman, J.A.; Finegold, D.N. Predicting scoliosis progression from skeletal maturity: A simplified classification during adolescence. *J. Bone Jt. Surg. Am.* **2008**, *90*, 540–553. [CrossRef]
38. Karol, L.A.; Johnston, C.; Mladenov, K.; Schochet, P.; Walters, P.; Browne, R.H. Pulmonary function following early thoracic fusion in non-neuromuscular scoliosis. *J. Bone Jt. Surg. Am.* **2008**, *90*, 1272–1281. [CrossRef]
39. Young-Hing, K.; Kalamchi, A.; MacEwen, G.D. Cervical spine abnormalities in neurofibromatosis. *J. Bone Jt. Surg. Am.* **1979**, *61*, 695–699. [CrossRef]
40. Gu, Y.; Shen, X.; Liu, Y.; Cao, P.; Yuan, W. Clinical outcomes of anterior correction and reconstruction for neurofibromatosis-associated severe cervical kyphotic deformity. *Int. Orthop.* **2019**, *43*, 639–646. [CrossRef]
41. Crawford, A.H.; Parikh, S.; Schorry, E.; von Stein, D. The immature spine in Type-1 neurofibromatosis. *J. Bone Jt. Surg.* **2007**, *89* (Suppl. S1), 123–142.
42. Campbell, R.M., Jr.; Smith, M.D.; Mayes, T.C.; Mangos, J.A.; Willey-Courand, D.B.; Kose, N.; Pinero, R.F.; Alder, M.E.; Duong, H.L.; Surber, J.L. The characteristics of thoracic insufficiency syndrome associated with fused ribs and congenital scoliosis. *J. Bone Jt. Surg. Am.* **2003**, *85*, 399–408. [PubMed]
43. Tauchi, R.; Kawakami, N.; Castro, M.A.; Ohara, T.; Saito, T.; Morishita, K.; Yamauchi, I. Long term surgical outcomes after early definitive spinal fusion for early onset scoliosis with NF Type-1 at mean follow-up of 14 years. *J. Pediatr. Orthop.* **2020**, *40*, 42–47. [CrossRef]
44. Jain, V.V.; Berry, C.A.; Crawford, A.H.; Emans, J.B.; Sponseller, P.D.; Growing Spine Study Group. Growing Rods Are an Effective Fusionless Method of Controlling Early-Onset Scoliosis Associated With Neurofibromatosis Type 1 (NF1): A Multicenter Retrospective Case Series. *J. Pediatr. Orthop.* **2017**, *37*, e612–e618. [PubMed]
45. Crawford, A.H. Pitfalls of spinal deformities associated with neurofibromatosis in children. *Clin. Orthop. Relat. Res.* **1989**, *245*, 29–42. [CrossRef]
46. Iwai, C.; Taneichi, H.; Inami, S.; Namikawa, T.; Takeuchi, D.; Kato, N.; Iida, T.; Shimizu, K.; Nohara, Y. Clinical outcomes of combined anterior and posterior spinal fusion for dystrophic thoracolumbar spinal deformities of neurofibromatosis-1: Fate of nonvascularized anterior fibular strut grafts. *Spine* **2013**, *38*, 44–50. [CrossRef] [PubMed]
47. Crawford, A.H.; Schorry, E.K. Neurofibromatosis update. *J. Pediatr. Orthop.* **2006**, *26*, 413–423.
48. Feldman, D.S.; Jordan, C.; Fonseca, L. Orthopaedic manifestations of neurofibromatosis type 1. *J. Am. Acad. Orthop. Surg.* **2010**, *18*, 346–357. [CrossRef] [PubMed]
49. Mladenov, K.V.; Spiro, A.S.; Krajewski, K.L.; Stücker, R.; Kunkel, P. Management of spinal deformities and tibial pseudarthrosis in children with neurofibromatosis type 1 (NF-1). *Childs Nerv. Syst.* **2020**, *36*, 2409–2425. [CrossRef]
50. Riccardi, C.; Perrone, L.; Napolitano, F.; Sampaolo, S. Understanding the Biological Activities of Vitamin D in Type 1 Neurofibromatosis: New Insights into Disease Pathogenesis and Therapeutic Design. *Cancers* **2020**, *12*, 2965. [CrossRef]
51. Gutmann, D.H.; Aylsworth, A.; Carey, J.C.; Korf, B.; Marks, J.; Pyeritz, R.E.; Rubenstein, A.; Viskochil, D. The diagnostic evaluation and multi disciplinary management of neurofibromatosis 1 and neurofibromatosis 2. *JAMA* **1997**, *278*, 51–57. [CrossRef]

cancers

MDPI

Article

A Mixed Methods Study of Medication Adherence in Adults with Neurofibromatosis Type 1 (NF1) on a Clinical Trial of Selumetinib

Millicent S. Curlee [1], Mary Anne Toledo-Tamula [1], Melissa Baker [1,†], Daniel Wikstrom [1], Cynthia Harrison [1,‡], Amanda Rhodes [1,§], Margaret Fagan [1], Cecilia Tibery [2], Pamela L. Wolters [1], Brigitte C. Widemann [1], Andrea M. Gross [1] and Staci Martin [1,*]

[1] Pediatric Oncology Branch, Center for Cancer Research, National Cancer Institute, 9030 Old Georgetown Road, Bethesda, MD 20892-8200, USA; milly.curlee@nih.gov (M.S.C.); maryanne.tamula@nih.gov (M.A.T.-T.); mb4341@mynsu.nova.edu (M.B.); dan.wikstrom@nih.gov (D.W.); cynthia.harrison@nyulangone.org (C.H.); margaret.fagan@nih.gov (M.F.); woltersp@mail.nih.gov (P.L.W.); widemanb@mail.nih.gov (B.C.W.); andrea.gross@nih.gov (A.M.G.)

[2] Clinical Research Directorate, Frederick National Laboratory for Cancer Research, Leidos Biomedical Research, Inc., Frederick, MD 21702, USA; cecilia.tibery@nih.gov

* Correspondence: martins@mail.nih.gov; Tel.: +1-240-760-6025

† Current address: College of Psychology, Nova Southeastern University, Fort Lauderdale, FL 33328, USA.

‡ Current address: New York University Grossman School of Medicine, New York University Langone Health, New York, NY 10016, USA.

§ Current address: Private Practice, Chevy Chase, MD 20815, USA.

Simple Summary: People with neurofibromatosis type 1 (NF1) may develop tumors called plexiform neurofibromas (PNs). Selumetinib was the first oral medication to gain FDA approval to treat PNs in children, and the drug also has activity in adults. Clinical observations suggest that people must continue taking selumetinib to maintain its effects. Therefore, it is important to research how well people take selumetinib as prescribed over a long period of time. We used electronic pill caps that record when the bottle is opened, pill counts, and self-report diaries to measure adherence over eighteen 28-day treatment cycles. We found that using the caps is feasible but presents some challenges. We also found evidence that depression and stress were related to lower adherence in our small sample. We also interviewed patients, who talked about things that make adherence easier (consistency, reminders, and social support) and more difficult (forgetting and dose timing).

Abstract: Background: Oral therapeutic options for plexiform neurofibromas (PNs) in individuals with neurofibromatosis type 1 (NF1) are receiving attention in clinical research. The MEK inhibitor (MEKi) Selumetinib is FDA-approved in children ages 2+ years with inoperable PNs, and shows activity in adults. Prolonged therapy with selumetinib is necessary to maintain tumor reduction. Therefore, investigating long-term adherence is vital to understand patterns of adherence over time and its impact on clinical outcomes. Mixed methods research offers rich information about adherence that can inform future intervention trials, and can assist practitioners in addressing medication adherence concerns. Methods: This mixed-method pilot study is the first examination of the feasibility of a technology-based adherence assessment method, the medication events monitoring system (MEMS^{TM}), among individuals with NF1-PN. Adherence was monitored in a small sample of patients (N = 12; mean age = 34.36 years; 58% male) with NF1 and PN across eighteen 28-day treatment cycles. Qualitative data were obtained from individual interviews using inductive and deductive techniques for thematic analysis. Results: The predetermined criterion was met, suggesting that using MEMS^{TM} is feasible despite some challenges with the caps. Depression and overall stress were significantly related to reduced adherence,

https://doi.org/10.3390/cancers17020295

although these results should be considered hypothesis-generating. Barriers to medication adherence included forgetting and the timing of doses related to eating. Facilitators included consistency, reminders, and social support. Conclusions: This study highlights patient characteristics that may be related to increased risk for nonadherence, as well as challenges with electronic pill caps that should be considered in future clinical trials for NF1-related PN. Results can inform future adherence interventions for adults with NF1 and PNs. Future research with larger samples is needed to fully explore factors related to long-term medication adherence among individuals with NF1.

Keywords: neurofibromatosis; plexiform neurofibroma; selumetinib; medication adherence; qualitative interview; medication event monitoring system; pill count; medication diary; clinical trial

1. Introduction

Neurofibromatosis Type 1 (NF1) is an autosomal dominant disorder that affects approximately 1 in 2132–4712 people [1] and can lead to the development of histologically benign peripheral nerve sheath tumors, known as plexiform neurofibromas (PNs). PNs occur in around 25–60% of people with NF1 (NF1-PN) and are most likely congenital [2]. Internal PNs often are not diagnosed until they are large and cause clinically relevant symptoms [3]. PNs are related to both morbidity and mortality in patients with NF1, as they can cause a wide variety of symptoms depending on the size and location of the tumor [4]. Other PN complications include airway obstruction, visual deficits, pain, and nerve function impairment [5–8]. Natural history studies show that the presence of PNs may impact psychosocial functioning and quality of life [9,10].

Until recently, the most common method for addressing PNs was resection; however, surgery is often contraindicated because tumors can extend into vital tissues [2,11] and can re-grow following partial resection [5,6,12]. To address this issue, clinical trials have focused increasingly on oral therapeutic options [13]. The first pediatric trial of the oral MEK 1/2 inhibitor selumetinib (the SPRINT trial; AZD6244) found that selumetinib resulted in PN reduction and clinical benefits in children [12], leading to the only FDA drug approval for children 2+ years with inoperable tumors [5,6,12]. An adult selumetinib trial also documented reduced tumor size and decreased tumor pain intensity and pain interference [14]. Medication adherence is crucial in clinical trials, where nonadherence can interfere with efficacy.

Although clinical trial participants tend to have greater medication adherence than the general population [15], poor adherence may under-power analyses and lead to incorrect conclusions [16,17]. In the SPRINT trial, adherence during the first three 28-day cycles was excellent per caregiver-completed diaries (99%) and staff-completed pill counts (98%) [13]. However, it has yet to be determined whether the dosing schedule or possible side effects (e.g., nausea, acneiform rash) may inhibit consistent medication-taking. In the phase 2 trial investigating selumetinib in adults, participants were initially prescribed 75 mg of selumetinib twice a day, approximately 12 h apart, for a 28-day cycle [14]. However, the study was amended following the first two participants' experience of dose-limiting skin toxicity. All other participants received a starting dose of 50 mg twice a day [14]. The medication was available in 10 mg or 25 mg capsules, so participants had to take several capsules for each dose. As complicated treatment regimens have been associated with worse adherence in other populations [18], it is necessary to investigate patients' adherence in a trial that requires both the specific timing of doses and food restriction. During the clinical trial, abstinence from eating two hours before and one hour after dosing was required, which may pose adherence challenges. Following the completion of this study, recent research led to changes in the FDA label [19]; selumetinib can now be taken with or without food [20].

Additionally, early clinical data suggested that prolonged treatment may be necessary to maintain efficacy [13]; therefore, research on long-term medication adherence is vital for assessing the impact on medical outcomes and implementing behavioral interventions targeting factors that put patients at risk for non-adherence. Studies examining other populations have found decreased medication adherence over time [21–24], suggesting the need to examine longitudinal adherence patterns in individuals with NF1-PN.

Compared to self-report and pill counts, a technology-based adherence assessment method is the medication events monitoring system (MEMS^{TM}), in which pill caps record dates and times of bottle openings [25]. MEMS^{TM} caps are useful for assessing adherence to medications with specific timing requirements (e.g., selumetinib). Some past research has shown electronic caps to be more reliable compared to self-report diaries [26,27], and have even been used to identify over-adherence (e.g., people who take more pills than prescribed) [28]. Further, the caps may be particularly suited to clinical trials, where reliable adherence data can help investigators have confidence in their findings related to efficacy. Thus, they may offer advantages over more traditional methods of adherence measurement. Challenges include changing medication-taking routines, transferring medication to the bottle fitted for the cap [29], and cap malfunctioning [26]. To date, no studies have assessed the feasibility of MEMS^{TM} caps for the NF1-PN population.

Study Rationale and Aims

The primary objective of this mixed method pilot study was to assess the feasibility of using MEMS^{TM} caps to monitor medication adherence in adults with NF1-PN on a clinical trial. Given the small sample size, all other objectives were considered exploratory. These include: (1) to document longitudinal patterns of adherence; (2) to identify patient characteristics and/or time periods during treatment that are related to poor adherence; (3) to compare adherence between MEMS^{TM} caps, pill counts, and diaries. The exploratory objective of the qualitative methods was to explore barriers and facilitators to adherence through semi-structured interviews with adults with NF1 on a clinical trial of selumetinib. Even with small sample sizes, qualitative data are vitally important to identify barriers and facilitators for adherence and can help inform adherence-promoting interventions for individuals enrolled in clinical trials.

2. Methods

2.1. Eligibility

Eligibility criteria included a confirmed diagnosis of NF1, aged 3–59 years, ability to understand and sign a written informed consent, ability to read and comprehend English, regular access to an electronic device with internet access, and enrollment on a clinical trial for selumetinib (manufactured by AstraZeneca/Alexion, Cambridge, UK) concomitantly with their participation in this adherence study. The clinical trial required participants to take selumetinib twice a day, twelve hours apart, and to abstain from eating for two hours before and one hour after the dose.

2.2. Measures

Baseline

Background Information. Participants provided information about demographic characteristics and medical status, and characterized their NF symptoms and their pain (separately) as mild, moderate, or severe.

Life Events Checklist (LEC). Participants completed the Life Events Checklist, adapted from Elliott-DeSorbo et al. [30], to document stressful events in the past three months. The score is the number of stressful events endorsed (range 0–22).

Rating of Overall Stress Scale (ROSS). Participants rated their stress in the past month from 0 (not stressed) to 10 (very stressed). This measure was adapted from Leidy et al. [31].

Quality of Life. The following PROMIS self-report short forms were administered: depression (8 items) [32], pain interference (6 items) [33], and cognitive function (8 items) [34]. Raw scores were converted to T-scores (M = 50, SD = 10). Subscales had excellent internal reliability ($\alpha = 0.916$–0.972).

2.3. Adherence

Pill Counts. At re-staging visits, a study team member documented the number of returned capsules, drug holds, and dose changes. Adherence was calculated by dividing the doses correctly taken by the number prescribed. During drug holds, doses were considered adherent if they were *not* taken. Twice, a pill bottle was lost by participants, so the pill count was missing.

Medication Diary. For each dose, participants were instructed to record the date, the time, and any comments. If a diary listed the time or number of capsules taken, researchers coded the dose as adherent. Empty cells were coded as non-adherent. One participant lost a diary for one cycle, but all other diaries were returned.

MEMS^{TM} Cap. Participants' study drug bottles were fitted with a MEMS^{TM} cap at baseline. Having been given instructions to take the drug 12 h apart, adherence was defined as opening the bottle 11–13 h since their last dose. Data were considered missing if <50% of doses in the cycle were represented. A priori, the MEMS^{TM} feasibility target was $\geq$2 cycles monitored for $\geq$75% of participants.

Barriers to Adherence Questionnaire. The barriers to adherence measure was created by the study team; participants were asked to think of times they missed a dose of their study drug in the past month and marked which of 16 possible reasons caused them to miss a dose. Participants also could provide additional reasons for missing medication.

Qualitative Adherence Interview. Participants completed a 15–30 min structured interview between cycles 8 and 12 (cycle = 28 days). Questions were about adherence barriers, facilitators, and advice participants would give to others.

2.4. Procedures

This study was approved by the National Institute of Health Intramural Institutional Review Board. Patients were approached and consented during their baseline visit on a selumetinib clinical trial [35] and provided informed consent for this adherence study (NCT03531814). For the clinical trial, participants completed 28-day treatment cycles and were instructed to take medication approximately 12 h apart. Routine protocol re-staging visits were performed before cycles 5, 13, and 19, and included the collection of adherence data. At each follow-up visit on the clinical trial, diaries and pill bottles (including empty ones) were collected, and MEMS^{TM} cap data were uploaded to Aardex MEMS^{TM} Adherence Software (ElectronReader 0.9.9). If adherence was <80% by any method, the team alerted the PI of the clinical trial, and adherence was discussed with the patient. Qualitative interviews were conducted by a licensed psychologist or trained psychology associate in a private clinic room (except for one that was over the telephone) and recorded for transcription. Participants completed the Barriers to Adherence questionnaire around the time of the interview.

2.5. Analyses

Quantitative. Quantitative analyses were conducted in SPSS 29.0.1. Pill count, diary, and MEMS^{TM} cap data were grouped across cycles 1–4, 5–8, 9–12, and 13–18. Adherence data were positively skewed, so non-parametric tests were used (i.e., Spearman correlations). Alpha was 0.05. As the primary outcome was feasibility, a power analysis was not conducted a priori. Given the small sample size, we were under-powered to perform some of the quantitative analysis. However, we report exploratory Spearman correlation results, as these require less power than analyses of variance comparing multiple groups (e.g., differences in adherence over time and differences between adherence assessment methods). Therefore, data comparing multiple groups are presented descriptively.

Qualitative. For qualitative data, thematic analysis was conducted using both deductive and inductive techniques. As the qualitative portion of this study was an exploratory aim, analyzing data for saturation was not part of the a priori methods. However, post hoc methods were conducted with thematic saturation defined as the point at which no new categories or codes were uncovered [36]. Retrospectively, the interview transcripts were reviewed in the order in which they were conducted to assess for new themes or subthemes. The initial coding dictionary was developed with broad themes that aligned with interview questions. The first two transcripts were coded by the last author, and subthemes were added to the dictionary as they arose. Next, themes and subthemes were discussed as a team (a licensed psychologist with extensive experience in qualitative research, a master's level psychology associate, a postdoctoral fellow, and a post-baccalaureate fellow) while reviewing transcripts together, and modifications to the dictionary were made as needed to reach consensus. Subsequent transcripts were divided among the team and discussed collaboratively. All transcripts were reviewed by at least two team members.

3. Results

3.1. Participants

All 12 participants (M age = 34.36, SD = 8.91) who were approached agreed to enroll on this study (see Table 1 for demographics). Although the adherence study was open to ages 3+ years, the only treatment protocol open at our institution during data collection was for adults. All participants provided complete data with one exception: one participant was not given the Barriers to Adherence questionnaire due to researcher error. After the first 12 participants were enrolled on this protocol, the clinical trial of selumetinib closed to enrollment; thus, we were unable to enroll more participants on this adherence study.

Table 1. Participant characteristics.

Participant Characteristics	N (%)
Age (Mean (SD))	34.36 (8.91), N = 12
Education (Mean (SD))	14.83 (1.80), N = 12
Sex Assigned at Birth	
Female	5 (41.6%)
Male	7 (58.3%)
Race/Ethnicity	
White	8 (66.7%)
Black	2 (16.7%)
Asian	1 (8.3%)

Table 1. *Cont.*

Participant Characteristics	N (%)
American Indian/Alaskan Native	1 (8.3%)
Not Hispanic/Latino/a/e	12 (100%)
Marital Status	
Single	10 (83.3%)
Married	2 (16.7%)
Occupational Status	
Unemployed	3 (25%)
Employed, (Full-time/Part-time)	7 (58.3%)/2 (16.7%)
Psychological/Neurological History	
Attention Deficit (ADHD)	2 (16.7%)
Learning Disability	4 (33.3%)
Depression	2 (16.7%)
Anxiety	3 (25%)

3.2. Quantitative Findings

Feasibility of MEMS™. Eleven of twelve participants (91.7%) completed at least the first two cycles; the 80% and 95% confidence intervals of the proportion are (75.8%, 98.1%) and (64.6%, 99.6%) based on Wilson's method, respectively [37]. Due to battery expiration between restaging visits (n = 5), forgetting to replace the cap on the next bottle (n = 1), or forgetting to return the cap (n = 1), at least one cycle was unable to be collected for some participants. Additionally, one participant withdrew because they did not like using the MEMS™ cap. One other participant's cap malfunctioned, resulting in no data collected for that participant across any cycles. One participant was taken off the drug trial at cycle 9; therefore, their adherence data were only grouped for cycles 1–4 and 5–8.

Adherence Over Time. Adherence was above 90% over all time points, as measured by pill counts and diaries (Table 2; Figure 1). According to MEMS™ caps, adherence remained relatively stable and ranged from 83.39% at cycles 1–5 to 79.68% during cycles 13–18. Pill count adherence rates ranged from 97.53% to 99.50%, while diary rates ranged from 96.14% to 99.22%.

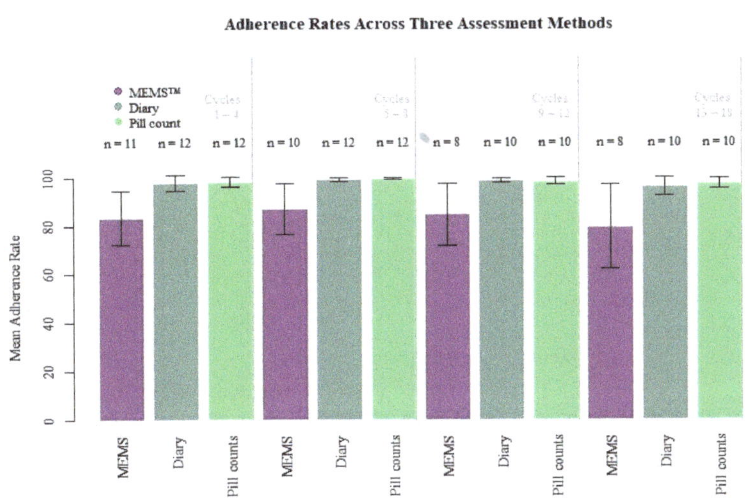

Figure 1. Adherence rates across three assessment methods.

Table 2. Adherence rates across three assessment methods.

Cycle	Method	Mean	Standard Deviation	95% Confidence Interval
	MEMS^{TM} (n = 11)	83.39	16.71	72.16–94.62
1–4	Diary (n = 12)	97.88	5.02	94.69–101.07
	Pill counts (n = 12)	98.25	3.22	96.20–100.30
	MEMS^{TM} (n = 10)	87.01	14.62	76.55–97.47
5–8	Diary (n = 12)	99.22	1.54	98.24–100.20
	Pill counts (n = 12)	99.50	0.82	98.98–100.02
	MEMS^{TM} (n = 8)	84.77	15.44	71.86–97.68
9–12	Diary (n = 10)	98.84	1.19	97.99–99.69
	Pill counts (n = 10)	98.51	2.14	96.98 -100.04
	MEMS^{TM} (n = 8)	79.68	20.85	62.25–97.11
13–18	Diary (n = 10)	96.14	5.35	92.31–99.97
	Pill counts (n = 10)	97.53	2.99	95.39–99.67

Comparison of Adherence Assessment Methods. Given the lack of sufficient power to have confidence in results of statistical comparisons, these results are presented descriptively. As shown in Table 2, the mean MEMS^{TM} adherence rates over most cycles are lower than for diaries and pill counts, while the means for diaries and pill counts are fairly close to each other.

Patient Characteristics and Time Periods Related to Adherence Differences. Poorer MEMS^{TM} adherence rates were correlated with higher depression scores (Table 3). The better adherence from MEMS^{TM} and pill count data in cycles 1–4 is related to lower baseline overall stress. When examining differences in MEMS^{TM} adherence levels by baseline NF1 symptom severity and pain intensity, those with mild and moderate (vs. severe) symptoms and pain were grouped. Descriptively, there was not a clear pattern of differences in mean MEMS^{TM} adherence based on NF1 severity (Cycles 1–4: Mild/Moderate = 84.55, Severe = 82.01. Cycles 5–8: Mild/Moderate = 85.19, Severe = 89.73. Cycles 9–12: Mild/Moderate = 81.61, Severe = 90.03. Cycles 13–18: Mild/Moderate = 77.96, Severe = 82.54.). There was also no discernible pattern in differences in adherence based on pain intensity (Cycles 1–4: No pain/Mild/Moderate = 79.58, Severe = 90.07. Cycles 5–8: No pain/Mild/Moderate = 84.52, Severe = 90.74. Cycles 9–12: No pain/Mild/Moderate = 83.85, Severe = 87.50. Cycles 13–18: No pain/Mild/Moderate = 80.55, Severe = 77.08.).

Table 3. Relationship between participant characteristics and adherence.

	MEMS^{TM} Cap	Medication Diary	Pill Count
	Number of Stressful Life Events at Baseline		
Cycles 1–4	$r = -0.035, p = 0.919$	$r = -0.546, p = 0.066$	$r = -0.399, p = 0.199$
Cycles 5–8	$r = 0.227, p = 0.528$	$r = -0.304, p = 0.337$	$r = -0.320, p = 0.310$
Cycles 9–12	$r = 0.179, p = 0.672$	$r = -0.494, p = 0.147$	$r = -0.086, p = 0.813$
Cycles 13–18	$r = 0.041, p = 0.923$	$r = -0.186, p = 0.606$	$r = -0.246, p = 0.494$
	Rating of Overall Stress at Baseline		
Cycles 1–4	$r = -0.638, p = 0.035$ *	$r = -0.472, p = 0.121$	$r = -0.617, p = 0.033$ *
Cycles 5–8	$r = -0.361, p = 0.306$	$r = -0.325, p = 0.302$	$r = -0.323, p = 0.306$
Cycles 9–12	$r = -0.407, p = 0.317$	$r = -0.106, p = 0.772$	$r = 0.198, p = 0.584$
Cycles 13–18	$r = -0.180, p = 0.670$	$r = 0.108, p = 0.766$	$r = 0.136, p = 0.708$
	PROMIS Depression at Baseline		
Cycles 1–4	$r = -0.607, p = 0.048$ *	$r = 0.062, p = 0.848$	$r = 0.124, p = 0.701$
Cycles 5–8	$r = -0.658, p = 0.038$ *	$r = -0.489, p = 0.107$	$r = -0.563, p = 0.057$
Cycles 9–12	$r = -0.708, p = 0.050$ *	$r = -0.556, p = 0.095$	$r = -0.503, p = 0.138$
Cycles 13–18	$r = -0.878, p = 0.004$ **	$r = -0.617, p = 0.057$	$r = -0.553, p = 0.097$

Table 3. *Cont.*

	MEMS™ Cap	Medication Diary	Pill Count
	PROMIS Cognitive Function at Baseline		
Cycles 1–4	$r = 0.293, p = 0.382$	$r = -0.255, p = 0.424$	$r = -0.326, p = 0.302$
Cycles 5–8	$r = 0.278, p = 0.436$	$r = 0.088, p = 0.784$	$r = 0.108, p = 0.737$
Cycles 9–12	$r = 0.229, p = 0.586$	$r = 0.019, p = 0.959$	$r = 0.100, p = 0.784$
Cycles 13–18	$r = 0.530, p = 0.177$	$r = 0.147, p = 0.686$	$r = 0.181, p = 0.617$
	PROMIS Pain Interference at Baseline		
Cycles 1–4	$r = -0.215, p = 0.526$	$r = 0.047, p = 0.884$	$r = 0.018, p = 0.955$
Cycles 5–8	$r = 0.049, p = 0.894$	$r = -0.077, p = 0.813$	$r = -0.125, p = 0.698$
Cycles 9–12	$r = -0.048, p = 0.911$	$r = 0.130, p = 0.721$	$r = 0.374, p = 0.287$
Cycles 13–18	$r = -0.167, p = 0.693$	$r = 0.178, p = 0.622$	$r = 0.239, p = 0.506$

* $p < 0.05$, ** $p < 0.01$.

3.3. *Qualitative Findings*

After coding all transcripts from the qualitative interviews, we reviewed them retrospectively to assess for saturation. The data reached saturation since no new subthemes were generated after the tenth participant.

3.4. *Adherence Themes*

A combined inductive and deductive thematic analysis resulted in subthemes spanning two major themes aligned with the interview questions: barriers to medication adherence (nine subthemes) and facilitators to medication adherence (10 subthemes).

3.5. *Barriers to Adherence*

Forgetting

Multiple patients described forgetting to take their study medication. One individual said, "Sometimes I forget", and another replied, "Just forgetting".

3.6. *Memory/Cognitive Difficulties*

Trouble remembering to take medication was a barrier distinct from momentary forgetfulness. Many individuals with NF1 have cognitive difficulties like attention deficits [38] and memory weakness [39]. One individual said "what has made it hard for me to take my meds is my memory. I have a really, really hard time remembering it. Um, like, ADHD, I guess".

3.6.1. Too Busy

One participant's work schedule made it difficult to take their medication: "if I'm busy for work and I can't eat at the same time that kind of messes up when I can take [the drug]".

3.6.2. Timing of Doses

The timing of doses made adherence challenging. Even participants who adhered well faced challenges complying with the drug's required eating window (which has recently been removed from the FDA label [20]). One individual noted, "planning taking my medicine around social events, like if I'm going to go get dinner with friends or go out that night. Um, sort of timing it appropriately". Another mentioned difficulty with timing medication during work, but followed this by sharing "It's more like the issue also comes with the food aspect of the drug so… [the eating window] makes it really hard to plan activities. So sometimes I find myself having to, you know, take the drug two hours earlier than I planned". Another participant described how social engagements can act as barriers, saying "I'm doing an activity with friends and I know I'm gonna eat. And I can't just tell them, we can only do it at this time. So it's more like life kinda gets in the way of the strict structure for the drug".

3.6.3. Being Away from Home

Not being home during dose times was a barrier, with one individual reporting, "The only time I've had a hard time is if I was out and I wasn't home". Another person shared, "if I'm on weekend and I try to go places and all, then I'll... need to remember to take my medication with me [sic]".

3.6.4. Medical Symptoms

One participant's stomach pain impacted their ability to follow the protocol's eating requirements, saying, "figuring out my stomach is different, because I have a little bit of gastroparesis, so I have to wait a little bit, uh different time frames. So, figuring that out was a little bit challenging".

3.6.5. Keeping Pills in MEMS Bottle

For one participant, use of the MEMS caps was identified as a barrier if it conflicted with their preference for organizing medications. One participant described their concerns, "the pills were inside the bottle, my mind just didn't associate that bottle with taking my meds because I didn't see the pills so I would forget about it". The patient further stated, "with the MEMS cap, I missed like two weeks' worth of pills". This patient withdrew from the adherence protocol early due to their difficulties with the MEMS cap.

3.6.6. Sleep Schedule

Another barrier related to participants' sleep schedules. One participant noted, "one time I overslept [past my dose time]". Another elaborated, "sometimes it's hard to stick to the exact times because, I mean, forcing yourself, in my case, to wake up at 4 in the morning—4 in the afternoon, it's hard".

3.6.7. No Barriers

Two participants did not report any barriers; one participant replied, "What situations make it... I mean, there's really no, no problem. I mean I take it as prescribed".

3.7. Adherence Facilitators

3.7.1. Consistency/Routine

A consistent schedule facilitated adherence. One individual said "Yeah, I have a schedule... basically I have a built-in alarm clock, basically. I'm always already up at a certain time and go to bed at 7, and that's right when I take it". Another said, "every single night I prep my pills for the next day, and I have them all out of their bottles".

3.7.2. Reminders

Participants reported that reminders were helpful. One participant described visual cues, stating "I put [a sticky note] on my computer and it stays there, you know, for a while. Now I remember". Another participant reported that physical cues helped reinforce adherence, as they remembered when "it starts hurting". Participants' social support also served as reminders, with one person saying, "Uh, it's my mom. She always says, 'Did you take your medication?'".

3.7.3. Technology

Many participants used adherence-promoting technology. Some used a phone alarm as a reminder for medication ("Setting my alarm, you know, on my phone and just taking it... at a certain—at time") and eating ("I have it—an alarm set for food"). Others used medication adherence apps, e.g., "My daily reminder on my phone, which is the app called Medisafe".

3.7.4. Support from Others

Participants described social support as helpful for adherence. One participant shared, "tell family and friends, so they know, 'hey, [NAME] can't eat at this time'. Or '[NAME] can only do this at this time'. So, they are aware". Another described their work environment as supportive, saying, "Everybody knows at 5 PM my phone rings, I am out of the meeting. I go take my medication and I come back".

3.7.5. Distraction

One participant described distracting themselves during food abstinence windows, noting, "I often, like, will plan things around [dose times]. Just so if I take the medicine, I'll go for a walk, so I have an hour [before I can eat]. It helps the time pass by faster". Another patient said, "Just trying to plan things around that time. I often have to, you know either, go longer without food than I'd like".

3.7.6. Planning for Side Effects

Planning for medication side effects helped one participant adhere to the selumetinib. This participant said, "And planning for those side effects. So, whether, like I said, knowing ahead of time that I get nauseous, I'll take Zofran first".

3.7.7. Belief the Drug Is Helping

Believing that the study drug was helping was another facilitator of adherence. One participant who had experienced a drug hold said, "because they took me off the drugs for a brief period of time, and I felt, again, what it was like not to be on it, I can definitely say, pain wise, it is definitely worth it to be on the drug".

3.7.8. Wanting to Help Research

For one patient, being a study participant was a facilitator. The patient said, "I want to be a good, I guess, guinea pig, so I'm trying to do my best".

3.7.9. Memory/Remembering

One individual described their memory as a facilitator. This person said, "And my memory—I still remember that I need to take it".

3.7.10. Keeping Medication with Them

Finally, keeping medication with the participants was an identified facilitator. One person commented, "Since with that [MEMS] cap and all, I cannot split it. Like I cannot put one in my pocket or leave some at home, leave some at work, you know. So, I have to carry the bottle with me all the time". Another described, "I usually did take the bottle with me, or I just excused myself, I get to home so I can take it on time".

3.8. Barriers to Adherence Questionnaire

Consistent with findings from the qualitative interviews, the most endorsed barrier on the Barriers to Adherence Questionnaire was "forgetting" (54.55% of participants). Both "busy with other things" and "changes in daily routine" were endorsed by 36.36% of participants. Less frequent barriers were "being away from home" (27.2%), "too tired or slept through dose time" (27.27%), "ran out of pills" (9.09%), and "didn't feel like it/needed a break" (9.09%). Wanting to avoid side effects, having too many pills to take, feeling sick, or feeling stressed were not endorsed by any participants. Two participants added a barrier in the "other" category, with one describing a drug hold and one describing a specific instance of forgetting.

4. Discussion

This pilot study used mixed methods to examine adherence in adults with NF1-PN, with a primary aim of investigating MEMS™ cap feasibility for adherence assessment in adults on a clinical trial of selumetinib. The predetermined target of obtaining data from $\geq$75% of participants over $\geq$2 cycles was exceeded, suggesting that MEMS™ caps are feasible. However, unexpected challenges resulted in missing data, including the cap's battery expiring, cap malfunction, patients forgetting to return the cap, and failure to replace the cap on the next cycles' bottle. Additionally, one participant withdrew from the adherence protocol because of their difficulties with the MEMS™ caps. Future research may circumvent some of these challenges by using wireless MEMS™ caps [40], which transmit data remotely and display the last opening to the participant.

Contrary to some prior research [21–24], our study did not find an obvious pattern of reduced longitudinal adherence over time, although we were underpowered to perform statistical comparisons here. Perhaps patients were encouraged to maintain high adherence due to the decreased PN volume and reduced pain documented in this clinical trial [35]. The trial also may have attracted patients more likely to adhere, or provided increased support for adherence compared to other settings. The qualitative results revealed many adherence facilitators in this sample, including consistency and routine, reminders, technology, and support from others. Although two participants identified no barriers to adherence, others described forgetting, being too busy, and the timing of doses as barriers.

As research increasingly focuses on treating PN with oral medications such as selumetinib [41,42] and mirdametinib [43], understanding patient experiences of barriers and facilitators to adherence is vitally important. Future research and clinical uses of MEK inhibitors targeting PN reduction may consider these patient experiences when discussing adherence strategies with patients. For example, researchers should encourage patients to develop consistent routines around medication, to set reminders, and to elicit social support. Additionally, medication timing was a common barrier; therefore, future randomized controlled trials could investigate the influence of timing on medication efficacy to determine the necessity of strict timing windows.

Higher depression and stress scores were associated with reduced adherence. These results were statistically significant despite our small sample size. Previous studies of other populations have reported similar findings, relating depressive symptoms (e.g., among people with cardiovascular disease [44], asthma [45], and type 2 diabetes [46]) and stress (e.g., among people with hypertension [47] and HIV [48]) to adherence. It is unsurprising that adherence in individuals with NF1 would be related to these factors. Preventative screening and treatment for depression and stress as strategies to increase adherence are worth considering; if interventions targeting these individuals could be started before or concurrently with drug initiation, adherence problems may be circumvented. With that said, adherence in this small sample was consistently high. Future studies with larger samples are needed to confirm these findings and explore factors that predict nonadherence in more depth.

Adherence interventions have been developed for several illnesses and therapies with varying efficacy [49,50]. While adherence-promoting strategies can be used effectively (e.g., health education, reminders), more research is necessary in the NF population [51]. Using patient-centered data sources, such as qualitative interviews, may help tailor interventions to specific patient populations. Future qualitative research also should examine facilitators and barriers for subpopulations of participants who may be at risk of poorer adherence, such as adults with depressive symptoms or high levels of stress.

Mean MEMS™ adherence rates in our sample were lower than the other methods by at least 12 points across all time periods. Future NF1 clinical trials should use MEMS™ caps to understand patterns of long-term adherence, while considering the challenges of battery expiration, cost, and error. Despite these challenges, MEMS™ caps may have use clinically in identifying people whose adherence drops below a pre-specified level.

Limitations

The current research was part of a pilot study investigating medication adherence in a trial of selumetinib; therefore, the sample size was intentionally (and necessarily) small. This limits generalizability to the larger NF1 population and was a barrier to exploring medical variables associated with adherence. However, pilot studies are necessary steps in the scientific process to evaluate feasibility and to inform future directions in research [52]. Additionally, the characteristics of individuals who participate in clinical trials tend to be different than those in the general population [53]. Further research is needed to explore facilitators and barriers for larger samples of people with NF1 as more oral medications become available for use outside of clinical trials. Future research should recruit larger samples to further explore MEMS™ feasibility, as well as the baseline characteristics that may predispose individuals to low adherence. Additionally, problems with missing MEMS™ data could be minimized through planning more frequent reminders, such as through a smartphone app. Documenting changes in perceived barriers and facilitators over the course of a trial and determining patient characteristics associated with particular barriers and facilitators are also worthwhile aims for future NF1 studies.

5. Conclusions

This pilot study is the first investigation using electronic pill caps to assess medication adherence among adults with NF1. MEMS™ caps proved a feasible method, and our results can inform future clinical trials studying oral medications with an NF1 population. Given the preliminary associations found in this study, providers may consider screening and treatment for depression and stress to increase adherence in both research and clinical settings. Additionally, qualitative data suggest that providers should encourage their patients to elicit social support, create a consistent routine, and use reminders to promote adherence. As medication adherence can be challenging, the continued exploration of factors related to adherence and the identification of other intervention targets to increase adherence among NF1 populations are warranted in larger samples. Larger samples will address potential biases inherent in pilot studies with small sample sizes.

Author Contributions: Conceptualization, S.M. and A.M.G.; methodology, M.A.T.-T., A.R. and S.M.; formal analysis, M.S.C., A.R., C.H., D.W., M.A.T.-T. and S.M.; data curation, A.R., M.S.C., D.W., M.B., C.H., M.F. and C.T.; writing—original draft preparation, M.S.C., S.M., D.W. and M.A.T.-T.; writing—review and editing, A.M.G., P.L.W., B.C.W., M.B. and M.F.; supervision, S.M.; funding acquisition, S.M. and A.M.G. All authors have read and agreed to the published version of the manuscript.

Funding: This publication was supported by a Sub-agreement from the Johns Hopkins University via the Neurofibromatosis Therapeutic Acceleration Program (NTAP) with funds provided by Grant Agreement from Bloomberg Philanthropies. Its contents are solely the responsibility of the authors and do not necessarily represent the official views of the Johns Hopkins University (Award ID: 182007).

This project was also supported by the Intramural Research Program of the National Institutes of Health, National Cancer Institute, Center for Cancer Research.

Institutional Review Board Statement: All procedures performed in studies involving human participants were in accordance with the ethical standards of the institutional and/or national research committee, and with the 1964 Helsinki declaration and its later amendments or comparable ethical standards.

Informed Consent Statement: Informed consent was obtained from all individual participants included in the study.

Data Availability Statement: Deidentified data are available in the NF Data Portal (https://nf.synapse.org (accessed on 12 January 2025)).

Acknowledgments: We would like to thank the participants who contributed to this study.

Conflicts of Interest: Author Cecilia Tibery was employed by the company Leidos Biomedical Research, Inc. The remaining authors declare that the research was conducted in the absence of any commercial or financial relationships that could be construed as a potential conflict of interest.

References

1. Lee, T.-S.J.; Chopra, M.; Kim, R.H.; Parkin, P.C.; Barnett-Tapia, C. Incidence and prevalence of neurofibromatosis type 1 and 2: A systematic review and meta-analysis. *Orphanet J. Rare Dis.* **2023**, *18*, 292. [CrossRef] [PubMed]
2. Prada, C.E.; Rangwala, F.A.; Martin, L.J.; Lovell, A.M.; Saal, H.M.; Schorry, E.K.; Hopkin, R.J. Pediatric Plexiform Neurofibromas: Impact on Morbidity and Mortality in Neurofibromatosis Type 1. *J. Pediatr.* **2012**, *160*, 461–467. [CrossRef] [PubMed]
3. Gross, A.M.; Dombi, E.; Widemann, B.C. Current status of MEK inhibitors in the treatment of plexiform neurofibromas. *Child's Nerv. Syst.* **2020**, *36*, 2443–2452. [CrossRef]
4. Fisher, M.J.; Blakeley, J.O.; Weiss, B.D.; Dombi, E.; Ahlawat, S.; Akshintala, S.; Belzberg, A.J.; Bornhorst, M.; Bredella, M.A.; Cai, W.; et al. Management of neurofibromatosis type 1-associated plexiform neurofibromas. *Neuro Oncol.* **2022**, *24*, 1827–1844. [CrossRef] [PubMed]
5. Anderson, M.K.; Johnson, M.; Thornburg, L.; Halford, Z. A Review of Selumetinib in the Treatment of Neurofibromatosis Type 1–Related Plexiform Neurofibromas. *Ann. Pharmacother.* **2022**, *56*, 716–726. [CrossRef]
6. Casey, D.; Demko, S.; Sinha, A.; Mishra-Kalyani, P.S.; Shen, Y.-L.; Khasar, S.; Goheer, M.A.; Helms, W.S.; Pan, L.; Xu, Y.; et al. FDA Approval Summary: Selumetinib for Plexiform Neurofibroma. *Clin. Cancer Res.* **2021**, *27*, 4142–4146. [CrossRef]
7. Nguyen, R.; Kluwe, L.; Fuensterer, C.; Kentsch, M.; Friedrich, R.E.; Mautner, V.-F. Plexiform Neurofibromas in Children with Neurofibromatosis Type 1: Frequency and Associated Clinical Deficits. *J. Pediatr.* **2011**, *159*, 652–655.e2. [CrossRef]
8. Gross, A.M.; Singh, G.; Akshintala, S.; Baldwin, A.; Dombi, E.; Ukwuani, S.; Goodwin, A.; Liewehr, D.J.; Steinberg, S.M.; Widemann, B.C. Association of plexiform neurofibroma volume changes and development of clinical morbidities in neurofibromatosis 1. *Neuro Oncol.* **2018**, *20*, 1643–1651. [CrossRef]
9. Wolters, P.L.; Burns, K.M.; Martin, S.; Baldwin, A.; Dombi, E.; Toledo-Tamula, M.A.; Dudley, W.N.; Gillespie, A.; Widemann, B.C. Pain interference in youth with neurofibromatosis type 1 and plexiform neurofibromas and relation to disease severity, social-emotional functioning, and quality of life. *Am. J. Med. Genet. Part A* **2015**, *167*, 2103–2113. [CrossRef]
10. Lai, J.-S.; Jensen, S.E.; Charrow, J.; Listernick, R. Patient Reported Outcomes Measurement Information System and Quality of Life in Neurological Disorders Measurement System to Evaluate Quality of Life for Children and Adolescents with Neurofibromatosis Type 1 Associated Plexiform Neurofibroma. *J. Pediatr.* **2019**, *206*, 190–196. [CrossRef]
11. Friedman, J.M. Review Article: Neurofibromatosis 1: Clinical Manifestations and Diagnostic Criteria. *J. Child Neurol.* **2002**, *17*, 548–554. [CrossRef]
12. Gross, A.M.; Wolters, P.L.; Dombi, E.; Baldwin, A.; Whitcomb, P.; Fisher, M.J.; Weiss, B.; Kim, A.; Bornhorst, M.; Shah, A.C.; et al. Selumetinib in Children with Inoperable Plexiform Neurofibromas. *N. Engl. J. Med.* **2020**, *382*, 1430–1442. [CrossRef] [PubMed]
13. Dombi, E.; Baldwin, A.; Marcus, L.J.; Fisher, M.J.; Weiss, B.; Kim, A.; Whitcomb, P.; Martin, S.; Aschbacher-Smith, L.E.; Rizvi, T.A.; et al. Activity of Selumetinib in Neurofibromatosis Type 1–Related Plexiform Neurofibromas. *N. Engl. J. Med.* **2016**, *375*, 2550–2560. [CrossRef]
14. Gross, A.M.; O'Sullivan Coyne, G.; Dombi, E.; Tibery, C.; Herrick, W.G.; Martin, S.; Angus, S.P.; Shern, J.F.; Rhodes, S.D.; Foster, J.C.; et al. Selumetinib in adults with NF1 and inoperable plexiform neurofibroma: A phase 2 trial. *Nat. Med.* **2025**. [CrossRef] [PubMed]

15. van Onzenoort, H.A.; Menger, F.E.; Neef, C.; Verberk, W.J.; Kroon, A.A.; de Leeuw, P.W.; van der Kuy, P.H. Participation in a clinical trial enhances adherence and persistence to treatment: A retrospective cohort study. *Hypertension* **2011**, *58*, 573–578. [CrossRef]
16. Boima, V.; Doku, A.; Agyekum, F.; Tuglo, L.S.; Agyemang, C. Effectiveness of digital health interventions on blood pressure control, lifestyle behaviours and adherence to medication in patients with hypertension in low-income and middle-income countries: A systematic review and meta-analysis of randomised controlled trials. *EClinicalMedicine* **2024**, *69*, 102432. [CrossRef] [PubMed]
17. Matsui, D. Strategies to Measure and Improve Patient Adherence in Clinical Trials. *Pharm. Med.* **2009**, *23*, 289–297. [CrossRef]
18. Pantuzza, L.L.; Ceccato, M.D.G.B.; Silveira, M.R.; Junqueira, L.M.R.; Reis, A.M.M. Association between medication regimen complexity and pharmacotherapy adherence: A systematic review. *Eur. J. Clin. Pharmacol.* **2017**, *73*, 1475–1489. [CrossRef]
19. Viskochil, D.; Wysocki, M.; Learoyd, M.; Sun, P.; So, K.; Evans, A.; Lai, F.; Hernàndez, H.S. Effect of food on selumetinib pharmacokinetics and gastrointestinal tolerability in adolescents with neurofibromatosis type 1-related plexiform neurofibromas. *Neuro Oncol. Adv.* **2024**, *6*, vdae036. [CrossRef] [PubMed]
20. AstraZeneca Pharmaceuticals LP. KOSELUGO® (Selumetinib) Capsules, for Oral Use [Label]. U.S. Food and Drug. Revised January 2024. Available online: https://www.accessdata.fda.gov/drugsatfda_docs/label/2024/213756s004lbl.pdf (accessed on 16 October 2024).
21. Bourdin, A.; Schneider, M.P.; Locatelli, I.; Schluep, M.; Bugnon, O.; Berger, J. Longitudinal analysis of safety and medication adherence of patients in the Fingolimod patient support program: A real-world observational study. *Sci. Rep.* **2021**, *11*, 4107. [CrossRef]
22. Smith, A.W.; Mara, C.A.; Modi, A.C. Adherence to antiepileptic drugs in adolescents with epilepsy. *Epilepsy Behav.* **2018**, *80*, 307–311. [CrossRef] [PubMed]
23. Ofori-Asenso, R.; Ilomäki, J.; Tacey, M.; Zomer, E.; Curtis, A.J.; Bell, J.S.; Zoungas, S.; Liew, D. Patterns of statin use and long-term adherence and persistence among older adults with diabetes. *J. Diabetes* **2018**, *10*, 699–707. [CrossRef]
24. Bhatia, S.; Landier, W.; Hageman, L.; Kim, H.; Chen, Y.; Crews, K.R.; Evans, W.E.; Bostrom, B.; Casillas, J.; Dickens, D.S.; et al. 6MP adherence in a multiracial cohort of children with acute lymphoblastic leukemia: A Children's Oncology Group study. *Blood* **2014**, *124*, 2345–2353. [CrossRef]
25. Hartman, L.; Lems, W.F.; Boers, M. Outcome measures for adherence data from a medication event monitoring system: A literature review. *J. Clin. Pharm. Ther.* **2019**, *44*, 1–5. [CrossRef]
26. Martin, S.; Elliott-Desorbo, D.K.; Calabrese, S.; Wolters, P.L.; Roby, G.; Brennan, T.; Wood, L.V. A Comparison of Adherence Assessment Methods Utilized in the United States: Perspectives of Researchers, HIV-Infected Children, and their Caregivers. *AIDS Patient Care STDs* **2009**, *23*, 593–601. [CrossRef]
27. Mosnaim, G.S.; Stempel, D.A.; Gonzalez, C.; Adams, B.; BenIsrael-Olive, N.; Gondalia, R.; Kaye, L.; Shalowitz, M.; Szefler, S. Electronic medication monitoring versus self-reported use of inhaled corticosteroids and short-acting beta(2)-agonists in uncontrolled asthma. *J. Asthma* **2022**, *59*, 2024–2027. [CrossRef]
28. Le Saux, O.; Bourmaud, A.; Rioufol, C.; Colomban, O.; Guitton, J.; Schwiertz, V.; Regnier, V.; You, B.; Ranchon, F.; Maraval-Gaget, R.; et al. Over-adherence to capecitabine: A potential safety issue in breast and colorectal cancer patients. *Cancer Chemother. Pharmacol.* **2018**, *82*, 319–327. [CrossRef] [PubMed]
29. Shellmer, D.A.; Zelikovsky, N. The challenges of using medication event monitoring technology with pediatric transplant patients. *Pediatr. Transplant.* **2007**, *11*, 422–428. [CrossRef] [PubMed]
30. Elliott-DeSorbo, D.K.; Martin, S.; Wolters, P.L. Stressful life events and their relationship to psychological and medical functioning in children and adolescents with HIV infection. *J. Acquir. Immune Defic. Syndr.* **2009**, *52*, 364–370. [CrossRef] [PubMed]
31. Leidy, N.K.; Margolis, M.K.; Marcin, J.P.; Flynn, J.A.; Frankel, L.R.; Johnson, S.; Langkamp, D.; Simoes, E.A.F. The Impact of Severe Respiratory Syncytial Virus on the Child, Caregiver, and Family During Hospitalization and Recovery. *Pediatrics* **2005**, *115*, 1536–1546. [CrossRef]
32. Pilkonis, P.A.; Choi, S.W.; Reise, S.P.; Stover, A.M.; Riley, W.T.; Cella, D.; Group, P.C. Item banks for measuring emotional distress from the Patient-Reported Outcomes Measurement Information System (PROMIS®): Depression, anxiety, and anger. *Assessment* **2011**, *18*, 263–283. [CrossRef]
33. Amtmann, D.; Cook, K.F.; Jensen, M.P.; Chen, W.-H.; Choi, S.; Revicki, D.; Cella, D.; Rothrock, N.; Keefe, F.; Callahan, L. Development of a PROMIS item bank to measure pain interference. *Pain* **2010**, *150*, 173–182. [CrossRef] [PubMed]
34. Lai, J.S.; Wagner, L.I.; Jacobsen, P.B.; Cella, D. Self-reported cognitive concerns and abilities: Two sides of one coin? *Psycho Oncol.* **2014**, *23*, 1133–1141. [CrossRef]
35. Gross, A.M.; O'Sullivan Coyne, G.; Dombi, E.; Tibery, C.; Herrick, W.G.; Martin, S.; Angus, S.P.; Shern, J.F.; Rhodes, S.D.; Foster, J.C.; et al. Clinical Responses and Pharmacodynamics of Selumetinib in a Phase 2 Study for Adults with NF1 and Inoperable, Symptomatic, or Growing Plexiform Neurofibromas. *Nat. Med.* **2025**.

36. Guest, G.; Namey, E.; McKenna, K. How Many Focus Groups Are Enough? Building an Evidence Base for Nonprobability Sample Sizes. *Field Methods* **2017**, *29*, 3–22. [CrossRef]
37. Wilson, E.B. Probable inference, the law of succession, and statistical inference. *J. Am. Stat. Assoc.* **1927**, *22*, 209–212. [CrossRef]
38. Hyman, S.L.; Shores, A.; North, K.N. The nature and frequency of cognitive deficits in children with neurofibromatosis type 1. *Neurology* **2005**, *65*, 1037–1044. [CrossRef]
39. Loucas, C.; Wolters, P.; Toledo-Tamula, M.A.; Rhodes, A.; Baldwin, A.; Goodwin, A.; Widemann, B.; Martin, S. Verbal learning and memory in youth with neurofibromatosis type 1 and plexiform neurofibromas: Relationships with disease severity. *Eur. J. Paediatr. Neurol.* **2022**, *38*, 7–12. [CrossRef]
40. Robiner, W.N.; Flaherty, N.; Fossum, T.A.; Nevins, T.E. Desirability and feasibility of wireless electronic monitoring of medications in clinical trials. *Transl. Behav. Med.* **2015**, *5*, 285–293. [CrossRef] [PubMed]
41. Gross, A.M.; Glassberg, B.; Wolters, P.L.; Dombi, E.; Baldwin, A.; Fisher, M.J.; Kim, A.; Bornhorst, M.; Weiss, B.D.; Blakeley, J.O.; et al. Selumetinib in children with neurofibromatosis type 1 and asymptomatic inoperable plexiform neurofibroma at risk for developing tumor-related morbidity. *Neuro Oncol.* **2022**, *24*, 1978–1988. [CrossRef] [PubMed]
42. Gross, A.M.; Dombi, E.; Wolters, P.L.; Baldwin, A.; Dufek, A.; Herrera, K.; Martin, S.; Derdak, J.; Heisey, K.S.; Whitcomb, P.M.; et al. Long-term safety and efficacy of selumetinib in children with neurofibromatosis type 1 on a phase 1/2 trial for inoperable plexiform neurofibromas. *Neuro Oncol.* **2023**, *25*, 1883–1894. [CrossRef]
43. Weiss, B.D.; Wolters, P.L.; Plotkin, S.R.; Widemann, B.C.; Tonsgard, J.H.; Blakeley, J.; Allen, J.C.; Schorry, E.; Korf, B.; Robison, N.J.; et al. NF106: A Neurofibromatosis Clinical Trials Consortium Phase II Trial of the MEK Inhibitor Mirdametinib (PD-0325901) in Adolescents and Adults With NF1-Related Plexiform Neurofibromas. *J. Clin. Oncol.* **2021**, *39*, 797–806. [CrossRef]
44. Kronish, I.M.; Rieckmann, N.; Halm, E.A.; Shimbo, D.; Vorchheimer, D.; Haas, D.C.; Davidson, K.W. Persistent Depression Affects Adherence to Secondary Prevention Behaviors After Acute Coronary Syndromes. *J. Gen. Intern. Med.* **2006**, *21*, 1178–1183. [CrossRef]
45. Krauskopf, K.A.; Sofianou, A.; Goel, M.S.; Wolf, M.S.; Wilson, E.A.H.; Martynenko, M.E.; Halm, E.A.; Leventhal, H.; Feldman, J.M.; Federman, A.D.; et al. Depressive Symptoms, Low Adherence, and Poor Asthma Outcomes in the Elderly. *J. Asthma* **2013**, *50*, 260–266. [CrossRef] [PubMed]
46. Hoogendoorn, C.J.; Shapira, A.; Roy, J.F.; Walker, E.A.; Cohen, H.W.; Gonzalez, J.S. Depressive Symptom Dimensions and Medication Non-adherence in Suboptimally Controlled Type 2 Diabetes. *J. Diabetes Complicat.* **2019**, *33*, 217–222. [CrossRef] [PubMed]
47. Krousel-Wood, M.; Joyce, C.; Holt, E.; Muntner, P.; Webber, L.S.; Morisky, D.E.; Frohlich, E.D.; Re, R.N. Predictors of Decline in Medication Adherence: Results From the Cohort Study of Medication Adherence Among Older Adults. *Hypertension* **2011**, *58*, 804–810. [CrossRef]
48. Mugavero, M.J.; Raper, J.L.; Reif, S.; Whetten, K.; Leserman, J.; Theilman, N.M.; Pence, B.W. Overload: Impact of Incident Stressful Events on Antiretroviral Medication Adherence and Virologic Failure in a Longitudinal, Multisite Human Immunodeficiency Virus Cohort Study. *Psychosom. Med.* **2009**, *71*, 920–926. [CrossRef]
49. Galo, J.S.; Mehat, P.; Rai, S.K.; Avina-Zubieta, A.; De Vera, M.A. What are the effects of medication adherence interventions in rheumatic diseases: A systematic review. *Ann. Rheum. Dis.* **2016**, *75*, 667–673. [CrossRef] [PubMed]
50. Wilhelmsen, N.C.; Eriksson, T. Medication adherence interventions and outcomes: An overview of systematic reviews. *Eur. J. Hosp. Pharm.* **2019**, *26*, 187–192. [CrossRef] [PubMed]
51. Tolley, A.; Hassan, R.; Sanghera, R.; Grewal, K.; Kong, R.; Sodhi, B.; Basu, S. Interventions to promote medication adherence for chronic diseases in India: A systematic review. *Front. Public Health* **2023**, *11*, 1194919. [CrossRef]
52. Malmqvist, J.; Hellberg, K.; Möllås, G.; Rose, R.; Shevlin, M. Conducting the Pilot Study: A Neglected Part of the Research Process? Methodological Findings Supporting the Importance of Piloting in Qualitative Research Studies. *Int. J. Qual. Methods* **2019**, *18*, 160940691987834. [CrossRef]
53. Storms, W. Clinical trials: Are these your patients? *J. Allergy Clin. Immunol.* **2003**, *112*, 5. [CrossRef] [PubMed]

cancers

MDPI

Article

Genetic Alterations in Patients with *NF2*-Related Schwannomatosis and Sporadic Vestibular Schwannomas

Jules P. J. Douwes [1,*], Ronald van Eijk [2], Sybren L. N. Maas [2,3], Jeroen C. Jansen [1], Emmelien Aten [4] and Erik F. Hensen [1]

1 Department of Otorhinolaryngology—Head and Neck Surgery, Leiden University Medical Center, 2333 ZA Leiden, The Netherlands; j.c.jansen@lumc.nl (J.C.J.); e.f.hensen@lumc.nl (E.F.H.)

2 Department of Pathology, Leiden University Medical Center, 2333 ZA Leiden, The Netherlands; r.van_eijk@lumc.nl (R.v.E.); s.l.n.maas@lumc.nl (S.L.N.M.)

3 Department of Pathology, Erasmus MC Cancer Institute, University Medical Center Rotterdam, 3015 CN Rotterdam, The Netherlands

4 Department of Clinical Genetics, Leiden University Medical Center, 2333 ZA Leiden, The Netherlands; e.aten@lumc.nl

* Correspondence: j.p.j.douwes@lumc.nl

Simple Summary: Vestibular schwannomas are tumors that occur on the nerve responsible for hearing and balance, the vestibulocochlear nerve. These benign tumors may appear on one side (unilateral) or both sides (bilateral), with bilateral cases often linked to a condition called *NF2*-related schwannomatosis. This study explored the genetic causes of vestibular schwannomas in three groups: patients with NF2, younger patients with a unilateral tumor, and older patients with a unilateral tumor. By analyzing DNA from the tumors and blood, we aimed to understand the genetic mutations that drive tumor development and how the genetics differed between the three groups. In all patients, it was found that one gene, *NF2*, played a major role in the development of vestibular schwannomas. However, there were also differences found in the types of genetic mutations and mechanisms involved, offering new insights into how these tumors form and progress.

Abstract: Background: Unilateral (uVS) and bilateral vestibular schwannoma (bVS) are distinct disease types, yet share tumorigenic features. This study examined causative genetic alterations in three groups: patients with *NF2*-related schwannomatosis (NF2), young patients with uVS ($\leq$30 years), and older patients with uVS ($\geq$40 years). **Methods**: Lymphocyte and vestibular schwannoma DNA was genetically analyzed. Outcomes included gene involvement, pathogenicity classification, variant type, effect, and location, and loss of heterozygosity (LOH) of chromosome 22. **Results**: Among 93 patients, 17% had NF2, 39% were $\leq$30 years with uVS, and 44% were $\geq$40 years with uVS. In all patients with NF2 (100%), two or more hits were detected in the tumor DNA, whereas patients with uVS had a slightly lower detection rate (89–98%). NF2-related tumors had a higher frequency of nucleotide variants (76%), while LOH events were more common in uVS (64–69%). Variants were mostly identified in *NF2*, with nonsense variants over-represented in patients with NF2 (38%) and frameshift variants more prevalent in uVS (44–51%). **Conclusions**: Biallelic *NF2* inactivation primarily drives vestibular schwannoma tumorigenesis. In patients with NF2, two pathogenic *NF2* variants or one *NF2* variant with LOH are common, whereas patients with uVS often exhibit one *NF2* variant with LOH. Additionally, variant types differ between patient groups.

Keywords: acoustic neuroma; cerebellopontine angle tumor; clinical genetics; *NF2*-related schwannomatosis; schwannomatosis; skull base surgery; tumor genetics; vestibular schwannoma

1. Introduction

Vestibular schwannomas (VSs) are benign nerve sheath tumors affecting the vestibular branch of the eighth (vestibulocochlear) cranial nerve. Globally, the annual incidence of vestibular schwannomas has been estimated at 1 in 64,000 to 92,000 people, resulting in a lifetime risk of 1 in every 1000 individuals [1–3]. Common symptoms that vestibular schwannomas present with are hearing loss, tinnitus, and vestibular complaints [4,5]. These may be impacted by determinants such as tumor size, intrameatal and/or extrameatal tumor location, cystic elements, and involvement of the cochlea and brainstem [6]. Management options include active surveillance, surgical resection, and radiotherapy [7]. Therapeutic interventions achieve overall adequate tumor control; however, vestibular schwannomas are associated with morbidity and a reduced quality of life because of the sequalae of the disease itself and/or the interventions performed [8–10].

Sporadic vestibular schwannomas typically arise unilaterally (uVSs). Bilateral vestibular schwannomas (bVSs), in contrast, are the hallmark lesion for *NF2*-related schwannomatosis (NF2) [11], a tumor syndrome predisposing one to multiple central nervous system tumors, including schwannomas, meningiomas, and ependymomas [11,12]. In the majority of cases, vestibular schwannoma is unilateral and solitary, but in 5% to 7%, it is associated with NF2 [1,13]. In contrast to uVS, NF2-related bVS may develop at a younger age, show a higher tumor progression rate, and respond less favorably to standard treatment options. As a result, patients with NF2 experience a higher morbidity, a higher mortality, and a more substantial decline in their quality of life [14–16]. The clinical severity of NF2, however, is highly variable. According to classical phenotype models, NF2 can present as a more severe (Wishart) phenotype with an early age of onset and a milder (Feiling–Gardner) phenotype with a later onset [17]. More detailed genotype–phenotype correlations have been proposed to predict the clinical severity of NF [16,18,19]. Other molecular measures, such as dysregulated cellular pathways and tumor microenvironment, are also coming to the forefront to provide greater prognostic insight [20–22].

The tumorigenesis of both uVS and bVS is hypothesized to be the result of a two-hit mutational mechanism, most frequently caused by inactivation of the neurofibromatosis type 2 (*NF2*) tumor suppressor gene, either by mutation of the *NF2* or loss of chromosome 22q (LOH) [23–26]. In the majority of tumors, a pathogenic nucleotide variant in *NF2* is detected together with the loss of the *NF2* wildtype copy of chromosome 22q. In *NF2*-related schwannomatosis, constitutional frameshift and nonsense (truncating) variants are linked to an aggressive phenotype originating at an adolescent age. Missense, in-frame, and silent variants have been associated with a milder phenotype and greater life expectancy, while splice-site and (multiple) exon-deleting variants result in a more variable clinical severity [16,18,27]. Vestibular schwannomas have also been associated with variants in several other genes, such as *CDC27*, *CDKN2A*, *LZTR1*, *MDM2*, *PRKAR1A*, *SMARCB1*, *TSC1*, and *TSC2* [20,24,26–35].

Although they are distinct disease types, there is both a clinical and genetic overlap between patients with uVS and patients with NF2-related bVS. It seems logical to suggest that young patients with NF2 develop uVS before they develop bVS, while patients under 30 years old presenting with uVS have a greater risk of developing bVS at a later point in life [36,37]. Testing for NF2 is therefore imperative in young patients less than 30 years of age with schwannomas of any location. It has also been suggested that uVS can be a milder phenotypical expression of NF2, as mosaicism rates of de novo NF2 have been found to be 60%, substantially higher than previously expected [19,38]. At the same time, true uVS typically develops after the age of 40 years [1,39]. Therefore, differences in the phenotype of patients with NF2 and patients with uVS, but also within-group differences for uVS, may be the result of distinct mutational mechanisms [40].

The aim of this study was to evaluate the causative genetic alterations of vestibular schwannomas in different patient groups, i.e., patients with confirmed NF2, young patients with uVS ($\leq$30 years), and older patients with uVS ($\geq$40 years).

2. Materials and Methods

2.1. Participants and Study Design

The present study included patients that were surgically treated for a vestibular schwannoma at the Leiden University Medical Center (LUMC) in The Netherlands, a tertiary skull base and NF2 referral center, between 1 December 1997 and 31 December 2023. The inclusion criteria comprised patients $\geq$ 18 years old with NF2-related or unilateral vestibular schwannoma and for whom frozen or fixated paraffine tumor material was available for retrospective genetic analysis. The diagnosis of NF2 was confirmed using the updated clinical and radiologic criteria [12]. The exclusion criteria comprised insufficient demographic or clinical data, tumor material with a lack of qualitative or quantitative DNA for genetic analysis, and other schwannomatosis-related disease types.

Following ethical approval and informed consent, electronic patient files were retrospectively examined for demographic, clinical, and genetic characteristics. Tumor specimens for variant analysis were collected from the Department of Pathology (LUMC), stored for long-term safekeeping in accordance with national guidelines. A secured online database was set up for the collection and storage of data. The study protocol was conducted in compliance with the ethical standard of The Declaration of Helsinki (2013).

2.2. Demographics and Clinical Assessment

The demographics included vital status, sex, age at the time of diagnosis, and age at the time of surgical intervention. For the present analysis, patients were divided into three groups: patients with clinically or genetically confirmed diagnosis of *NF2*-related schwannomatosis, patients $\leq$ 30 years old when diagnosed with uVS, and patients $\geq$ 40 years old when diagnosed with uVS. Clinical outcomes of interest included tumor characteristics, treatment history, family history of NF2 or uVS, and genetic germline diagnostics (in the case of NF2 or individuals at risk of NF2 [41]).

2.3. DNA Extraction and Analysis

Germline DNA was extracted from peripheral blood lymphocytes, and vestibular schwannoma DNA was extracted from micro-dissected frozen or paraffine tumor specimens, using standard diagnostic procedures. In some cases, a genetic analysis had already been performed on lymphocyte DNA and/or tumor specimens prior to this study at the discretion of the treating multidisciplinary team or in compliance with patient preferences [42].

Since 2017, next-generation sequencing (NGS) has been used as the golden standard for detecting pathogenic variants in clinical settings [43]. Prior to that, direct Sanger sequencing and multiple ligation-dependent probe amplification (MLPA) were employed. Although NGS is favored over Sanger sequencing, we included all individuals that had received germline and/or tumor analysis to deal with sample size constraints. All the included samples were sequenced and analyzed according to a globally recognized standard for quality management and handled according to medical ethical guidelines described in the Code Proper Secondary Use of Human Tissue established by the Dutch Federation of Medical Sciences [44].

The LUMC Department of Pathology (section Molecular Diagnostics) designed an Ion-Torrent-based NGS Ampliseq gene panel (Thermo Scientific, Waltham, MA, USA), named Rare Cancer PaneL (RCPL) [45]. The RCPL sequences genes and hotspot regions in rare tumors that frequently express distinct mutational profiles. For vestibular schwannomas, the RCPL includes, among others, the following relevant genes: *CDC27*, *CDKN2A*, *LZTR1*, *MDM2/CDK4*, *NF2*, *PRKAR1A*, *SMARCB1*, *SMARCE1*, *TSC1*, and *TSC2*. Additionally, LOH were assessed for chromosome 22. The sequencing criteria have been described in more detail in the RCPL guideline [45].

Outcomes of interest included the affected gene, pathogenicity classification according to the American College of Medical Genetics and Genomic [46], variant type, variant effect, location of the variants according to predetermined *NF2* gene domains (exon 1, exon 2–7, exon 8–13, and exon 14–17) [16,18], and presence of LOH. If applicable, a genetic severity score was established [18].

2.4. Statistics

For the statistical analyses, IBM SPSS Statistics for Windows (version 27.0. Armond, NY, USA: IBM Corp) was used. Descriptive statistics were used to describe patient characteristics. Non-normally distributed data were reported using median, range, frequency count, and percentages. Missing, unused, and incorrect data were documented and adjusted for during data collection and study analysis.

3. Results

3.1. Patient Characteristics

Ninety-three patients were included. Of these, 16 patients (17%) were diagnosed with NF2, 36 patients (39%) were ≤30 years old with uVS, and 41 patients (44%) were ≥40 years old with uVS (Table 1). The median age at diagnosis was 33.7 years (12.6–61.9) for NF2, 27.1 (16.7–30.6) for young patients with uVS, and 55.5 (40.0–79.5) for older patients with uVS. Fifteen patients with NF2 (94%) presented with bilateral vestibular schwannomas. Three patients with NF2 (19%) passed away after being diagnosed, and no deaths were recorded among the patients with uVS.

Table 1. Demographics and treatment characteristics of the study cohort.

Patient Characteristics	Patients with NF2, *n* = 16	Patients with uVS ≤ 30 Years, *n* = 36	Patients with uVS ≥ 40 Years, *n* = 41
Female, *n* (%)	11 (68.8)	24 (66.7)	20 (48.8)
Age, years, median (range)			
Diagnosis	33.7 (12.6–61.9)	27.1 (16.7–30.6)	55.5 (40.0–79.5)
Time of treatment	35.0 (20.7–62.7)	28.0 (17.0–38.4)	56.4 (43.7–81.0)
Current	54 (25–79)	32 (18–44)	58 (45–84)
Family history of NF2 or uVS, *n* (%)	1 (6.7)	0 (0.0)	1 (2.4)
Previous treatment on target tumor, *n* (%)			
Surgical resection	2 (12.5)	2 (5.6)	0 (0.0)
Radiotherapy	0 (0.0	5 (13.9)	0 (0.0)
Bevacizumab	2 (12.5)	n.a.	n.a.
Surgical indication, *n* (%)			
Large tumor size	10 (71.4)	22 (61.1)	11 (26.8)
Tumor progression	2 (14.3)	9 (25.0)	23 (56.1)
Symptoms	2 (14.3)	5 (13.9)	7 (17.1)

Legend: NF2 = *NF2*-related schwannomatosis; *n* = number of patients; uVS = unilateral vestibular schwannoma; and n.a. = not applicable.

3.2. Germline Analysis

Germline sequencing of *NF2* was performed in twelve patients with NF2 (75%) prior to this study. Variant analysis was primarily performed with a combination of Sanger sequencing and MLPA (8/12, 67%), followed by Sanger sequencing alone (2/12, 17%) and NGS (1/12, 8%). For one case, the sequencing technique was unknown.

In five patients with NF2 (42%), a pathogenic germline variant was detected. Their median age at presentation was 24.3 years (12.5–30.6). Patient 7 had a large deletion of 19 genes on chromosome 22, including exon 1 of the *NF2* gene. No pathogenic variants were detected in *LZTR1* and *SMARCB1*. The other four patients had different nucleotide variants of *NF2*, all classified as likely pathogenic (Human Genome Variation Society Nomenclature class 4) [47]. The molecular details are described in Table 2.

Table 2. Pathogenic germline variants in five patients with *NF2*-related schwannomatosis.

No.	Age at Pres.	Exon	DNA Sequence	Protein Sequence	Variant Type	Genetic Severity
02	24.3	12	c.1132G > T	p.Glu378*	Nonsense	2B
04	16.5	8	c.702dupT	p.Gly235Trpfs*	Frameshift	3
06	12.6	13	c.1341-2A > G	p.?	Splice site	2A
07	30.6	1	c.del22q12.1q12.2	p.?	Large deletion	2A
15	27.2	10	c.892C > T	p.Gln298*	Nonsense	2B

Legend: No. = patient study number; and Pres. = presentation.

Twenty-three young patients with uVS (66%) underwent germline NF2 screening [36]. We deployed Sanger sequencing with MLPA in fifteen cases (65%), NGS in seven cases (30%), and a sequencing technique of unknown origin in a single case (4%). All patients (100%) were tested for *NF2*, while fourteen patients (61%) were additionally tested for *LZTR1* and five (22%) for *SMARCB1* alterations. One patient (4%) harbored an *LZTR1* variant (NM_006767.3 (exon 13): c.1433G > A, p.Arg478Gln), yet pathogenicity was unknown (class 3, variant of unknow significance (VUS)). No other variants were detected.

3.3. Tumor Analysis

Tumor samples were primarily analyzed using NGS (NF2: 94%; uVS $\leq$ 30 years: 92%; and uVS $\geq$ 40 years: 100%), specifically with the RCPL (NF2: 89%; uVS $\leq$ 30 years: 94%; and uVS $\geq$ 40 years: 100%). The remaining samples were sequenced using Sanger sequencing and MLPA.

In all patients with NF2 (100%), two or more hits were detected in the tumor DNA. The detection rate was marginally lower for patients with uVS: at least 1 hit in 32 out of 36 tumors (89%) among young patients with uVS and 40 out of 41 tumors (98%) in older patients with uVS. Patients with *NF2*-related schwannomatosis harbored an even distribution of tumor samples with either two distinct nucleotide variants or one variant as the presumed first hit and the LOH of chromosome 22 as the second hit. The majority of patients with uVS possessed the latter (Figure 1).

Two patients with NF2 harbored three hits: a germline *NF2* variant, a second hit in *NF2*, and a third *SMARCB1* VUS or LOH of chromosome 22, respectively. Among the patients with uVS, three individuals aged $\leq$30 years and four aged $\geq$40 years showed a three- or four-hit mechanism in the tumor sample. A relatively high number of nucleotide variants were found in the NF2-related samples, whereas the samples from patients with uVS showed more LOH events (Figure 2). The screening details are available online in the Supplementary Materials.

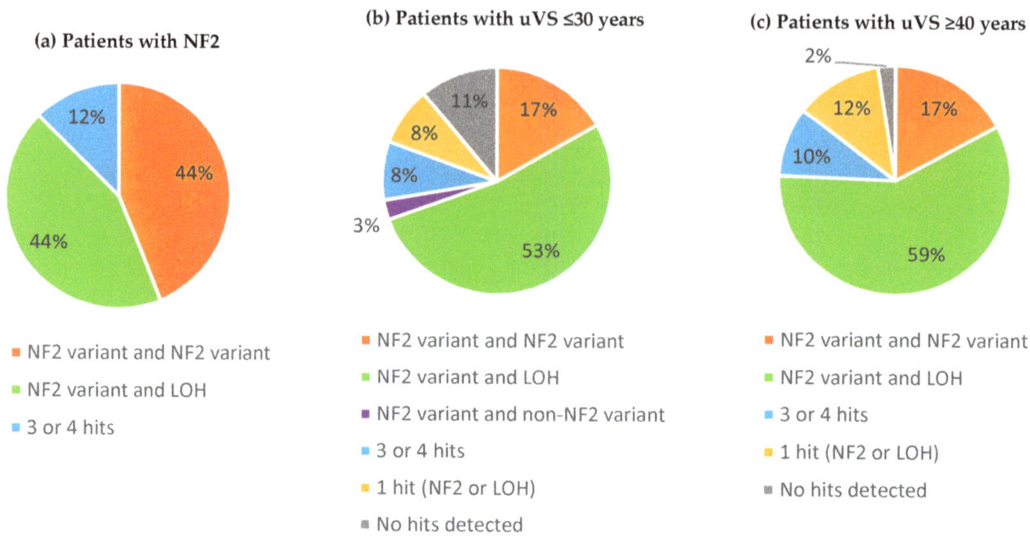

Figure 1. Multi-hit mechanism for the development of vestibular schwannoma in (**a**) patients with NF2 (n = 16), (**b**) young patients with uVS (≤30 years) (n = 36), and (**c**) older patients with uVS (≥40 years) (n = 41). Legend: patients with NF2 = patients with *NF2*-related schwannomatosis; uVS = unilateral vestibular schwannoma; and LOH = loss of heterozygosity.

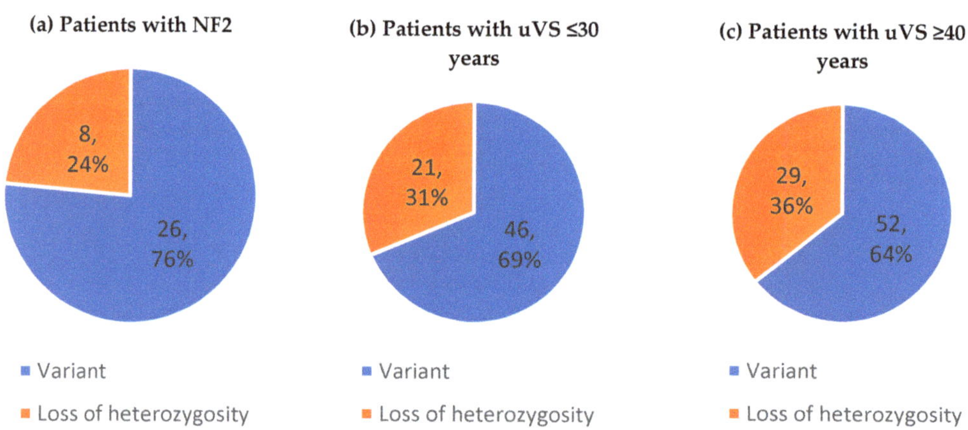

Figure 2. Total number of mutational events detected in vestibular schwannomas in (**a**) patients with NF2, (**b**) young patients with uVS (≤30 years), and (**c**) older patients with uVS (≥40 years). Legend: NF2 = *NF2*-related schwannomatosis; and uVS = unilateral vestibular schwannoma.

Nucleotide variants were primarily identified in *NF2* in comparison to other genes (Table 3). Tumors from younger patients with uVS harbored the greatest diversity of variants, namely in *NF2* (n = 40; 85%), *SMARCB1* (n = 3; 6%), *TSC1* (n = 2; 4%), *LZTR1* (n = 1; 2%), and *NF1* (n = 1; 2%). In the *NF2* gene, a substitution was predominant in patients with NF2 compared to a frameshift deletion in older patients with uVS. Nonsense variants were most frequently identified in NF2-related tumors, while frameshift variants predominated in patients with uVS.

Table 3. Detailed description of nucleotide variants identified in vestibular schwannomas.

Variants	Patients with NF2	Patients with uVS ≤30 Years	Patients with uVS ≥40 Years
Gene, *n* (%)			
NF2	25 (96.2)	40 (85.1)	48 (92.3)
LZTR1	0	1 (2.1)	0
SMARCB1	1 (3.8)	3 (6.4)	2 (3.8)
Other	0	3 (6.4)	2 (3.8)
Type of *NF2* variant, *n* (%)			
Substitution	14 (56.0)	17 (48.6)	18 (38.3)
Duplication	1 (4.0)	2 (5.7)	3 (6.4)
Insertion	0	0	1 (2.1)
Deletion	8 (32.0)	14 (40.0)	23 (48.9)
Deletion/insertion	1 (4.0)	2 (5.7)	2 (4.3)
Large deletion	1 (4.0)	0	0
Unknown (c.?)	0	4	1
Effect of *NF2* variant, *n* (%)			
Missense	2 (8.3)	1 (2.9)	2 (4.4)
Splice site	5 (20.8)	4 (11.8)	6 (13.3)
Frameshift	7 (29.2)	15 (44.1)	23 (51.1)
Nonsense	9 (37.5)	13 (38.2)	12 (26.7)
Deletion	1 (4.2)	0	0
Deletion/insertion	0	1 (2.9)	1 (2.2)
Silent	0	0	1 (2.2)
Unknown (p.?)	0	5	3
Variant location on *NF2*, *n* (%)			
Exon 1	1 (4.0)	2 (5.1)	4 (8.3)
Exons 2–7	12 (48.0)	16 (41.0)	22 (45.8)
Exons 8–13	11 (44.0)	15 (38.5)	15 (31.3)
Exons 14–16	1 (4.0)	6 (15.4)	7 (14.6)

Pathogenicity classification according to the American College of Medical Genetics and Genomics [47]. Legend: NF2 = *NF2*-related schwannomatosis; uVS = unilateral vestibular schwannoma; and *n* = number of cases.

All five patients with NF2 that had an identifiable germline variant also had a second NF2-related pathogenic hit in the tumor (Table 4). In two out of the five tumors (40%), a truncation was identified.

Table 4. Pathogenic tumor variants in patients with *NF2*-related schwannomatosis with identified germline NF2 variants.

No.	First (Germline) *NF2* Hit [1]	Second Hit in Tumor	Third Hit in Tumor
02	c.1132G>, p.Glu378*	NF2 (exon 12): c.558_561delGAGA, p.Arg187Leufs*	LOH
04	c.702dupT, p.Gly235Trpfs*	*NF2* (exon 12): c.1331C > A, p.Ser444*	n.a.
06	c.1341-2A > G, p.?	LOH	n.a.
07	c.del22q12.1q12.2, p.?	*NF2* (exon 7): c.632C > A, p.Ala211Asp	n.a.
15	c.892C > T, p.Gln298*	LOH	n.a.

[1] Germline details in Table 2. Legend: No. = patient number; LOH = loss of heterozygosity; and n.a. = not applicable.

3.4. Age Differences in NF2

An additional subgroup analysis was performed on the NF2 cohort, based on their age of diagnosis in relation to the group's median age. Young patients with NF2 (<33.7 years) had a more severe clinical phenotype compared to older patients with NF2 (>33.7 years) with respect to their vital status (deceased, % = 38 vs. 0), the presence of meningiomas (patients, % = 100 vs. 38), and the total tumor load (tumor count, median = 15 vs. 5).

The genetic analysis showed that younger patients with NF2 were more likely to harbor a nucleotide variant in *NF2* as the second hit (patients, % = 63 vs. 38), had a higher variant pathogenicity (classification, mean = 4.1 vs. 3.8), and carried more truncating variants in the tumor (variants, % = 73 vs. 50). On the other hand, LOH was less prevalent in the younger NF2 subgroup (patients, % = 50 vs. 71).

3.5. Sequencing Statistics

An average sequencing coverage of 94.6% (range 92.3–98.9%) for the coding sequences of *NF2*, *LZTR1*, and *SMARCB1* was achieved. Targeted bases were sequenced at least 150 times with an average of >1000 reads. Further details are provided in the RCPL source file [45].

4. Discussion

In the present study, causative genetic alterations of vestibular schwannomas were investigated from patients with NF2, young patients with uVS (age $\leq$ 30 years), and older patients with uVS (age $\geq$ 40 years). All patients showed pathogenic gene variants located in *NF2*, underlining its central role as a driver in the pathogenesis of NF2-related and sporadic vestibular schwannomas [24,27].

However, our results also show genetic differences between the study groups. Patients with *NF2*-related schwannomatosis had an even distribution of samples with either two distinct *NF2* variants or one *NF2* variant and LOH of chromosome 22 (44%), whereas patients with uVS predominantly possessed one *NF2* variant with LOH (53–59%). The frequency of LOH also varied across study groups. Previously reported rates in patients with uVS ranged between 53% and 75% [24,27,31,37,48]. In patients with NF2, a slightly lower range of 45% to 67% was described [26,27,49]. Here, we detected similar rates of LOH: 62% for NF2-related tumors, 68% for young patients with uVS, and up to 73% in older patients with uVS. These findings support the hypothesis that biallelic inactivation of the *NF2* gene is required for the tumorigenesis of vestibular schwannoma, yet they also point out possible different mutational pathways observed in patients with NF2 and patients with uVS [24–26,31]. One possible explanation may be the unique timing of mutational events, as patients with NF2 already harbor pathogenic *NF2* variants during the embryonic stage. However, other explanations such as intronic variants, copy-neutral LOH, or technical limitations of panel-based NGS should also be considered.

In total, nucleotide variants constituted 76% of the mutational hits in patients with NF2, 69% in younger patients with uVS, and 64% in older patients with uVS. As with most tumor-suppressor genes, most mutations in *NF2* were predicted to truncate (by nonsense or frameshift) or shorten (by incorrect splicing) the protein product. Truncating variations were most prevalent across all three study groups, yet a difference was observed in the truncation type. Nonsense variants were predominant over frameshift variants in patients with NF2, in line with previous studies on patients with NF2 [19,50]. On the other hand, frameshift variants were more prevalent in patients with uVS and the ratio of frameshift to nonsense variants substantially increased with an older age in patients with uVS [26,37,48]. This is in agreement with the hypothesis that age-related increase in mutagenesis and decreased potential for DNA repair lead to an altered mutational pattern [37,41,48]. Splice-site *NF2* variants are the second most common mutational hit after truncation. This was also visible in our data. Interestingly, substantial phenotypic variability can be observed between splice-site variants [16,18,51,52]. Our sample size was too small to test for such phenotypic differences. Missense variants are less common, but occur somewhat more frequently in NF2-related tumors than their unilateral counterpart [53,54].

The exon location of pathogenic variants alone has also been linked to specific NF2 genotype–phenotypes, with variants detected towards the 5′ end of *NF2* being associated with a more severe phenotype [18]. In uVS, a similar trend towards the 5′ end has been observed [55]. In all three our study groups, the majority of patients harbored nucleotide variants of *NF2* towards the 5′ end. A correlation with their clinical phenotype was beyond the scope of this research.

In a minority of tumors found across all patient subgroups, the pathogenic gene variants in *NF2* were accompanied by variants in other genes, such as *LZTR1* and *SMARCB1*, two candidate genes for an alternative diagnosis of 22q-related schwannomatosis (SWN), and tumor suppressor gene *TSC1*, which may function as a co-factor in tumorigenesis. While this highlights the genetic heterogeneity in the tumorigenesis of vestibular schwannomas [33,35], the detection rates of genetic variants in genes other than *NF2* remain low and vary across studies [33,35,48,50,56].

This study has several limitations. All patients in the present study received surgery, thus introducing selection bias towards a more severe phenotype which required surgical intervention. Additionally, the sample size of the groups of patients with NF2 was relatively small, inherent to the rarity of NF2. We performed statistical comparisons for all variables possible, yet, due to a lack of power, we were not able to demonstrate statistically significant results. Furthermore, the reliance on archival tumor samples (the oldest sample dating back to 1997) for genetic analysis may have introduced potential biases related to sample quality, tissue preservation methods, and variations in sequencing techniques over time. Lastly, variability in sequencing techniques across patients could have introduced underestimations or inconsistencies in variant detection and interpretation.

Despite these limitations, several strengths can also be identified. First, the inclusion of three distinct patient groups—patients with NF2, younger patients with uVS ($\leq$30 years), and older patients with uVS ($\geq$40 years)—provided a valuable evaluation of vestibular schwannomas across different age groups and disease subtypes. Second, the incorporation of both germline and tumor DNA analysis provided insights into both hereditary and somatic genetic events contributing to vestibular schwannoma tumorigenesis.

NF2-related schwannomatosis is a disease characterized by considerable clinical variation, with patients who present with progressive tumors at a young age and others who present with limited, slowly progressive disease at an older age. This is highlighted by the genetic differences found in the present young and old NF2 subgroups. In the present study, no young patient with uVS harbored a germline *NF2* variant. The mutational hits and number of mutational events appeared to be more similar to older patients with uVS than to patients with NF2. Therefore, the expectation is that few young patients with uVS actually harbored *NF2*-related schwannomatosis. A follow-up analysis with age-matched patients with uVS could provide further insights into the unique genetic characteristics of vestibular schwannomas across disease subtypes and severities, while it may also help predict the risk of developing bVS at a later point in life.

5. Conclusions

Our study contributes to a better understanding of the genetic alterations in vestibular schwannomas across different disease subtypes and age groups. In all three study groups, biallelic inactivation of the *NF2* gene was the main cause of vestibular schwannoma tumorigenesis. However, in patients with NF2, we found an even distribution of either pathogenic gene variants in both *NF2* copies or one pathogenic variant together with the LOH of chromosome 22. Meanwhile, in patients with uVS, we most frequently observed a single pathogenic *NF2* variant in combination with LOH. In addition, truncating variations were the most prevalent across subgroups, yet a difference was observed in the truncation type: nonsense variants were over-represented in patients with NF2, whereas frameshift variants were more prevalent in uVS.

Supplementary Materials: The following supporting information can be downloaded at https://www.mdpi.com/article/10.3390/cancers17030393/s1, Table S1: Patient characteristics and genetics.

Author Contributions: Conceptualization, J.P.J.D., E.A. and E.F.H.; methodology, J.P.J.D., R.v.E., S.L.N.M., E.A. and E.F.H.; validation, J.P.J.D. and R.v.E.; formal analysis, J.P.J.D.; investigation, J.P.J.D. and R.v.E.; resources, J.P.J.D., R.v.E., S.L.N.M., J.C.J., E.A. and E.F.H.; data curation, J.P.J.D. and R.v.E.; writing—original draft preparation, J.P.J.D.; writing—review and editing, J.P.J.D., R.v.E., S.L.N.M., J.C.J., E.A. and E.F.H.; visualization, J.P.J.D.; supervision, R.v.E., J.C.J., E.A. and E.F.H.; and project administration, J.P.J.D. All authors have read and agreed to the published version of the manuscript.

Funding: This research received no external funding.

Institutional Review Board Statement: This study was conducted in accordance with the Declaration of Helsinki and approved by the Institutional Review Board of Leiden University Medical Center (nWMO-div3, ref. 23-3032, 24 April 2023).

Informed Consent Statement: Informed consent was obtained from all the subjects involved in this study.

Data Availability Statement: The original contributions presented in this study are included in the Supplementary Materials. Further inquiries can be directed to the corresponding authors.

Conflicts of Interest: The authors declare no conflicts of interest.

References

1. Evans, D.G.; Moran, A.; King, A.; Saeed, S.; Gurusinghe, N.; Ramsden, R. Incidence of Vestibular Schwannoma and Neurofibromatosis 2 in the North West of England over a 10-year Period: Higher Incidence than Previously Thought. *Otol. Neurotol.* **2005**, *26*, 93–97. [CrossRef] [PubMed]
2. Kleijwegt, M.; Ho, V.; Visser, O.; Godefroy, W.; van der Mey, A. Real Incidence of Vestibular Schwannoma? Estimations From a National Registry. *Otol. Neurotol.* **2016**, *37*, 1411–1417. [CrossRef]
3. Kshettry, V.R.; Hsieh, J.K.; Ostrom, Q.T.; Kruchko, C.; Barnholtz-Sloan, J.S. Incidence of vestibular schwannomas in the United States. *J. Neurooncol.* **2015**, *124*, 223–228. [CrossRef]
4. Matthies, C.; Samii, M. Management of 1000 Vestibular Schwannomas (Acoustic Neuromas): Clinical Presentation. *Neurosurgery* **1997**, *40*, 1–10. [CrossRef] [PubMed]
5. Kentala, E.; Pyykkö, I. Clinical picture of vestibular schwannoma. *Auris Nasus Larynx* **2001**, *28*, 15–22. [CrossRef] [PubMed]
6. Kanzaki, J.; Tos, M.; Sanna, M.; Moffat, D.A. New and Modified Reporting Systems from the Consensus Meeting on Systems for Reporting Results in Vestibular Schwannoma. *Otol. Neurotol.* **2003**, *24*, 642–649. [CrossRef] [PubMed]
7. Goldbrunner, R.; Weller, M.; Regis, J.; Lund-Johansen, M.; Stavrinou, P.; Reuss, D.; Evans, D.G.; Lefranc, F.; Sallabanda, K.; Falini, A.; et al. EANO guideline on the diagnosis and treatment of vestibular schwannoma. *Neuro Oncol.* **2020**, *22*, 31–45. [CrossRef] [PubMed]
8. Robinett, Z.N.; Walz, P.C.; Miles-Markley, B.; Moberly, A.C.; Welling, D.B. Comparison of Long-term Quality-of-Life Outcomes in Vestibular Schwannoma Patients. *Otolaryngol. Head Neck Surg.* **2014**, *150*, 1024–1032. [CrossRef]
9. Carlson, M.L.; Tveiten, O.V.; Driscoll, C.L.; Goplen, F.K.; Neff, B.A.; Pollock, B.E.; Tombers, N.M.; Castner, M.L.; Finnkirk, M.K.; Myrseth, E.; et al. Long-term quality of life in patients with vestibular schwannoma: An international multicenter cross-sectional study comparing microsurgery, stereotactic radiosurgery, observation, and nontumor controls. *J. Neurosurg.* **2015**, *122*, 833–842. [CrossRef] [PubMed]
10. Soulier, G.; van Leeuwen, B.M.; Putter, H.; Jansen, J.C.; Malessy, M.J.A.; van Benthem, P.P.G.; van der Mey, A.G.L.; Stiggelbout, A.M. Quality of Life in 807 Patients with Vestibular Schwannoma: Comparing Treatment Modalities. *Otolaryngol. Head Neck Surg.* **2017**, *157*, 92–98. [CrossRef]
11. Evans, D.G. Neurofibromatosis 2. In *GeneReviews(R)*; Adam, M.P., Ardinger, H.H., Pagon, R.A., Wallace, S.E., Bean, L.J.H., Gripp, K.W., Mirzaa, G.M., Amemiya, A., Eds.; University of Washington: Seattle, WA, USA, 1993.

12. Plotkin, S.R.; Messiaen, L.; Legius, E.; Pancza, P.; Avery, R.A.; Blakeley, J.O.; Babovic-Vuksanovic, D.; Ferner, R.; Fisher, M.J.; Friedman, J.M.; et al. Updated diagnostic criteria and nomenclature for neurofibromatosis type 2 and schwannomatosis: An international consensus recommendation. *Genet. Med.* **2022**, *24*, 1967–1977. [CrossRef]
13. Evans, D.G.; Howard, E.; Giblin, C.; Clancy, T.; Spencer, H.; Huson, S.M.; Lalloo, F. Birth incidence and prevalence of tumor-prone syndromes: Estimates from a UK family genetic register service. *Am. J. Med. Genet. A* **2010**, *152A*, 327–332. [CrossRef]
14. Blakeley, J.O.; Evans, D.G.; Adler, J.; Brackmann, D.; Chen, R.; Ferner, R.E.; Hanemann, C.O.; Harris, G.; Huson, S.M.; Jacob, A.; et al. Consensus recommendations for current treatments and accelerating clinical trials for patients with neurofibromatosis type 2. *Am. J. Med. Genet. A* **2012**, *158A*, 24–41. [CrossRef]
15. Hornigold, R.E.; Golding, J.F.; Leschziner, G.; Obholzer, R.; Gleeson, M.J.; Thomas, N.; Walsh, D.; Saeed, S.; Ferner, R.E. The NFTI-QOL: A Disease-Specific Quality of Life Questionnaire for Neurofibromatosis 2. *J. Neurol. Surg. Part B Skull Base* **2012**, *73*, 104–111. [CrossRef]
16. Hexter, A.; Jones, A.; Joe, H.; Heap, L.; Smith, M.J.; Wallace, A.J.; Halliday, D.; Parry, A.; Taylor, A.; Raymond, L.; et al. Clinical and molecular predictors of mortality in neurofibromatosis 2: A UK national analysis of 1192 patients. *J. Med. Genet.* **2015**, *52*, 699–705. [CrossRef] [PubMed]
17. Ruggieri, M.; Iannetti, P.; Polizzi, A.; La Mantia, I.; Spalice, A.; Giliberto, O.; Platania, N.; Gabriele, A.L.; Albanese, V.; Pavone, L. Earliest clinical manifestations and natural history of neurofibromatosis type 2 (NF2) in childhood: A study of 24 patients. *Neuropediatrics* **2005**, *36*, 21–34. [CrossRef] [PubMed]
18. Halliday, D.; Emmanouil, B.; Pretorius, P.; MacKeith, S.; Painter, S.; Tomkins, H.; Evans, D.G.; Parry, A. Genetic Severity Score predicts clinical phenotype in NF2. *J. Med. Genet.* **2017**, *54*, 657–664. [CrossRef]
19. Evans, D.G.; Hartley, C.L.; Smith, P.T.; King, A.T.; Bowers, N.L.; Tobi, S.; Wallace, A.J.; Perry, M.; Anup, R.; Lloyd, S.K.W.; et al. Incidence of mosaicism in 1055 de novo NF2 cases: Much higher than previous estimates with high utility of next-generation sequencing. *Genet. Med.* **2020**, *22*, 53–59. [CrossRef]
20. de Vries, M.; van der Mey, A.G.L.; Hogendoorn, P.C.W. Tumor Biology of Vestibular Schwannoma: A Review of Experimental Data on the Determinants of Tumor Genesis and Growth Characteristics. *Otol. Neurotol.* **2015**, *36*, 1128–1136. [CrossRef]
21. Chiasson-MacKenzie, C.; Vitte, J.; Liu, C.-H.; Wright, E.A.; Flynn, E.A.; Stott, S.L.; Giovannini, M.; McClatchey, A.I. Cellular mechanisms of heterogeneity in NF2-mutant schwannoma. *Nat. Commun.* **2023**, *14*, 1559. [CrossRef] [PubMed]
22. Barrett, T.F.; Patel, B.; Khan, S.M.; Mullins, R.D.Z.; Yim, A.K.Y.; Pugazenthi, S.; Mahlokozera, T.; Zipfel, G.J.; Herzog, J.A.; Chicoine, M.R.; et al. Single-cell multi-omic analysis of the vestibular schwannoma ecosystem uncovers a nerve injury-like state. *Nat. Commun.* **2024**, *15*, 478. [CrossRef]
23. Woods, R.; Friedman, J.M.; Evans, D.G.R.; Baser, M.E.; Joe, H. Exploring the "two-hit hypothesis" in NF2: Tests of two-hit and three-hit models of vestibular schwannoma development. *Genet. Epidemiol.* **2003**, *24*, 265–272. [CrossRef]
24. Carlson, M.L.; Smadbeck, J.B.; Link, M.J.; Klee, E.W.; Vasmatzis, G.; Schimmenti, L.A. Next Generation Sequencing of Sporadic Vestibular Schwannoma: Necessity of Biallelic NF2 Inactivation and Implications of Accessory Non-NF2 Variants. *Otol. Neurotol.* **2018**, *39*, e860–e871. [CrossRef] [PubMed]
25. Kehrer-Sawatzki, H.; Farschtschi, S.; Mautner, V.-F.; Cooper, D.N. The molecular pathogenesis of schwannomatosis, a paradigm for the co-involvement of multiple tumour suppressor genes in tumorigenesis. *Hum. Genet.* **2017**, *136*, 129–148. [CrossRef] [PubMed]
26. Hadfield, K.D.; Smith, M.J.; Urquhart, J.E.; Wallace, A.J.; Bowers, N.L.; King, A.T.; Rutherford, S.A.; Trump, D.; Newman, W.G.; Evans, D.G. Rates of loss of heterozygosity and mitotic recombination in NF2 schwannomas, sporadic vestibular schwannomas and schwannomatosis schwannomas. *Oncogene* **2010**, *29*, 6216–6221. [CrossRef]
27. Hexter, A.T.; Evans, D.G. The Genetics of Vestibular Schwannoma. *Curr. Otorhinolaryngol. Rep.* **2014**, *2*, 226–234. [CrossRef]
28. Trofatter, J.A.; MacCollin, M.M.; Rutter, J.L.; Murrell, J.R.; Duyao, M.P.; Parry, D.M.; Eldridge, R.; Kley, N.; Menon, A.G.; Pulaski, K.; et al. A novel moesin-, ezrin-, radixin-like gene is a candidate for the neurofibromatosis 2 tumor suppressor. *Cell* **1993**, *72*, 791–800. [CrossRef]
29. Kim, H.; Kwak, N.-J.; Lee, J.Y.; Choi, B.H.; Lim, Y.; Ko, Y.J.; Kim, Y.-H.; Huh, P.-W.; Lee, K.-H.; Rha, H.K.; et al. Merlin Neutralizes the Inhibitory Effect of Mdm2 on p53. *J. Biol. Chem.* **2004**, *279*, 7812–7818. [CrossRef] [PubMed]
30. Jones, G.N.; Tep, C.; Towns, W.H.; Mihai, G.; Tonks, I.D.; Kay, G.F.; Schmalbrock, P.M.; Stemmer-Rachamimov, A.O.; Yoon, S.O.; Kirschner, L.S. Tissue-Specific Ablation of Prkar1a Causes Schwannomas by Suppressing Neurofibromatosis Protein Production. *Neoplasia* **2008**, *10*, 1213-IN1219. [CrossRef]
31. Lassaletta, L.; Torres-Martín, M.; Peña-Granero, C.; Roda, J.M.; Santa-Cruz-Ruiz, S.; Castresana, J.S.; Gavilan, J.; Rey, J.A. NF2 Genetic Alterations in Sporadic Vestibular Schwannomas: Clinical Implications. *Otol. Neurotol.* **2013**, *34*, 1355–1361. [CrossRef] [PubMed]
32. Piotrowski, A.; Xie, J.; Liu, Y.F.; Poplawski, A.B.; Gomes, A.R.; Madanecki, P.; Fu, C.; Crowley, M.R.; Crossman, D.K.; Armstrong, L.; et al. Germline loss-of-function mutations in LZTR1 predispose to an inherited disorder of multiple schwannomas. *Nat. Genet.* **2014**, *46*, 182–187. [CrossRef]

33. Agnihotri, S.; Jalali, S.; Wilson, M.R.; Danesh, A.; Li, M.; Klironomos, G.; Krieger, J.R.; Mansouri, A.; Khan, O.; Mamatjan, Y.; et al. The genomic landscape of schwannoma. *Nat. Genet.* **2016**, *48*, 1339–1348. [CrossRef]
34. Pathmanaban, O.N.; Sadler, K.V.; Kamaly-Asl, I.D.; King, A.T.; Rutherford, S.A.; Hammerbeck-Ward, C.; McCabe, M.G.; Kilday, J.-P.; Beetz, C.; Poplawski, N.K.; et al. Association of Genetic Predisposition with Solitary Schwannoma or Meningioma in Children and Young Adults. *JAMA Neurol.* **2017**, *74*, 1123–1129. [CrossRef] [PubMed]
35. Håvik, A.L.; Bruland, O.; Myrseth, E.; Miletic, H.; Aarhus, M.; Knappskog, P.-M.; Lund-Johansen, M. Genetic landscape of sporadic vestibular schwannoma. *J. Neurosurg.* **2018**, *128*, 911–922. [CrossRef] [PubMed]
36. Evans, D.; Ramsden, R.; Gokhale, C.; Bowers, N.; Huson, S.; Wallace, A. Should NF2 mutation screening be undertaken in patients with an apparently isolated vestibular schwannoma? *Clin. Genet.* **2007**, *71*, 354–358. [CrossRef] [PubMed]
37. Mohyuddin, A.; Neary, W.J.; Wallace, A.; Wu, C.L.; Purcell, S.; Reid, H.; Ramsden, R.T.; Read, A.; Black, G.; Evans, D.G.R. Molecular genetic analysis of the NF2 gene in young patients with unilateral vestibular schwannomas. *J. Med. Genet.* **2002**, *39*, 315–322. [CrossRef] [PubMed]
38. Evans, D.G.; Wallace, A.J.; Wu, C.L.; Trueman, L.; Ramsden, R.T.; Strachan, T. Somatic Mosaicism: A Common Cause of Classic Disease in Tumor-Prone Syndromes? Lessons from Type 2 Neurofibromatosis. *Am. J. Hum. Genet.* **1998**, *63*, 727–736. [CrossRef]
39. Marinelli, J.P.; Lohse, C.M.; Carlson, M.L. Incidence of Vestibular Schwannoma over the Past Half-Century: A Population-Based Study of Olmsted County, Minnesota. *Otolaryngol. Head Neck Surg.* **2018**, *159*, 717–723. [CrossRef] [PubMed]
40. Evans, D.G.; Maher, E.R.; Baser, M.E. Age related shift in the mutation spectra of germline and somatic NF2 mutations: Hypothetical role of DNA repair mechanisms. *J. Med. Genet.* **2005**, *42*, 630–632. [CrossRef]
41. Evans, D.G.; Raymond, F.L.; Barwell, J.G.; Halliday, D. Genetic testing and screening of individuals at risk of NF2. *Clin. Genet.* **2012**, *82*, 416–424. [CrossRef] [PubMed]
42. Halliday, D.; Emmanouil, B.; Evans, D.G.R. Updated protocol for genetic testing, screening and clinical management of individuals at risk of NF2-related schwannomatosis. *Clin. Genet.* **2023**, *103*, 540–552. [CrossRef]
43. Goodwin, S.; McPherson, J.D.; McCombie, W.R. Coming of age: Ten years of next-generation sequencing technologies. *Nat. Rev. Genet.* **2016**, *17*, 333–351. [CrossRef]
44. COREON. Code of Conduct for Health Research. 2022. Available online: https://www.coreon.org/wp-content/uploads/2023/06/Code-of-Conduct-for-Health-Research-2022.pdf (accessed on 2 December 2024).
45. Leiden University Medical Center. *Rare Cancer Panel*; Department of Pathology, Leiden University Medical Center: Leiden, The Netherlands, 2023; pp. 1–3. Available online: https://www.palga.nl/media/uploads/pdf/5/8/581_136-rcpl-lumc.pdf (accessed on 2 December 2024).
46. Richards, S.; Aziz, N.; Bale, S.; Bick, D.; Das, S.; Gastier-Foster, J.; Grody, W.W.; Hegde, M.; Lyon, E.; Spector, E.; et al. Standards and guidelines for the interpretation of sequence variants: A joint consensus recommendation of the American College of Medical Genetics and Genomics and the Association for Molecular Pathology. *Genet. Med.* **2015**, *17*, 405–423. [CrossRef]
47. Karbassi, I.; Maston, G.A.; Love, A.; DiVincenzo, C.; Braastad, C.D.; Elzinga, C.D.; Bright, A.R.; Previte, D.; Zhang, K.; Rowland, C.M.; et al. A Standardized DNA Variant Scoring System for Pathogenicity Assessments in Mendelian Disorders. *Hum. Mutat.* **2016**, *37*, 127–134. [CrossRef] [PubMed]
48. Sadler, K.V.; Bowers, N.L.; Hartley, C.; Smith, P.T.; Tobi, S.; Wallace, A.J.; King, A.; Lloyd, S.K.W.; Rutherford, S.; Pathmanaban, O.N.; et al. Sporadic vestibular schwannoma: A molecular testing summary. *J. Med. Genet.* **2021**, *58*, 227–233. [CrossRef]
49. Kluwe, L.; Friedrich, R.E.; Hagel, C.; Lindenau, M.; Mautner, V.-F. Mutations and Allelic Loss of the NF2 Gene in Neurofibromatosis 2-Associated Skin Tumors. *J. Investig. Dermatol.* **2000**, *114*, 1017–1021. [CrossRef] [PubMed]
50. Teranishi, Y.; Miyawaki, S.; Hongo, H.; Dofuku, S.; Okano, A.; Takayanagi, S.; Ota, T.; Yoshimura, J.; Qu, W.; Mitsui, J.; et al. Targeted deep sequencing of DNA from multiple tissue types improves the diagnostic rate and reveals a highly diverse phenotype of mosaic neurofibromatosis type 2. *J. Med. Genet.* **2021**, *58*, 701–711. [CrossRef] [PubMed]
51. Kluwe, L.; MacCollin, M.; Tatagiba, M.; Thomas, S.; Hazim, W.; Haase, W.; Mautner, V.-F. Phenotypic variability associated with 14 splice-site mutations in the NF2 Gene. *Am. J. Med. Genet.* **1998**, *77*, 228–233. [CrossRef]
52. Baser, M.E.; Kuramoto, L.; Woods, R.; Joe, H.; Friedman, J.M.; Wallace, A.J.; Ramsden, R.T.; Olschwang, S.; Bijlsma, E.; Kalamarides, M.; et al. The location of constitutional neurofibromatosis 2 (NF2) splice site mutations is associated with the severity of NF2. *J. Med. Genet.* **2005**, *42*, 540–546. [CrossRef] [PubMed]
53. Chen, H.; Zhang, X.; Zhang, Z.; Yang, T.; Wang, Z.; Wu, H. The role of NF2 gene mutations and pathogenesis-related proteins in sporadic vestibular schwannomas in young individuals. *Mol. Cell. Biochem.* **2014**, *392*, 145–152. [CrossRef] [PubMed]
54. Sadler, K.V.; Rowlands, C.F.; Smith, P.T.; Hartley, C.L.; Bowers, N.L.; Roberts, N.Y.; Harris, J.L.; Wallace, A.J.; Evans, D.G.; Messiaen, L.M.; et al. Re-evaluation of missense variant classifications in NF2. *Hum. Mutat.* **2022**, *43*, 643–654. [CrossRef] [PubMed]

55. Ahronowitz, I.; Xin, W.; Kiely, R.; Sims, K.; MacCollin, M.; Nunes, F.P. Mutational spectrum of the NF2 gene: A meta-analysis of 12 years of research and diagnostic laboratory findings. *Hum. Mutat.* **2007**, *28*, 1–12. [CrossRef] [PubMed]
56. Louvrier, C.; Pasmant, E.; Briand-Suleau, A.; Cohen, J.; Nitschké, P.; Nectoux, J.; Orhant, L.; Zordan, C.; Goizet, C.; Goutagny, S.; et al. Targeted next-generation sequencing for differential diagnosis of neurofibromatosis type 2, schwannomatosis, and meningiomatosis. *Neuro Oncol.* **2018**, *20*, 917–929. [CrossRef]

cancers

MDPI

Systematic Review

Efficacy and Toxicity of Bevacizumab in Children with NF2-Related Schwannomatosis: A Systematic Review

Annemijn L. Tops [1,*], Josefine E. Schopman [2], Radboud W. Koot [3], Hans Gelderblom [2], Nabila A. Putri [4], Latifah N. A. Rahmi [5], Jeroen C. Jansen [1] and Erik F. Hensen [1]

1 Department of Otorhinolaryngology—Head and Neck Surgery, Leiden University Medical Center, 2333 ZA Leiden, The Netherlands; e.f.hensen@lumc.nl (E.F.H.)
2 Department of Medical Oncology, Leiden University Medical Center, 2333 ZA Leiden, The Netherlands; j.e.schopman@lumc.nl (J.E.S.); a.j.gelderblom@lumc.nl (H.G.)
3 Department of Neurosurgery, Leiden University Medical Center, 2333 ZA Leiden, The Netherlands
4 School of Medicine and Health Sciences, Atma Jaya Catholic University of Indonesia, Jakarta 14440, Indonesia
5 Faculty of Medicine, Universitas Indonesia, Jakarta 10430, Indonesia
* Correspondence: a.l.tops@lumc.nl

Simple Summary: This systematic review investigates the effect of bevacizumab in pediatric patients with NF2-related schwannomatosis (NF2), a tumor predisposition syndrome characterized by the occurrence of multiple schwannomas, meningiomas, and/or ependymomas, with bilateral vestibular schwannomas as the hallmark lesion. While bevacizumab has demonstrated effectiveness in reducing the size of (vestibular) schwannomas and improving hearing in adults, its efficacy in children remains underexplored. Through a comprehensive review of the existing literature, we found that the majority of the reported pediatric patients experienced regression or stabilization of the target tumor. A considerable number of pediatric patients experienced hearing stabilization or even improvement. Bevacizumab was relatively well tolerated, with only a few reported severe adverse effects. These findings suggest that bevacizumab offers a promising, non-invasive therapeutic option for progressive (vestibular) schwannomas and/or hearing loss in children with NF2.

Abstract: Background/Objectives: NF2-related schwannomatosis (NF2) is a tumor predisposition syndrome that typically presents with bilateral vestibular schwannomas, together with other intracranial and spinal schwannomas, meningiomas, and/or ependymomas. Bevacizumab, a VEGF inhibitor, has the potential to decrease schwannoma volume and improve hearing in adults, but the literature on the effects in children is sparse. This narrative review aims to evaluate the use of bevacizumab in pediatric NF2 patients, focusing on hearing, tumor progression, and toxicity. Methods: A literature review was conducted following PRISMA guidelines. Articles were searched in PubMed, Embase, Web of Science, Cochrane Library, Emcare, and Academic Search Premier on 18 July 2024. Inclusion criteria were patients $\leq$ 18 years, diagnosed with NF2 and treated with bevacizumab. Two authors independently assessed the quality of the evidence and extracted relevant data from the included articles. Results: Seventeen articles including 62 pediatric NF2 patients met the inclusion criteria. Studies varied widely in treatment regimens and outcome parameters. Tumor regression was reported in 6/56 patients (11%) and 38/56 (68%) remained stable. Hearing improved in 15/45 patients (33%) and did not further deteriorate in 27/45 (60%). An improvement in other symptoms was seen in 6/29 patients (28%). Toxicity was reported in five studies, documenting 13 adverse events in 28 patients ranging from grade 1 to grade 3. Treatment was discontinued in both patients who experienced grade 3 toxicity. Conclusions: Bevacizumab seems to be a viable treatment option for pediatric NF2 patients. Tumor regression or stabilization is achieved in the majority of patients (77%). Moreover, a considerable number of pediatric patients experience hearing

https://doi.org/10.3390/cancers17030519

stabilization or improvement (93%). Bevacizumab appears to be relatively well tolerated, offering a non-invasive therapeutic option for children with NF2 suffering from progressive vestibular schwannomas and hearing loss.

Keywords: neurofibromatosis type 2; schwannomatosis; bevacizumab; vestibular schwannoma; children; tumor response; adverse events; hearing

1. Introduction

NF2-related schwannomatosis (NF2, formerly neurofibromatosis type 2) is a rare, autosomal dominant tumor predisposition syndrome caused by a mutation in the NF2 gene. The incidence is estimated to be between 1 in 25,000 to 33,000 in the United Kingdom and 1 in 87,410 in Finland [1,2]. NF2 typically presents with bilateral vestibular schwannomas but is associated with numerous other tumors, including meningiomas, ependymomas, and intracranial, intraspinal, and peripheral schwannomas [3]. The clinical phenotype varies widely, depending on the type of genetic mutation [4]. Symptoms can manifest at any age, but the peak incidence occurs during adolescence and early adulthood, while occurrences in young children are less common [5]. However, when NF2 manifests early in life, it tends to be more severe, with a higher likelihood of developing multiple and progressive tumors [6]. Consequently, optimal management of tumors in pediatric patients is of high importance. In adults, current management options comprise active surveillance, surgery, stereotactic radiotherapy, and pharmacotherapy, and the treatment strategy is tailored to individual patient and tumor characteristics [7–9]. In pediatric patients, however, treatment approaches may differ due to potential long-term adverse events, which are of greater concern in this population [10]. Additionally, because pediatric patients often present with a greater tumor burden, a systemic treatment that targets multiple tumors simultaneously—rather than addressing them individually through surgery or radiotherapy—may be more beneficial.

Bevacizumab, a VEGF inhibitor, has shown promise in reducing both hearing loss and tumor volume, primarily in adult populations [8]. However, evidence regarding its effects on hearing, tumor progression, and toxicity in children is limited. This study aims to provide a comprehensive review of the currently available evidence regarding the use of bevacizumab in pediatric patients with NF2-related schwannomatosis, with a focus on its effects on hearing, tumor progression, and treatment-related toxicity.

2. Materials and Methods

2.1. Search Strategy

Following the PRISMA guidelines, an extensive literature review was performed to analyze the effect and toxicity of bevacizumab in children. Relevant articles were identified in PubMed, Embase, Web of Science, Cochrane Library, Emcare, and Academic Search Premier through a computerized search conducted by an academic librarian. The search strategy included the MeSH terms 'Neurofibromatosis 2' and 'Bevacizumab' along with their corresponding entry terms. The limited amount of available literature allowed the search strategy to remain broad, without narrowing the search with terms such as 'child' or 'pediatric'. This approach ensured that studies comprising both adults and children were included in this search, and pediatric subgroups within these studies were not overlooked and could be included in this review when separate extraction of data for this population was possible. The complete search strategy is listed in Supplementary Table S1. The search was conducted on 18 July 2024, without restrictions on language or date of publication. After removing duplicates, the remaining abstracts were screened independently by two reviewers, and discrepancies were resolved by a third reviewer. Full texts were then assessed for eligibility. This systematic review was not registered and a protocol was not published.

2.2. Inclusion and Exclusion Criteria

Inclusion criteria were (1) patients aged ≤18 years, (2) diagnosed with NF2, (3) treated with bevacizumab, and (4) reported radiological, clinical, and/or hearing outcomes and/or toxicity. Exclusion criteria were (1) studies describing administration of bevacizumab via routes other than intravenous infusion and (2) studies that did not report outcomes specifically for children. Studies that included mixed populations were included if data of the pediatric subgroup could be extracted separately.

2.3. Data Extraction

Data were extracted by two reviewers using a data extraction form. Information collected from each study included the first author, year of publication, study design, total number of patients, and number of pediatric patients. Information collected from each eligible patient included age, gender, dosage, duration of treatment, baseline tumor size, previous treatments, radiographic response, hearing response, clinical response, and complications. In the study where the data were only presented in graphs, data points were extracted manually [11].

2.4. Assessment of Quality and Risk of Bias

Assessment of quality of evidence and risk of bias was assessed by two reviewers independently, and discrepancies were resolved by a third reviewer. The quality of the included cohort studies and case series was assessed using a version of the Newcastle Ottawa Scale, modified for non-comparative case series; see Supplementary Table S1. The quality of included case reports was assessed using the JBI Critical Appraisal Tool for case reports; see Supplementary Table S2.

2.5. Data Analysis

Due to the high level of heterogeneity of the included studies—such as differences in dosage, length of treatment, outcome measures and previous treatments—a meta-analysis on pooled data could not be performed. Consequently, a narrative synthesis was conducted, with an emphasis on summarizing and comparing the findings related to efficacy and toxicity.

3. Results

3.1. Overview of Main Characteristics of Eligible Studies

The search strategy yielded 465 studies. After removing the duplicates, 174 abstracts were screened for eligibility. Subsequently, 129 studies were excluded based on the predefined criteria. After assessing the 45 full articles, 17 articles comprising 62 pediatric NF2 patients remained that met the inclusion criteria. Details on reasons for exclusion are stated in Figure 1.

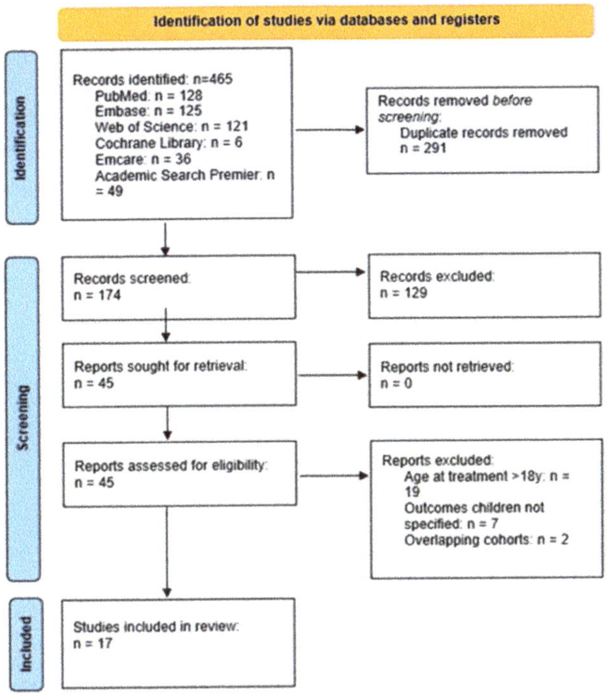

Figure 1. Flowchart illustrating the selection process of the studies according to the Preferred Reporting Items for Systematic Reviews and Meta-Analyses (PRISMA) guidelines.

3.2. Study Characteristics

The seventeen studies were published between 2009 and 2023 with baseline characteristics presented in Table 1. The total number of described patients per study varied between 1 and 61, and the number of pediatric patients fulfilling the inclusion criteria ranged between 1 and 17 per study. Dosage was variable and ranged from 5 to 15 mg/kg every 2 to 4 weeks. Duration of treatment ranged between 3 and 86 months. Baseline tumor size varied between 0.39 and 38.9 cm^3. Previous therapy, either systemic treatment or interventions targeting vestibular schwannomas specifically, was reported in eleven studies [8,11–20].

3.3. Methodological Quality

The results of the critical appraisal tools used are presented in Supplementary Tables S1 and S2. Overall quality was moderate in seven studies and high in ten.

3.4. Radiological Response

Radiological response, as shown in Table 2, was measured in all studies including 62 patients, although the methods for reporting varied widely. Some studies reported the response only in descriptive terms (tumor progression, stable disease, or tumor regression) while other studies included numerical measurements (volume change in percentage or in cm^3). In most studies, progressive disease was defined as >20% increase in tumor volume compared to baseline volume measurements of VS and tumor regression was defined as >20% reduction in tumor volume. One study used linear measurements to assess radiological response [19]. Three studies did not specify whether tumor size was measured using linear or volumetric measurements, nor did they provide baseline tumor measurements [13,15,18].

Table 1. Main characteristics of the studies included in the review.

Study	Design	Pediatric Patients (Total Patients)	Pediatric Patients with Radiological Outcome Reported	Pediatric Patients with Hearing Outcome Reported	Median Age at Treatment (Range; Years)	Gender F (%)	Initial Dosage	Median Duration of Treatment (Range; Months)	Median Baseline Tumor Size (Range)	Previous Treatment for VS
Ardern-Holmes et al., 2021 [21]	Retrospective cohort	4 (11)	4	3	14.5 (13–17)	NS	5–15 mg/kg/2–4 weeks (NS)	13.5 (9–47)	7.6 (1.45–37.9) cm^3	NS
Farschtschi et al., 2016 [22]	Retrospective cohort	2 (8)	2	0	15	0	7.5 mg/kg/3 weeks; 5 mg/kg/2 weeks	34.5 (11–58)	NR	NR
Fuji et al., 2020 [12]	Feasibility study	3 (10)	3	0	18 (12–18)	2 (66)	5 mg/kg/2 weeks	6	5.1 (0.81–16.16) cm^3	SRS (n = 1); SRT (n = 1)
Gugel et al., 2019 [11]	Retrospective cohort	2 (9)	2	1	17.5 (17–18)	2 (100)	5 mg/kg/2 weeks	28 (23–33)	0.4 (0.39–1.17) cm^3	Surgery (n = 2)
Hawasli et al., 2013 [13]	Case series	2 (6)	2	2	15 (14–16)	0	5–10 mg/kg/2–3 weeks (NS)	8.5 (5–12)	NR	Surgery + CI (n = 1); lovastatin (n = 1)
Hochart et al., 2015 [14]	Retrospective cohort	7 (7)	7	4	15.0 (11–18)	4 (57)	5–10 mg/kg/2 weeks	11.3 (3–55)	2.7 (0.4–13.5) cm^3	Surgery (n = 3)
Kim et al., 2022 [15]	Case report	1 (1)	1	0	NR	0	5 mg/kg/2 weeks	6	NR	None
Morris et al., 2016 [23]	Prospective cohort	6 (61)	6	0	NR	NS	5–10 mg/kg/2–3 weeks	NS	5.0 (1.6–8.9) cm^3	NS

Table 1. *Cont.*

Study	Design	Pediatric Patients (Total Patients)	Pediatric Patients with Radiological Outcome Reported	Pediatric Patients with Hearing Outcome Reported	Median Age at Treatment (Range; Years)	Gender F (%)	Initial Dosage	Median Duration of Treatment (Range; Months)	Median Baseline Tumor Size (Range)	Previous Treatment for VS
Nigro et al., 2020 [16]	Case report	1 (1)	1	1	13	0	5 mg/kg/ 3 weeks	108	NR	None
Plotkin et al., 2009 [8]	Retrospective cohort	3 (10)	3	3	18 (16–18)	1 (33)	5 mg/kg/ 2 weeks	13 (8–19)	24.9 (22.6-38.9) cm^3	Erlotinib (n = 2)
Plotkin et al., 2023 [24]	Prospective cohort	6 (20)	6	6	17 (12–18)	4 (67)	5 mg/kg/ 3 weeks *	17 (14.5–18)	NS	NS
Renzi et al., 2020 [17]	Retrospective cohort	17 (17)	17	17	15.8 (10–17)	9 (53)	5–10 mg/kg/ 2–3 weeks	14.6 (3.6–86.4)	NR	Surgery; SRS; RTx and erlotinib/sirolimus
Santoro et al., 2019 [18]	Case report	1 (1)	1	1	13	0	5 mg/kg/ 2 weeks	6	NR	None
Shepard et al., 2012 [19]	Case series	2 (5)	2	2	NR	1 (50)	NR	18	1.7 (1.5–3.9) cm **	Surgery (n = 2)
Subbiah et al., 2012 [25]	Case series	1 (5)	1	1	16	1 (100)	NR	10+	NR	NR
Sverak et al., 2019 [26]	Case series	3 (17)	3	3	17 (15–18)	2 (67)	5–10 mg/kg/ 2–6 weeks (NS)	9 (6–9)	0.3 (0.3–4.5 cm^3	NR
Tripathi et al., 2020 [20]	Case series	1 (2)	1	1	17	1 (100)	NR	8 cycles	10.21 cm^3	GKRS
Total patients		62	62	45						

NR = not reported, NS = not stated specifically for pediatric patients, VS = vestibular schwannoma, GKRS = gamma knife radiosurgery, SRS = stereotactic radiosurgery, SRT = stereotactic radiation therapy, RTx = radiotherapy. * Patients started with an induction dosage of 10q2 and after 6 months switched to maintenance dosage of 5q3; present study includes results on maintenance dosage of 5q3. ** Only linear measurements of tumor size were reported, instead of volumetric measurements.

Table 2. Reported radiological response after treatment with bevacizumab in pediatric patients with NF2-related schwannomatosis.

Study	Tumor Regression (Number of Patients; %)	Change in Tumor Volume (%)	Stable Disease (Number of Patients; %)	Change in Tumor Volume (L/R; %)	Tumor Progression (Number of Patients; %)	Change in Tumor Volume (L/R; %)	Stable Disease or Tumor Progression (Number of Patients; %)	Total Eligible Patients
Ardern-Holmes et al., 2021 [21]			2 (50%)	+17%; +14%	2 (50%)	+30%; +241%		4
Farschtschi et al., 2016 [22]							2 (100%)	2
Fuji et al., 2020 [12]			3 (100%)	+19/−15%; +13/+1%; +6/+2%				3
Gugel et al., 2019 [11]			2 (100%)	+0% *; +23%/+4% *				2
Hawasli et al., 2013 [13]			2 (100%)					2
Hochart et al., 2015 [14]	1 (14%)	−22%	4 (57%)	−17%; +12%; +0%; −3%/−6%	2 (29%)	+51%; +36%/+81%;		7
Kim et al., 2022 [15]			1 (100%)					1
Morris et al., 2016 [23]	1 (17%)						5 (83%)	6
Nigro et al., 2020 [16]			1 (100%)					1
Plotkin et al., 2009 [8]	1 (33%)	−44%	2 (67%)	−5%; −17%				3
Plotkin et al., 2023 [24]			5/10 tumors (50%)		5/10 tumors (50%)			0
Renzi et al., 2020 [17]	2 (12%)		15 (88%)					17

Table 2. *Cont.*

Study	Tumor Regression (Number of Patients; %)	Change in Tumor Volume (%)	Stable Disease (Number of Patients; %)	Change in Tumor Volume (L/R; %)	Tumor Progression (Number of Patients; %)	Change in Tumor Volume (L/R; %)	Stable Disease or Tumor Progression (Number of Patients; %)	Total Eligible Patients
Santoro et al., 2019 [18]			1 (100%)					1
Shepard et al., 2012 [19]			2 (100%)	0%; −15%				2
Subbiah et al., 2012 [25]			1 (100%)					1
Sverak et al., 2019 [26]	1 (33%)	−20%	1 (33%)	−15%	1 (33%)	+74%		3
Tripathi et al., 2020 [20]			1 (100%)					1
Total	6 patients (11%)		38 patients (68%)		5 patients (9%)		7 patients (13%)	56 patients

* = extracted manually from graph.

Radiological response was detailed per patient in all studies except one [24]. In that study, including six pediatric participants and ten corresponding VS, the response was reported per tumor. Of the ten VS, five (50%) showed tumor progression and five (50%) showed stable disease. Since no percentage of patients could be extracted from these data on the specific tumors, results are shown in Table 1 but could not be included in the calculation. In patients with two tumors with different radiological responses, the most favorable response was included [11].

In the sixteen remaining studies, 38 of 56 patients (68%) were reported to have stable disease. Regression in tumor size was reported in six (11%) patients and progressive disease was reported in five (9%). Two studies, comprising seven patients (13%), only reported 'no response', not specifying whether it meant tumor stability or progression of disease [22,23].

3.5. Hearing Response

Thirteen studies assessed hearing response, shown in Table 3. Hearing was described in various ways in these studies. Some reported changes in word recognition score (WRS) in percentage or change in pure tone average (PTA) in decibels (dB), or both. Other studies offered only descriptive outcomes, indicating whether patients experienced progressive hearing loss, stable hearing, or hearing improvement. In most studies, hearing improvement was defined as a >10 dB improvement in PTA or a significant increase in WRS compared to baseline scores. However, two studies adopted stricter definitions, requiring a >20 dB and >12 dB improvement in PTA, respectively [17,24]. Hearing was assessed according to the definition used in the study. In one study, in which hearing was assessed using both PTA and WRS, the best response was included [11]. In another study also assessing both PTA and WRS, only the response in PTA was included, since the assessment of WRS was solely provided per tumor and not per patient [24].

Table 3. Reported hearing response after treatment with bevacizumab in pediatric patients with NF2-related schwannomatosis. Only studies reporting data on hearing response are included.

Study	Hearing Improvement (Number of Patients; %)	Stable Hearing (Number of Patients; %)	Hearing Deterioration (Number of Patients; %)	Total Eligible Patients
Ardern-Holmes et al., 2021 [21]		2 (67%)	1 (33%)	3
Gugel et al., 2019 [11]		1 (100%) ***		1
Hawasli et al., 2013 [13]	1 (50%)	1 (50%)		2
Hochart et al., 2015 [14]	1 (25%)	3 (75%)		4
Nigro et al., 2020 [16]		1 (100%)		1
Plotkin et al., 2009 [8]	1 (33%)	2 (67%)		3
Plotkin et al., 2023 [24]	1 (17%) **	4 (67%) **	1 (17%) **	6
Renzi et al., 2020 [17]	8 (47%) *	9 (52%) *		17
Santoro et al., 2019 [18]		1 (100%)		1
Shepard et al., 2012 [19]	1 (50%)	1 (50%)		2
Subbiah et al., 2012 [25]		1 (100%)		1
Sverak et al., 2019 [26]	1 (33%)	1 (33%)	1 (33%)	3
Tripathi et al., 2020 [20]	1 (100%)			1
Total	15 (33%)	27 (60%)	3 (7%)	45

* = Alternate definition of hearing response PTA > 20 dB; ** = alternate definition of hearing response PTA > 12 dB; *** = extracted manually from graph.

The thirteen studies that reported on hearing outcomes comprised 45 patients. Hearing improved in 15 patients (33%), remained stable in 27 patients (60%), and worsened in 3 patients (7%).

3.6. Symptomatic Response

Symptomatic response was reported in six studies involving a total of 29 patients; however, the symptoms were not specified in the majority of these. In eight patients (28%), symptoms improved, while they remained stable in twenty-one patients (72%). Of these eight patients, one reported improved dysphagia and another reported improvement in sensory deficits and pain [21]. The remaining six patients were reported to have a mild improvement in subjective hearing and reduction in tinnitus [17]. In the 21 patients with stable symptoms, the stability was observed in different domains. Four patients were specifically described to have a stable neurological examination [13,15,16]. Eleven patients were only mentioned to have a stable clinical response, with no further details provided about the specific symptoms [17]. Six patients showed no clinically significant difference in questionnaires assessing tinnitus-related complaints (TRQs) and quality of life (NFTI-QoL) [24].

3.7. Toxicity

Toxicity was documented specifically for children in five studies comprising 28 patients. Thirteen adverse events were reported, ranging from grade 1 to grade 3 according to the Common Terminology Criteria for Adverse Events (Table 4). Two patients experienced a grade 3 adverse event (one osteomyelitis and one hypertension) and discontinued treatment because of it [14]. No other patients discontinued treatment due to toxicity. Grade 1 adverse events included chest pain, epistaxis, malaise, and a non-infectious wound complication. The grade 2 adverse events included intermenstrual bleeding, proteinuria, epistaxis, hypertension (n = 2), hypothyroidism, and secondary amenorrhea. Two studies reported no significant side effects [16,25].

Table 4. Reported toxicity of bevacizumab in pediatric patients with NF2-related schwannomatosis. Only studies reporting relevant data are included.

Study	Adverse Events (Frequency)	Grade	Consequence	Total Eligible Patients
Hawasli et al., 2013 [13]	Chest pain (1) Epistaxis (1)	1 1	None None	2
Hochart et al., 2015 [14]	Osteomyelitis (1) Intermenstrual bleeding (1) Hypertension (1) Proteinuria (1) Malaise (1) Non-infectious wound infection (1) Epistaxis (1)	3 2 3 2 1 1 2	Discontinuation of treatment None Discontinuation of treatment None None None None	7
Nigro et al., 2020 [16]	None		None	1
Renzi et al., 2020 [17]	Hypertension (2) Hypothyreoidism (1) Secondary amenorrhea (1)	2 2 2	None None None	17
Subbiah et al., 2012 [25]	None		None	1
Total	13			28

4. Discussion

This study reviews the published experience with bevacizumab treatment in children affected by NF2. While there is limited research on the efficacy of bevacizumab in adults, specific results for pediatric patients are even more scarce. This study addresses an important gap in the current literature regarding the treatment of NF2 in children, who often present with a more severe disease phenotype and limited treatment options. To date, only 62 pediatric patients receiving bevacizumab have been reported separately. There is considerable heterogeneity in the existing studies concerning the doses of bevacizumab administered, duration of treatment, and reported outcome parameters. This variability precludes a meta-analysis of the outcome of treatment on pooled data.

The therapeutic effect of bevacizumab appears to be less pronounced in children compared to adults. A 2021 meta-analysis by Shi et al. pooled data of 274 NF2 patients with 332 VS and reported tumor regression in 30% of patients [27]. A more recent systematic review by Chiranth et al., which assessed targeted therapy for VS in NF2 patients, included 10 studies with 200 patients aged 10 to 79 and found tumor regression in 38% and tumor progression in 9% of patients [28]. These results suggest that bevacizumab has a more significant effect on tumor volume in adult patients than in pediatric patients, as our review shows tumor regression in only 11% and progression in 9–22%. However, hearing outcomes appear more comparable between the age groups. Shi et al. reported a positive hearing response in 32% of patients, whereas Chiranth et al. documented hearing improvement in 45% and hearing decline in 10% of cases. Our review reveals hearing improvement in 33% of pediatric patients and a decline in 7%. This suggests that bevacizumab offers comparable hearing benefits in both children and adults. However, because of the small numbers and differences in patient characteristics, study design, and outcome parameters, comparisons between effectiveness in children and adults should be made with caution. Future studies including standardized outcome measures and larger patient cohorts will be necessary to adequately compare these patient groups. One possible explanation for the reduced effectiveness of bevacizumab on tumor progression in children may be attributed to the more progressive course of the disease in younger patients [29–31]. Another factor may be the definition of treatment success. This hypothesis is illustrated by the findings of Hochart et al. who described two patients with a persistent increase in tumor volume after bevacizumab, although the progression rate showed a substantial decrease [14]. The tumor progression rate in both patients decreased by more than threefold; for example, one patient's tumor progression rate decreased from 123% to 36%. Despite the decrease in progression rates, these tumors are still progressive and therefore labeled therapy failures, whereas the decrease in the tumor progression rate could also be considered a therapy success. This discrepancy illustrates that, when drawing conclusions from the most frequently used outcome parameters, the effect of bevacizumab might be underestimated.

Toxicity is a primary concern when considering bevacizumab treatment in children. Based on the adverse events reported in the included studies, bevacizumab appears to be reasonably well tolerated. Toxicity could be evaluated in 28 children, and whilst 13 adverse events were identified, most were mild to moderate. Only two grade 3 adverse events were found, both leading to treatment discontinuation. The incidence of severe adverse (grade 3 or 4) events in children (7%; 2 out of 28) appears lower than the rates reported in the two meta-analyses comprising predominantly adult patients (12% and 17%) [27,32]. Hypertension of all severities occurred in 11% of pediatric patients (3 out of 28), which is lower than the 29% and 33% observed in adults. Additionally, proteinuria is less common in children (4%; 1 out of 28) compared to adults (30–43%). These lower rates of adverse events may in part be attributed to the reduced presence of comorbidities in children. However, comparisons between adult and pediatric patients are hampered by the limited number of pediatric patients for which toxicities are specified, thus precluding definite conclusions.

Long-term toxicity is of particular importance in children receiving bevacizumab. While more data on long-term toxicity in this group of patients is needed, four studies in this review included treatment durations exceeding two years. Notably, 11 out of 13 reported adverse events were observed in the studies with the longest treatment durations. This observation suggests a correlation between cumulative dosage and the incidence of adverse events. A study by Slusarz et al., investigating long-term toxicity in adults, found that while overall toxicity was manageable, the cumulative dose of bevacizumab was associated with increased blood pressure [33]. Although hypertension, one of the most prevalent adverse events, was observed in 58% of patients at a median treatment duration of 34 months, it was successfully managed with medication in 39% of adult patients, and no patients required interruption in therapy. Proteinuria had an incidence of 62% in adult patients but was not associated with cumulative bevacizumab dosage. Farschtschi et al. found that by decreasing the dosage in a study of three long-term bevacizumab users, toxicity could be managed and effectiveness maintained [34]. No other studies have been published to date investigating the effects and toxicity of smaller doses than 2.5 mg/kg every 3 weeks. This could be a potential solution worth exploring, especially given the increasing number of patients requiring long-term bevacizumab treatment. This possibility is further supported by the meta-analysis conducted by Shi et al., which separately analyzed low-dose and high-dose effectiveness. The analysis confirms that high-dose regimen increases the risk of adverse events in adult patients without improving radiological or hearing response. Another possible way to manage adverse events is introducing treatment breaks, allowing for resolution of treatment toxicities in between cycles. It has been shown that bevacizumab treatment can be restarted successfully after discontinuation in NF2 patients; however, this has not yet been studied in children specifically [34,35].

The limitations of this review include the limited number of retrospective cohort studies and case series and the absence of randomized controlled trials. In addition, some studies only reported on short observation periods, precluding adequate evaluation of long-term effects and toxicities. In general, there is a lack of detailed information regarding the course of the treatment response per patient over time, including specific time points at which tumor progression or stability were assessed. It is well established that tumors may respond differently with each treatment cycle, initially causing a reduction in tumor size, followed by no effect, or vice versa [35]. Therefore, data on tumor size at multiple time points and the impact of treatment breaks would provide valuable insights into the overall response. Another limitation of the study is the heterogeneity in outcome measures across studies, which hampers comparability between studies and precludes the pooling of data. To draw clear conclusions, particularly in small populations affected by rare diseases, it is essential that study design and outcomes are reported in a standardized manner. Evaluation of the therapeutic interventions in NF2 should encompass effect on tumor size, hearing, toxicity, and symptomatic response, including vestibular symptoms. The current literature contains data on substantially more children than the 62 patients in this review; however, these outcomes are often not stratified by age. As this review shows that there may be distinct differences in the effects of bevacizumab in pediatric and adult patients, we argue that when studies include both patient subgroups, results should be presented separately.

5. Conclusions

Bevacizumab appears to be a viable treatment option for pediatric patients with NF2. Stabilization or regression of the target tumor is achieved in the majority of patients (77%), which is especially important since children often have faster growing tumors. Moreover, following treatment with bevacizumab, hearing did not further deteriorate in a remarkable 93%, and in 33%, hearing even improved. Bevacizumab appears to be relatively well tolerated, offering a non-invasive therapeutic option for children facing multiple growing tumors and hearing loss. Future research on the effects and long-term toxicity in pediatric patients is needed and should include the use of uniform treatment regimens and standardized outcome measures.

Supplementary Materials: The following supporting information can be downloaded at https://www.mdpi.com/article/10.3390/cancers17030519/s1: Table S1: Quality of evidence assessment of non-comparative cohorts and case series; Table S2: Quality of evidence assessment of case reports.

Funding: The study was financially supported by the Stichting het Heinsius-Houbolt Fonds.

Data Availability Statement: No new data were created or analyzed in this study. Data sharing is not applicable to this article.

Conflicts of Interest: The authors declare no conflicts of interest.

References

1. Evans, D.G.R.; Moran, A.; King, A.; Saeed, S.; Gurusinghe, N.; Ramsden, R. Incidence of Vestibular Schwannoma and Neurofibromatosis 2 in the North West of England over a 10-year period: Higher incidence than previously thought. *Otol. Neurotol.* **2005**, *26*, 93–97. [CrossRef] [PubMed]
2. Antinheimo, J.; Sankila, R.; Carpén, O.; Pukkala, E.; Sainio, M.; Jaaskelainen, J. Population-based analysis of sporadic and type 2 neurofibromatosis-associated meningiomas and schwannomas. *Neurology* **2000**, *54*, 71–76. [CrossRef] [PubMed]
3. Asthagiri, A.R.; Parry, D.M.; Butman, J.A.; Kim, H.J.; Tsilou, E.T.; Zhuang, Z.; Lonser, R.R. Neurofibromatosis type 2. *Lancet* **2009**, *373*, 1974–1986. [CrossRef]
4. Evans, D.G.; Trueman, L.; Wallace, A.; Collins, S.; Strachan, T. Genotype/phenotype correlations in type 2 neurofibromatosis (NF2): Evidence for more severe disease associated with truncating mutations. *J. Med. Genet.* **1998**, *35*, 450–455. [CrossRef]
5. Evans, D.; Huson, S.; Donnai, D.; Neary, W.; Blair, V.; Newton, V.; Harris, R. A clinical study of type 2 neurofibromatosis. *QJM Int. J. Med.* **1992**, *84*, 603–618. [CrossRef]
6. Ruggieri, M.; Pratico, A.D.; Serra, A.; Maiolino, L.; Cocuzza, S.; Di Mauro, P.; Licciardello, L.; Milone, P.; Privitera, G.; Belfiore, G.; et al. Childhood neurofibromatosis type 2 (NF2) and related disorders: From bench to bedside and biologically targeted therapies. *Acta Otorhinolaryngol. Ital.* **2016**, *36*, 345. [CrossRef]
7. Evans, D.G. Neurofibromatosis type 2 (NF2): A clinical and molecular review. *Orphanet J. Rare Dis.* **2009**, *4*, 16. [CrossRef]
8. Plotkin, S.R.; Stemmer-Rachamimov, A.O.; Barker, F.G., II.; Halpin, C.; Padera, T.P.; Tyrrell, A.; Sorensen, A.G.; Jain, R.K.; di Tomaso, E. Hearing improvement after bevacizumab in patients with neurofibromatosis type 2. *N. Engl. J. Med.* **2009**, *361*, 358–367. [CrossRef]
9. Ren, Y.; A Chari, D.; Vasilijic, S.; Welling, D.B.; Stankovic, K.M. New developments in neurofibromatosis type 2 and vestibular schwannoma. *Neuro-Oncol. Adv.* **2020**, *3*, vdaa153. [CrossRef]
10. Ardern-Holmes, S.; Fisher, G.; North, K. Neurofibromatosis type 2. *J. Child Neurol.* **2017**, *32*, 9–22. [CrossRef] [PubMed]
11. Gugel, I.; Kluwe, L.; Zipfel, J.; Teuber, C.; Tatagiba, M.; Mautner, V.-F.; Schuhmann, M.U.; Grimm, F. Minimal Effect of Bevacizumab Treatment on Residual Vestibular Schwannomas after Partial Resection in Young Neurofibromatosis Type 2 Patients. *Cancers* **2019**, *11*, 1862. [CrossRef]
12. Fujii, M.; Ichikawa, M.; Iwatate, K.; Bakhit, M.; Yamada, M.; Kuromi, Y.; Sato, T.; Sakuma, J.; Saito, K. Bevacizumab Therapy of Neurofibromatosis Type 2 Associated Vestibular Schwannoma in Japanese Patients. *Neurol. Med. -Chir.* **2020**, *60*, 75–82. [CrossRef] [PubMed]
13. Hawasli, A.H.; Rubin, J.B.; Tran, D.D.; Adkins, D.R.; Waheed, S.; Hullar, T.E.; Gutmann, D.H.; Evans, J.; Leonard, J.R.; Zipfel, G.J.; et al. Antiangiogenic agents for nonmalignant brain tumors. *J. Neurol. Surg. Part B Skull Base* **2013**, *74*, 136–141. [CrossRef]
14. Hochart, A.; Gaillard, V.; Baroncini, M.; André, N.; Vannier, J.-P.; Vinchon, M.; Dubrulle, F.; Lejeune, J.-P.; Vincent, C.; Nève, V.; et al. Bevacizumab decreases vestibular schwannomas growth rate in children and teenagers with neurofibromatosis type 2. *J. Neuro-Oncol.* **2015**, *124*, 229–236. [CrossRef] [PubMed]
15. Kim, B.-S.; Jung, T.-Y.; Jang, W.-Y.; Baek, H.-J.; Kim, S.-K.; Lee, K.-H. Multiple craniospinal tumors in a pediatric patient with neurofibromatosis type 2: A case report. *Child's Nerv. Syst.* **2022**, *38*, 2205–2209. [CrossRef]

16. Nigro, O.; Coppola, A.; Tartaro, T.; Tuzi, A.; Vallini, I.; Pinotti, G. Long-term therapy with Bevacizumab in a young patient affected by NF2. Stop or continue treatment? An update of a case report and review of the literature. *Anti-Cancer Drugs* **2020**, *31*, 754–757. [CrossRef] [PubMed]
17. Renzi, S.; Michaeli, O.; Salvador, H.; Alderete, D.; Ponce, N.F.; Zapotocky, M.; Hansford, J.R.; Malalasekera, V.S.; Toledano, H.; Maguire, B.; et al. Bevacizumab for NF2-associated vestibular schwannomas of childhood and adolescence. *Pediatr. Blood Cancer* **2020**, *67*, e28228. [CrossRef]
18. Santoro, C.; Palladino, F.; Bernardo, P.; Cinalli, G.; Mirone, G.; Giugliano, T.; Piluso, G.; Perrotta, S. Report on a child with neurofibromatosis type 2 and unilateral moyamoya: Further evidence of cerebral vasculopathy in NF2. *Neurol. Sci.* **2019**, *40*, 1475–1476. [CrossRef] [PubMed]
19. Shepard, T.H.; Tucci, D.L.; Grant, G.A.; Kaylie, D.M. Management of Hearing in Pediatric NF2. *Otol. Neurotol.* **2012**, *33*, 1066–1070. [CrossRef] [PubMed]
20. Tripathi, M.; Deora, H.; Kumar, N.; Batish, A.; Dutta, P.; Gurnani, J.; Mohindra, S.; Hussain Shahid, A.; Kataria, K.; Agrahari, A.; et al. Role of Bevacizumab as a prophylactic and rehabilitative treatment modality in cases of sporadic and syndromic vestibular schwannoma: Fifty shades of grey! *Interdiscip. Neurosurg. Adv. Tech. Case Manag.* **2020**, *19*, 100607. [CrossRef]
21. Ardern-Holmes, S.; White, C.; Bahure, S.; So, S.; McCowage, G.; Hovey, E.; Troon, S.; De Souza, P.; Simes, J.; Slancar, M.; et al. The Effect of Bevacizumab on Vestibular Schwannoma Related to Neurofibromatosis Type 2. *Australas. J. Neurosci.* **2021**, *31*, 5–14. [CrossRef]
22. Farschtschi, S.; Merker, V.L.; Wolf, D.; Schuhmann, M.; Blakeley, J.; Plotkin, S.R.; Hagel, C.; Mautner, V.F. Bevacizumab treatment for symptomatic spinal ependymomas in neurofibromatosis type 2. *Acta Neurol. Scand.* **2016**, *133*, 475–480. [CrossRef]
23. Morris, K.A.; Golding, J.F.; Axon, P.R.; Afridi, S.; Blesing, C.; Ferner, R.E.; Halliday, D.; Jena, R.; Pretorius, P.M.; Evans, D.G.; et al. Bevacizumab in neurofibromatosis type 2 (NF2) related vestibular schwannomas: A nationally coordinated approach to delivery and prospective evaluation. *Neuro-Oncol. Pract.* **2016**, *3*, 281–289. [CrossRef] [PubMed]
24. Plotkin, S.R.; Allen, J.; Dhall, G.; Campian, J.L.; Clapp, D.W.; Fisher, M.J.; Jain, R.K.; Tonsgard, J.; Ullrich, N.J.; Thomas, C.; et al. Multicenter, prospective, phase II study of maintenance bevacizumab for children and adults with NF2-related schwannomatosis and progressive vestibular schwannoma. *Neuro-Oncology* **2023**, *25*, 1498–1506. [CrossRef] [PubMed]
25. Subbiah, V.; Slopis, J.; Hong, D.S.; Ketonen, L.M.; Hamilton, J.; McCutcheon, I.E.; Kurzrock, R. Treatment of patients with advanced neurofibromatosis type 2 with novel molecularly targeted therapies: From bench to bedside. *J. Clin. Oncol.* **2012**, *30*, e64–e68. [CrossRef]
26. Sverak, P.; Adams, M.E.; Haines, S.J.; Levine, S.C.; Nascene, D.; Sommer, K.; Dusenbery, K.; Huang, T.C.; Moertel, C. Bevacizumab for Hearing Preservation in Neurofibromatosis Type 2: Emphasis on Patient-Reported Outcomes and Toxicities. *Otolaryngol. Head. Neck Surg.* **2019**, *160*, 526–532. [CrossRef] [PubMed]
27. Shi, J.; Lu, D.; Gu, R.; Sun, H.; Yu, L.; Pan, R.; Zhang, Y. Reliability and toxicity of bevacizumab for neurofibromatosis type 2-related vestibular schwannomas: A systematic review and meta-analysis. *Am. J. Otolaryngol.* **2021**, *42*, 103148. [CrossRef] [PubMed]
28. Chiranth, S.; Langer, S.W.; Poulsen, H.S.; Urup, T. A systematic review of targeted therapy for vestibular schwannoma in patients with *NF2*-related schwannomatosis. *Neuro-Oncol. Adv.* **2023**, *5*, vdad099. [CrossRef]
29. Picry, A.; Bonne, N.-X.; Ding, J.; Aboukais, R.; Lejeune, J.-P.; Baroncini, M.; Dubrulle, F.; Vincent, C. Long-term growth rate of vestibular schwannoma in neurofibromatosis 2: A volumetric consideration. *Laryngoscope* **2016**, *126*, 2358–2362. [CrossRef] [PubMed]
30. Li, P.; Li, S.; Wang, Y.; Zhao, F.; Wang, Z.; Wang, X.; Wang, B.; Yang, Z.; Liu, P. Clinical risk factor analysis of bilateral vestibular schwannoma's growth pattern inconsistency in individual NF2 patients. *Clin. Neurol. Neurosurg.* **2021**, *200*, 106365. [CrossRef]
31. Kang, H.; Ji, S.Y.; Hwang, K.; Kim, C.-Y.; Han, J.H. Different Growth Pattern of Vestibular Schwannomas in Neurofibromatosis Type 2 Patients According to Age. *Neuro-Oncology* **2024**, *26*, viii38. [CrossRef]
32. Lu, V.M.; Ravindran, K.; Graffeo, C.S.; Perry, A.; Van Gompel, J.J.; Daniels, D.J.; Link, M.J. Efficacy and safety of bevacizumab for vestibular schwannoma in neurofibromatosis type 2: A systematic review and meta-analysis of treatment outcomes. *J. Neuro-Oncol.* **2019**, *144*, 239–248. [CrossRef] [PubMed]
33. Slusarz, K.M.; Merker, V.L.; Muzikansky, A.; Francis, S.A.; Plotkin, S.R. Long-term toxicity of bevacizumab therapy in neurofibromatosis 2 patients. *Cancer Chemother. Pharmacol.* **2014**, *73*, 1197–1204. [CrossRef]

34. Farschtschi, S.; Kollmann, P.; Dalchow, C.; Stein, A.; Mautner, V.-F. Reduced dosage of bevacizumab in treatment of vestibular schwannomas in patients with neurofibromatosis type 2. *Eur. Arch. Otorhinolaryngol.* **2015**, *272*, 3857–3860. [CrossRef] [PubMed]
35. Douwes, J.P.J.; Hensen, E.F.; Jansen, J.C.; Gelderblom, H.; Schopman, J.E. Bevacizumab Treatment for Patients with *NF2*-Related Schwannomatosis: A Single Center Experience. *Cancers* **2024**, *16*, 1479. [CrossRef] [PubMed]

cancers

MDPI

Article

Bevacizumab Treatment for Patients with *NF2*-Related Schwannomatosis: A Single Center Experience

Jules P. J. Douwes [1,*], Erik F. Hensen [1], Jeroen C. Jansen [1], Hans Gelderblom [2] and Josefine E. Schopman [2]

[1] Department of Otorhinolaryngology–Head and Neck Surgery, Leiden University Medical Center, 2333 ZA Leiden, The Netherlands; e.f.hensen@lumc.nl (E.F.H.); j.c.jansen@lumc.nl (J.C.J.)

[2] Department of Medical Oncology, Leiden University Medical Center, 2333 ZA Leiden, The Netherlands; a.j.gelderblom@lumc.nl (H.G.); j.e.schopman@lumc.nl (J.E.S.)

* Correspondence: j.p.j.douwes@lumc.nl

Simple Summary: In this study, we explored the use of bevacizumab as a treatment for *NF2*-related schwannomatosis, a condition characterized by the development of schwannomas on both vestibulocochlear nerves. This study revealed that the majority of patients experienced either improved or preserved hearing and effective control of the targeted vestibular schwannoma with bevacizumab. However, common adverse events included hypertension and fatigue, and severe adverse events led to treatment discontinuation in a quarter of the patients. Thus, while bevacizumab demonstrates positive effects on hearing, tumor control, and symptomatology in *NF2*-related schwannomatosis, careful consideration of potential side effects is crucial.

Abstract: (1) Background: *NF2*-related schwannomatosis, characterized by the development of bilateral vestibular schwannomas, often necessitates varied treatment approaches. Bevacizumab, though widely utilized, demonstrates variable effectiveness on hearing and tumor growth. At the same time, (serious) adverse events have been frequently reported. (2) Methods: A single center retrospective study was conducted, on *NF2*-related schwannomatosis patients treated with bevacizumab from 2013 to 2023, with the aim to assess treatment-related and clinical outcomes. Outcomes of interest comprised hearing, radiologic response, symptoms, and adverse events. (3) Results: Seventeen patients received 7.5 mg/kg bevacizumab for 7.1 months. Following treatment, 40% of the patients experienced hearing improvement, 53%, stable hearing, and 7%, hearing loss. Vestibular schwannoma regression occurred in 31%, and 69% remained stable. Further symptomatic improvement was reported by 41%, stable symptoms by 47%, and worsened symptoms by 12%. Treatment discontinuation due to adverse events was observed in 29% of cases. Hypertension (82%) and fatigue (29%) were most frequently reported, with no occurrences of grade 4/5 toxicities. (4) Conclusion: Supporting previous studies, bevacizumab demonstrated positive effects on hearing, tumor control, and symptoms in *NF2*-related schwannomatosis, albeit with common adverse events. Therefore, careful consideration of an appropriate management strategy is warranted.

Keywords: acoustic neuroma; adverse events; bevacizumab; cerebellopontine angle tumor; hearing; neurofibromatosis type 2; schwannomatosis; tumor response; vestibular schwannoma

1. Introduction

NF2-related schwannomatosis (NF2) is a rare autosomal dominant tumor predisposition syndrome caused by mutations in the NF2 tumor suppressor gene located on chromosome 22. The disease is characterized by the development of bilateral vestibular schwannomas, along with other schwannomas, meningiomas, and ependymomas, in the central and peripheral nervous system [1,2]. The clinical presentation of NF2 is highly variable. While the associated vestibular schwannomas are benign and usually slow growing, they may lead to symptoms such as hearing loss, tinnitus, and vestibular complaints.

Without appropriate intervention, the progression of vestibular schwannomas can result in severe cranial nerve deficits, intracranial hypertension, and brainstem compression [2,3].

Most current treatment paradigms for NF2-related vestibular schwannomas consider (micro)surgery, radiotherapy, and pharmacotherapeutic treatment with bevacizumab [4–6]. Microsurgery generally achieves satisfactory tumor mass reduction; however, tumor recurrence and hearing loss occur in half of the cases [7]. Radiotherapy offers good tumor control in most NF2 patients but frequently results in hearing loss and other cranial nerve deficits [7,8]. Moreover, the inherent tumor susceptibility of NF2 patients has been linked to a 6% increased risk of malignant transformation or new tumor growth on the irradiated tissues [9].

Bevacizumab, a monoclonal antibody, acts to inhibit vascular endothelial growth factor (VEGF) expressed in tumors like vestibular schwannomas [10,11]. Bevacizumab has demonstrated the ability to halt or reverse nervous system tumor progression, particularly in schwannomas. In addition, previous studies have reported improvements in objective and subjective hearing, tinnitus, balance problems, and overall quality of life with bevacizumab treatment [10–18]. Bevacizumab has therefore become a widespread treatment for NF2-related schwannomas. Even so, the efficacy and durability of its therapeutic effects can vary between schwannomas and between patients. At the same time, side effects of bevacizumab, including hypertension, proteinuria, and several blood disorders, are frequently reported [18,19]. There is still no international consensus about the optimal treatment dosage, frequency, and duration. Even now that patents have expired, bevacizumab remains an expensive treatment and creates a burden on healthcare costs.

Variable treatment regimens and clinical outcomes, frequent side effects, and cost of bevacizumab treatment were reasons to conduct a retrospective analysis on the clinical effectiveness and adverse effects of bevacizumab treatment for vestibular schwannoma in NF2 patients in our institution.

2. Materials and Methods

2.1. Participants and Study Design

The present study included NF2 patients eligible for medical treatment with bevacizumab at Leiden University Medical Center (LUMC), a tertiary NF2 referral center in Leiden, The Netherlands, between 1 January 2013 and 31 October 2023. Inclusion criteria comprised a patient age ≥18 years, a confirmed diagnosis of NF2 [20], administration of at least one dose of bevacizumab, and written informed consent. Exclusion criteria comprised insufficient demographic or clinical data.

Following informed consent, we conducted a retrospective, single center, non-blinded data-analysis using electronic patient charts to explore demographics, treatment regimens, and clinical characteristics. A highly secure online database was set up for data storage and analysis. The study protocol was approved by the institutional review board and conducted in full compliance with the ethical standard of the 2013 Declaration of Helsinki.

2.2. Treatment Protocol and Outcomes

As per standard-of-care in The Netherlands, 7.5 mg/kg bevacizumab was intravenously administered every three weeks for at least six months or until there was a clinically relevant event, as judged by the treating oncologist and/or NF2 multidisciplinary team. At any time point, treatment with bevacizumab could be discontinued or modified at the discretion of the treating specialist or in accordance with patient preference. Likewise, bevacizumab treatment could be restarted if signs or symptoms required reintervention after a prolonged period of discontinuation.

Hematologic and urinary evaluations were performed prior to the start of bevacizumab treatment and repeated regularly until treatment was discontinued. Vital functions were taken at every admission for bevacizumab treatment. Toxicity was recorded at every visit at the outpatient clinic while treatment was ongoing. In case of an adverse event, this was recorded in the patient chart and reported to the treating specialist. Action was taken if deemed medically necessary and likewise recorded in the patient chart. All adverse events were classified according to the Common Terminology Criteria for Adverse Events (CTCAE), version 5.0 [21].

2.3. Clinical Assessment

Demographic characteristics included vital status, sex, age at the time of NF2 diagnosis, and age at the initiation of treatment. Clinical outcomes of interest comprised the treatment history associated with NF2 and vestibular schwannoma, diagnostic NF2 criteria [20], tumor burden and localization, family history of NF2, vestibulocochlear manifestations (hearing, tinnitus, vertigo, and/or imbalance), cranial nerve functionality, and peripheral neurology. Clinical evaluations were conducted at four distinct timepoints: upon initial presentation after referral, at the patient visit preceding start of bevacizumab treatment, at the conclusion of bevacizumab treatment, and at most recent patient visit during the extended follow-up period. In the event a patient underwent surgery or radiotherapy due to NF2-related disease progression, the last patient visit prior to re-intervention was deemed the termination point for follow-up after bevacizumab treatment.

The primary outcome of interest was hearing at the side of the target tumor at the end of bevacizumab treatment. Hearing was examined with pure tone audiometry (PTA) and the word recognition score (WRS). The PTA was measured as average hearing threshold at 0.5, 1, 2, and 3 kilo Hertz [22,23]. Hearing was defined as improved ($\geq$10% increase in WRS), stable (no significant change in WRS), or worsened ($\geq$10% decrease in WRS) in relation to hearing at the start of bevacizumab treatment. In case of 100% WRS at both times of measurement, a $\geq$10 decibel (dB) change in average PTA was considered significant. Secondary audiological outcomes of interest included subjective hearing and presence of tinnitus.

As NF2 patients often suffer from other symptoms than those related to the vestibular schwannomas, overall neurological symptoms were assessed to evaluate disease burden due to NF2-related lesions. We report subjectively improved, stable, or worsened overall symptoms related to NF2. Symptoms were divided in functioning of the trigeminal nerve, the facial nerve, and other cranial nerves (excluding the vestibulocochlear nerve) and peripheral neurology. Facial nerve function was graded according to the House Brackmann scale (HB) [24]. Other cranial nerves functions and peripheral neuropathy were collected using patient records.

2.4. Radiological Assessment

Radiological evaluations were limited to vestibular schwannomas. Target tumor characteristics were evaluated using routine clinical thin-slice ($\leq$1.5 mm) gadolinium-enhanced T1-weighted Magnetic Resonance Images (MRIs) of the cerebellopontine angle [25,26]. The primary outcome of interest was radiologic response of the target vestibular schwannoma, defined as improved ($\geq$20% decrease in extrameatal tumor volume), stable (no significant change in extrameatal tumor volume, $>-20\%$ to $<20\%$), or worsened ($\geq$20% increase in extrameatal tumor volume) at the end of bevacizumab treatment [25,27]. Secondary outcomes of interest were extrameatal tumor volume (cm^3) and tumor growth rate. Tumor volume and growth rate were calculated using the largest linear dimensions in three planes (anterior–posterior; medial–lateral; cranial–caudal) from consecutive MRI scans [28–30]. Other intracranial lesions were not evaluated.

Similar to the clinical assessment, four standardized timepoints were used to assess radiologic characteristics of the target tumor: upon initial presentation after referral, at imaging preceding start of bevacizumab treatment, at the conclusion of bevacizumab treatment, and at most recent imaging during radiological surveillance after treatment.

2.5. Statistical Analysis

For statistical analyses, IBM SPSS Statistics for Windows (version 27.0. Armond, NY, USA: IBM Corp) was used. Median, range, frequency count, and percentage were used to report on non-normally distributed data. Standard descriptive statistics were used to describe patient and treatment characteristics. Missing, unused, and incorrect data were documented in the data collection and study report.

3. Results

3.1. Patient Characteristics

Seventeen patients were included in the present analysis. Demographics, treatment history, and disease characteristics are listed in Table 1. The median age was 39.1 (16.5–67.3) years at time of diagnosis and 48.1 (22.9–70.7) years at the start of initial bevacizumab treatment. Prior to bevacizumab therapy, two patients underwent partial surgical resection of the target vestibular schwannoma. Three patients received radiotherapy prior to bevacizumab but none of these on the tumor of interest. No patient was under treatment with bevacizumab at the time of data collection.

Table 1. Demographics and disease characteristics of *NF2*-related schwannomatosis patient cohort.

Patient Characteristics		**Patients, *n* = 17**
Alive, *n* (%)		16 (94.1)
Age, years, median (range)	Time of diagnosis	39.1 (16.5–67.3)
	Start of treatment	48.1 (22.9–70.7)
Female, *n* (%)		9 female (52.9)
Family history of NF2, *n* (%)		2 (11.8)
Previous treatment, yes, *n* (%)	Total	11 (64.7)
	Surgical resection	10 (58.8)
	Target vestibular schwannoma	2 (11.8)
	Non-target tumor(s)	10 (58.8)
	Radiotherapy	3 (17.6)
	Target vestibular schwannoma	0 (0.0)
	Non-target tumor(s)	3 (17.6)
NF2 classification, *n* (%) [1]	Class 1	15 (88.2)
	Class 2	0 (0.0)
	Class 3	2 (11.8)
Tumor localization, *n* (%)	Unilateral vestibular schwannoma	2 (11.8)
	Bilateral vestibular schwannoma	15 (88.2)
	Non-vestibular schwannoma	12 (70.6)
	Central nervous system	12 (70.6)
	Peripheral nervous system	3 (17.6)
Total tumor count, median (range)		12 (2–40)

[1] According to the updated diagnostic criteria [20]. Legend: *n* = number of patients; NF2 = *NF2*-related schwannomatosis.

Four patients were excluded from the study for the following reasons: Three patients received bevacizumab at a different institute, and their data were incomplete. One patient passed away shortly after treatment was started, so follow-up data were not available. The cause of death in this case was unrelated to bevacizumab treatment.

3.2. Bevacizumab Treatment

Bevacizumab treatment was started a median of 57.5 (13.3–311.7) months after first presentation. Patients received a median dose of 7.5 (5.6–7.5) mg/kg every 3 (3.0–4.4) weeks. The duration of bevacizumab treatment ranged from 2.1 to 23.9 months, with a median of 7.1 months. The primary reason for bevacizumab therapy was progressive hearing loss in the majority of cases (59%). Other indications included symptoms related to other NF2-related schwannomas (35%) and target tumor size (6%).

Three patients deviated from the standard-of-care protocol. In two patients, bevacizumab dose was lowered to a maintenance dosage (orange bar, Figure 1). Patient 7 received a lower dosage of 5.0 mg/kg every 4 weeks for 2.9 months, while patient 12 received a dosage of 7.5 mg/kg every 6 weeks for 6.7 months. Patient 14 skipped one injection after 12 months to allow for a minor surgical intervention.

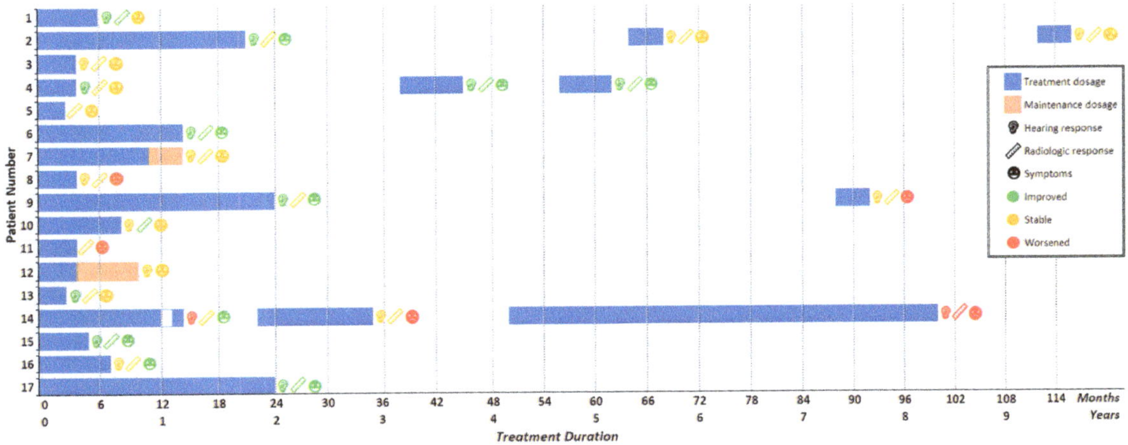

Figure 1. Treatment regimens and response of individual patients in the cohort. Duration and dosage of treatment is indicated by bar length and coloring, respectively. At the end of each treatment course, hearing, radiologic, and symptomatic response were recorded. Symbols indicate the outcome of interest, coloring indicates an improved, stable, or worsened response. Four patients received more than one bevacizumab treatment course. Time interval between consecutive treatments corresponds to the white area between the horizontal bars.

The most common reason to stop treatment was the achievement of the treatment goal(s): radiologic tumor stability or regression (29%), radiologic tumor stability or regression plus stable or improved hearing (24%), and improved symptoms (6%). Adverse events were the second most common reason to discontinue treatment (29%), and response failure was less frequently reported (6%). A single patient (6%) preferred to stop treatment despite the physician's advice to continue.

For six patients, the end of treatment coincided with the last available patient visit. The eleven patients remaining were followed up after treatment for a median of 29.2 (2.7–52.4) months. After an extended time period, bevacizumab was reintroduced in four patients (Figure 1). Three patients also received bevacizumab a third time. Time between consecutive treatment courses varied from 7 to 64 months. Reasons to reintroduce bevacizumab were hearing loss ($n = 2$, 50%), vestibular complaints ($n = 1$, 25%), and tumor progression of other NF2-related schwannomas ($n = 1$, 25%).

3.3. Adverse Events

Out of seventeen patients, sixteen patients (94%) experienced at least one adverse event. One patient (6%) reported no treatment-related sequelae. A total of 50 adverse events were reported: 31 of grade 1 (62%), 17 of grade 2 (34%), and 2 of grade 3 (4%). Grade 4 toxicities or treatment-related deaths did not occur. The most commonly reported adverse events were hypertension (82%) and fatigue (29%). Five of fourteen patients with hypertension (36%) required antihypertensive medication during active treatment. An overview of all adverse events is shown in Table 2.

Table 2. Adverse events and laboratory abnormalities during treatment with bevacizumab, graded according to Common Terminology Criteria for Adverse Events (version 5.0) [21].

Adverse Event [1]	Patients, *n* (%)	Grade 1, *n* (%)	Grade 2, *n* (%)	Grade 3, *n* (%)
Total	16 (94.1)	13 (76.5)	12 (70.6)	2 (11.8)
Hypertension	14 (82.4)	3 (17.6)	9 (52.9)	2 (11.8)
Fatigue	5 (29.4)	5 (29.4)		
Elevated liver enzymes	3 (17.6)	3 (17.6)		
Diarrhea	2 (11.8)	2 (11.8)		
Dry skin	2 (11.8)	2 (11.8)		
Epistaxis	2 (11.8)	2 (11.8)		
Headache	2 (11.8)	1 (5.9)	1 (5.9)	
Hyperkalemia	2 (11.8)	1 (5.9)	1 (5.9)	
Impaired wound healing	2 (11.8)	2 (11.8)		
Infection	2 (11.8)	2 (11.8)		
Irregular menses [2]	2 (22.2)	1 (11.1)	1 (11.1)	
Myalgia	2 (11.8)	2 (11.8)		
Nausea	2 (11.8)	1 (5.9)	1 (5.9)	
Allergic dermatologic reaction	1 (5.9)	1 (5.9)		
Dysphonia	1 (5.9)	1 (5.9)		
Edema of limbs	1 (5.9)		1 (5.9)	
Erectile dysfunction	1 (5.9)	1 (5.9)		
Hyperglycemia	1 (5.9)	1 (5.9)		
Proteinuria	1 (5.9)		1 (5.9)	
Thrombocytopenia	1 (5.9)	1 (5.9)		
Vertigo	1 (5.9)		1 (5.9)	

[1] Number of patients and percentages taken from entire cohort. [2] Based on total of female patients ($n = 9$). Legend: n = number.

Treatment was discontinued (29%) due to an allergic dermatologic reaction after injection ($n = 1$), vertigo after injection ($n = 1$), edema of the limbs ($n = 1$), and a cluster of complications ($n = 2$). Patient 9 stopped bevacizumab after 24 months due to delayed medication-related adverse events. The majority of patients who had to stop bevacizumab (patients 4, 5, 11, and 13) experienced serious adverse events shortly after starting treatment.

All four individuals subjected to multiple courses of bevacizumab experienced more than one adverse event. During the second and third treatment courses, a total of 30 adverse events were documented: 21 classified as grade 1 (70%), 8 as grade 2 (27%), and 1 as grade 3 (3%). As observed in patients receiving only one course, the most common adverse event was hypertension. No instances of more severe toxicities were observed after multiple courses of bevacizumab.

3.4. Hearing Response

Between first presentation and the start of bevacizumab treatment, two patients experienced total hearing loss due to surgical resection of the target tumor. Consequently, hearing assessment in the target ear was feasible for fifteen of seventeen patients (Figures 1 and 2). Three patients (patients 2, 9, and 12) already had maximum speech recognition at the start of treatment.

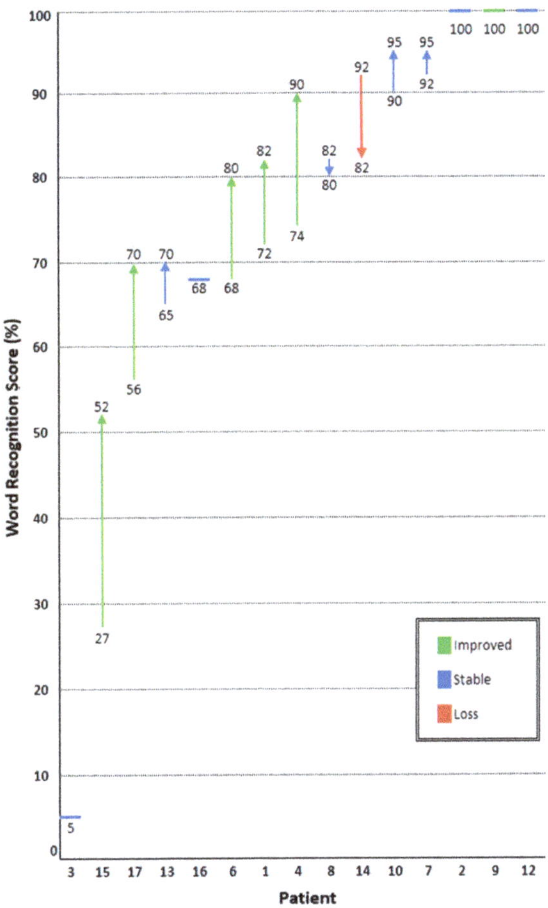

Figure 2. Change in maximum word recognition score (WRS) after treatment with bevacizumab. Patients are represented on the horizontal axis. Individual WRS before and after bevacizumab are stated above and below the arrows. Percentage change in WRS is represented by the length of the arrow, with the direction representing hearing improvement or loss. Six patients (40%) experienced improved hearing, eight patients (53%) had stable hearing, and one patient (7%) experienced hearing loss. Three patients (patients 2, 9, and 12) already had maximum speech recognition at the start of treatment.

Improved hearing was detected in six of fifteen patients (40%), eight patients (53%) had stable hearing, and one patient (7%) experienced hearing loss. At the start of treatment, the median WRS was 74% (5–100) and PTA 57 (10–100) dB. After treatment, the median WRS improved to 82% (5–100), and the PTA slightly increased to 61 (10–88) dB. For patients 1, 4, 6, 15, and 17, the WRS increased ≥10%, but the PTA remained stable (>−10 dB to <10 dB). In patients 9 and 13, a stable WRS was reported, while the PTA improved from 41 to 21 dB and 100 to 73 dB, respectively. As patient 9 already had maximum speech recognition, hearing was regarded as improved based on the PTA. Both the WRS and PTA remained stable after treatment in patients 2, 3, 7, 8, 10, 12, and 16. Patient 14 experienced hearing loss, with a WRS of −10% and an increased PTA from 60 to 67 dB.

Audiometric follow-up after treatment discontinuation was available for eleven patients, with a median follow-up of 7.4 (2.7–63.3) months. Stable hearing was observed in nine of eleven patients (82%), while two patients (18%) experienced hearing loss. These two patients and two others underwent a second course of bevacizumab. Following the second treatment course, one patient experienced hearing improvement and three patients had stable hearing. Hearing loss during surveillance after the second treatment course prompted three patients to resume bevacizumab treatment for a third time. In two of three patients hearing stabilized, while in the third patient, hearing loss progressed.

3.5. Radiologic Response

One patient was excluded as only repeated Computed Tomography (CT) images were available. Radiologic tumor response could therefore be evaluated in sixteen patients (Table 3) (Figures 1 and 3). Two patients had a partial resection of the target vestibular schwannoma before treatment with bevacizumab. Their tumor characteristics prior to bevacizumab were disregarded, but the radiologic responses of the tumor residue following bevacizumab treatment were included.

Table 3. Radiological characteristics of the target vestibular schwannomas before, during, and after treatment with bevacizumab.

Radiologic Characteristics		n =
First presentation		16
Extrameatal extension, n (%)	13 (81.3)	
Extrameatal volume, cm^3, median (range)	2.07 (0.09–24.45)	
Start of bevacizumab treatment		16
Extrameatal extension, n (%)	14 (87.5)	
Extrameatal volume, cm^3, median (range)	1.24 (0.05–12.67)	
Relative change, % (range)	43 (−61–816)	
End of bevacizumab treatment		16
Extrameatal extension, n (%)	13 (81.3)	
Extrameatal volume, cm^3, median (range)	1.15 (0.0 [1]–10.52)	
Relative change, % (range)	−12 (−100 [1]–6)	
Most recent radiologic surveillance		12
Extrameatal extension, n (%)	11 (91.7)	
Extrameatal volume, cm^3, median (range)	1.52 (0.03–8.25)	
Relative change, % (range)	27 (−22–275)	

[1] Full regression of extracanicular tumor component. Legend: n = number of patients, max. = maximum, cm = centimeters.

Five patients (31%) showed extrameatal tumor regression, while eleven (69%) showed a stable tumor. No patient experienced tumor progression ($\geq$20%) on active treatment. Median extrameatal tumor volume shrunk from 1.24 (0.06–12.67) cubic centimeters (cm^3) at the start of treatment to 1.15 (0.0–10.52) cm^3 after treatment. At the start of treatment, extrameatal tumor growth was 43% (−61~+816) overall or 15% (−5~+150) annually (median follow-up 55.9 months; 16.2–218.5). During treatment, tumor growth lowered to −12% (−100~+6) overall or −13% (−161~+5) annually (median follow-up 12.6 months; 4.3–28.8).

Data on radiologic surveillance after bevacizumab were available in twelve patients (median follow-up 19.3 months; 4.0–52.4). Continued tumor regression was detected in one patient (9%), four patients (36%) had stable target tumors, and six patients (55%) showed tumor progression.

After the second course of bevacizumab, one patient experienced tumor regression, while three patients had stable tumors. One vestibular schwannoma remained stable for at least 10.6 months. This patient did not receive another course of bevacizumab. The other three patients received a third reintroduction of bevacizumab. In between the second and third treatment course, all patients experienced tumor progression. During the third course of bevacizumab, tumor regression, stabilization, and growth were observed in one patient each.

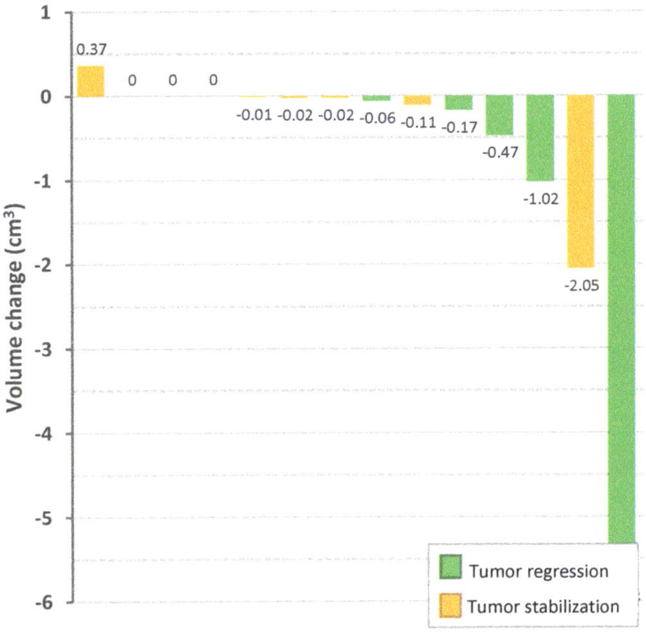

Figure 3. Change in absolute extracanicular volume (cm^3) of vestibular schwannomas after bevacizumab treatment. Vertical bars represent the target vestibular schwannoma of a patient. Coloring of the bars indicate the corresponding tumor response: green for tumor regression (volume change $\geq$20%), yellow for stable tumor (volume change between -20% and 20%). Three target vestibular schwannomas are not shown: one tumor was confined to the internal auditory canal, two other tumors were not followed up with MRI at the end of treatment.

3.6. Symptomatic Response

Symptoms could be evaluated in all seventeen patients (Figure 1). At the start of treatment, all patients ($n = 17$, 100%) reported vestibulocochlear complaints: sixteen patients (94%) experienced hearing loss, fourteen patients (82%) reported tinnitus, and ten patients (59%) suffered from imbalance. Paresis of the facial nerve was present in six patients (35%). Of these, three patients experienced a mild paresis (HB3; 50%), one patient a severe paresis (HB5; 17%), and two a total paralysis (HB6; 33%). Neuropathy of the trigeminal nerve and other cranial nerves was present in four (24%) and six (35%) patients, respectively. Seven patients (41%) experienced peripheral neuropathy.

Following treatment with bevacizumab, seven patients (41%) experienced an improvement of symptoms, eight patients (47%) maintained stable symptoms, and two patients (12%) experienced a deterioration in symptoms. Improved symptoms included hearing ($n = 5$), tinnitus ($n = 1$), balance ($n = 2$), vision ($n = 2$), and/or peripheral nerve functioning ($n = 2$). One patient reported a new tingling sensation of the hand but also reported improved hearing and vision and was therefore categorized as an overall improvement of symptoms. Similarly, another patient experienced increased unsteadiness but likewise demonstrated improved hearing and vision and was consequently considered to have experienced an overall improvement. Both patients who reported symptomatic deterioration experienced greater imbalance.

Clinical surveillance after discontinuation of bevacizumab was available in eleven patients, with a median time of 29.2 (2.7–52.4) months. After treatment was stopped, no patient experienced further improvement of symptoms, three patients (27%) experienced stable symptoms, and eight (73%) had increased symptomatology. All four patients that received a second or third treatment course had experienced worsened symptoms after initial treatment discontinuation. Following the second treatment course, one patient experienced symptom improvement, one experienced stable symptoms, and two patients experienced worsened symptoms. Three patients, one with stable symptoms and two with worsened symptoms, received a third course of bevacizumab. Thereafter, symptoms improved in one patient, remained stable in one, and worsened in another.

4. Discussion

An overall positive response to bevacizumab was found in the present cohort of NF2 patients, using a treatment regimen of 7.5 mg/kg bevacizumab every three weeks. Notably, hearing preservation was observed in 93% of the patients (improved in 40%; stable in 53%). Similar responses were found for tumor size, as 31% of the target tumors exhibited regression, and 69% remained stable. In addition, NF2-related symptoms improved in 88% of the patients.

Comparable findings were reported in a recent systematic review including 200 NF2 patients treated with bevacizumab [18]. The pooled data in the study indicated hearing improvement in 45% and stabilization in 55% of the patients. Moreover, tumor regression was observed in 38%, while stabilization occurred in 53% of the patients. It is important to note, however, that the present cohort differed from the pooled population in the systematic review. In our study, a higher median age and a shorter treatment duration were found. Additionally, the systematic review included two studies focused on pediatric patients, which was beyond the scope of the present study. On the other hand, a greater variability in dosage regimens was reported in the systematic review. A multicenter, prospective study of 22 NF2 patients (15 adult; 7 pediatric) also evaluated the efficacy and toxicity of bevacizumab for vestibular schwannoma at a higher dosage (10 mg/kg every two weeks for six months) [31]. In the study, hearing improved in 41% of the patients. Tumor regression was observed in 32%.

In our study cohort, adverse events, particularly hypertension (82%) and fatigue (29%), were frequently observed. The incidence of hypertension was higher than in previous studies (33–58%) [18,19,31,32]. A possible explanation may be the higher median age in our cohort and differences in dosage regimens between studies, as both factors have been found to be predictors of developing hypertension during bevacizumab treatment [19]. The frequency of measuring blood pressure during treatment may also account for differences between studies. Even so, grade 3 hypertension was infrequent (12% of patients) and aligned with the rates reported in other studies [11,15,19,33].

Fatigue stands out as a frequently documented complication arising from the administration of bevacizumab. The incidence in our study (29%) was comparable to the previously reported incidence (23–64%) [11,15,19,31,33].

The prevalence of proteinuria was relatively low in the present cohort. It was observed in only 6% of the patients during the initial treatment with bevacizumab. Other studies have reported higher rates (43–62%) [18,19]. It has been hypothesized that proteinuria is a late complication of bevacizumab treatment, with intervals between start of treatment and proteinuria onset of 10.7 to 23.7 months [19,32]. The lower rate of proteinuria in our study may therefore be explained by the shorter treatment duration of 7.1 months. An alternative explanation could be differences in execution of urinalysis. In our institute, the evaluation of proteinuria during treatment with bevacizumab was performed at variable time intervals.

Early termination of bevacizumab treatment occurred in 29% of patients in the present study, which falls within the upper range of dropout rates observed in other studies (9–28%) [11,13,15,33]. The notable rate of treatment discontinuation underscores that bevacizumab is not well-tolerated by a significant number of patients. The nature of toxicity leading to treatment discontinuation varies across studies and appears to be highly patient-specific. Notably, the way in which treatment toxicities are reported is diverse and often lacks standardization, with the Common Terminology Criteria for Adverse Events (CTCAE) being a frequently employed classification system [21]. However, the use of other national or international guidelines further complicates the comparison of adverse event rates between studies. Careful monitoring of adverse effects, according to a standardized format, should remain a relevant treatment parameter in future studies on bevacizumab for NF2 patients.

In the present study, only two patients were partly treated with bevacizumab under a maintenance regimen. Both patients showed a stable response despite the variation from the standard treatment protocol. In a small case series, patients restarted bevacizumab at a reduced dosage (2.5 mg/kg every two weeks), resulting in stable hearing and tumor size during the maintenance phase, though limited data were available [34]. Other studies have also used a maintenance regimen to enable long-term treatment of NF2 patients that showed a stable clinical response, but an optimal dosage threshold remains to be determined [15,31,35].

Limited data exist on NF2 patients resuming bevacizumab after an initial course, and the available literature mainly addresses treatment breaks due to factors such as toxicity, surgical interventions, or patient preference, with most breaks lasting only a few months. Insight into the within-subject variability of bevacizumab efficacy and toxicity after extended treatment gaps is scant. Extended breaks ($\geq$3 months) have been associated with tumor (re)growth and hearing decline, consistent with our findings [15,33,34]. We found notable variability in the response after reintroduction of bevacizumab, encompassing both between-subject and within-subject differences in efficacy and toxicity during consecutive treatment courses (Figure 1). As with other associated symptoms, hearing may restabilize or improve after the restart of bevacizumab therapy, but further progression is also observed. The same holds true for tumor progression. This implies that successful restart of bevacizumab is feasible if symptoms or tumor progression recur after prolonged treatment stops; however, previous positive effects do not reliably predict future treatment success.

The present study has several strengths. Firstly, the data analysis provides an extensive longitudinal examination of NF2 patients receiving bevacizumab. This study extends beyond assessing the efficacy and toxicity of bevacizumab during active initial treatment, incorporating a clinical analysis of NF2 patients from their initial presentation at the expert center through the first administration of bevacizumab, spanning over 4.8 years. Post treatment, patients continued to be monitored for a median duration of 2.5 years. Secondly, in addition to audiometric and radiologic follow-up, symptoms were included in the analysis. Thirdly, this study also assessed the effect of sequential courses of bevacizumab in patients that resumed treatment after extended treatment gaps.

Study limitations include the retrospective design and the small sample size, inherent to the rarity of this disease. This is illustrated by a recent systematic review on this topic, in which only 10 patient cohorts totaling 200 patients could be identified, with a median number of 16.5 included patients per cohort.

Tumor volume measurements were calculated using three linear dimensions. These are therefore an estimate of the actual tumor volumes. Additionally, variations in the timing of follow-up measurements for hearing, radiology, and symptoms among patients introduce variability. This makes it difficult to draw conclusions about the timing and durability of the response after treatment. In the present study, four general timepoints were used to assess outcome measurements, yet the clinic's follow-up regimen has evolved over time. Nowadays, our patients are followed up every six months.

The management of NF2 remains challenging, despite successful therapeutic interventions. Bevacizumab provides an effective alternative to surgery or radiotherapy for vestibular schwannoma and related symptoms. However, its effect on target tumors is variable. Moreover, different bevacizumab regimens and surveillance protocols are used across institutes, and the effect of dosage on reported efficacy and toxicity remains uncertain. It appears that lower dosages of bevacizumab result in a similar treatment efficacy compared to higher dosages, while toxicity may be less substantial [18]. This study identified an overall positive response to 7.5 mg/kg bevacizumab every three weeks, consistent with these findings [18]. Nevertheless, adverse effects were common, and a quarter of all NF2 patients eligible for bevacizumab discontinued treatment prematurely due to toxicity. Therefore, we carefully suggest an updated treatment dosage of 7.5 mg/kg every three weeks for three months, followed by a maintenance dosage of 5 mg/kg every four weeks for three months.

Limited attention is still given to the overall disease burden and patient-reported outcomes. While hearing and tumor volumetrics are paramount, symptoms related to NF2-related tumors and quality of life in relation to different management options are often overlooked. Given the chronic and progressive nature of NF2, patients often undergo multiple and repeated interventions over time. While some respond favorably to multiple courses of bevacizumab, the response is not universal. Both tumor and clinical responses show noticeable between-subject and within-subject variability. Predicting the response to bevacizumab treatment would be valuable for developing a more effective and personalized treatment plan. Future studies in a multicenter, randomized format with larger cohorts would be ideal to evaluate the effectiveness of different treatment regimens and gain insight into factors that predict the outcome. Still, these may remain elusive due to the rarity of the disease and the inherent complexities of study design and execution. Reporting experiences with large case series such as these will therefore continue to be important in furthering our understanding of the disease and the treatment.

5. Conclusions

The majority of *NF2*-related schwannomatosis patients treated with bevacizumab had an overall positive therapeutic response. After treatment, all target vestibular schwannomas showed tumor stabilization or regression, and the large majority of patients experienced improvement or stabilization of hearing and other NF2-related symptoms. However, adverse events were common, and a quarter of all patients treated with bevacizumab discontinued treatment prematurely due to toxicity. Therefore, careful consideration of treatment benefits and risks is warranted to provide patients with an appropriate management strategy.

Author Contributions: Conceptualization, J.P.J.D., E.F.H. and J.E.S.; methodology, J.P.J.D., E.F.H. and J.E.S.; validation, J.P.J.D.; formal analysis, J.P.J.D.; investigation, J.P.J.D.; resources, J.P.J.D., E.F.H., J.C.J., H.G. and J.E.S.; data curation, J.P.J.D.; writing—original draft preparation, J.P.J.D.; writing—review and editing, J.P.J.D., E.F.H., J.C.J., H.G. and J.E.S.; visualization, J.P.J.D.; supervision, E.F.H., J.C.J. and J.E.S.; project administration, J.P.J.D. All authors have read and agreed to the published version of the manuscript.

Funding: This research received no external funding.

Institutional Review Board Statement: The study was conducted in accordance with the Declaration of Helsinki, and approved by the Institutional Review Board of Leiden University Medical Center (nWMODIV2_2023028, 14 September 2023).

Informed Consent Statement: Informed consent was obtained from all subjects involved in the study.

Data Availability Statement: The data presented in this study are available on request from the corresponding author. The data are not publicly available due to privacy restrictions.

Conflicts of Interest: The authors declare no conflicts of interest.

References

1. Evans, D. Chapter 5—Neurofibromatosis type 2. In *Neurocutaneous Syndromes*; Islam, M.P., Roach, E.S., Eds.; Elsevier: Amsterdam, The Netherlands, 2015; Volume 132, pp. 87–96.
2. Asthagiri, A.R.; Parry, D.M.; Butman, J.A.; Kim, H.J.; Tsilou, E.T.; Zhuang, Z.; Lonser, R.R. Neurofibromatosis type 2. *Lancet* **2009**, *373*, 1974–1986. [CrossRef]
3. Evans, D.; Huson, S.; Donnai, D.; Neary, W.; Blair, V.; Newton, V.; Harris, R. A Clinical Study of Type 2 Neurofibromatosis. *QJM Int. J. Med.* **1992**, *84*, 603–618. [CrossRef]
4. Evans, D. Neurofibromatosis type 2 (NF2): A clinical and molecular review. *Orphanet J. Rare Dis.* **2009**, *4*, 16. [CrossRef]
5. Blakeley, J.O.; Evans, D.G.; Adler, J.; Brackmann, D.; Chen, R.; Ferner, R.E.; Hanemann, C.O.; Harris, G.; Huson, S.M.; Jacob, A.; et al. Consensus recommendations for current treatments and accelerating clinical trials for patients with neurofibromatosis type 2. *Am. J. Med. Genet. A* **2012**, *158A*, 24–41. [CrossRef]

6. Goldbrunner, R.; Weller, M.; Regis, J.; Lund-Johansen, M.; Stavrinou, P.; Reuss, D.; Evans, D.G.; Lefranc, F.; Sallabanda, K.; Falini, A.; et al. EANO guideline on the diagnosis and treatment of vestibular schwannoma. *Neuro Oncol.* **2020**, *22*, 31–45. [CrossRef]
7. Maniakas, A.; Saliba, I. Neurofibromatosis Type 2 Vestibular Schwannoma Treatment: A Review of the Literature, Trends, and Outcomes. *Otol. Neurotol.* **2014**, *35*, 889–894. [CrossRef]
8. Tosi, U.; Maayan, O.; An, A.; Lavieri, M.E.T.; Guadix, S.W.; DeRosa, A.P.; Christos, P.J.; Pannullo, S.; Stieg, P.E.; Brandmaier, A.; et al. Stereotactic radiosurgery for vestibular schwannomas in neurofibromatosis type 2 patients: A systematic review and meta-analysis. *J. Neurooncol.* **2022**, *156*, 431–441. [CrossRef]
9. Evans, D.; Halliday, D.; Obholzer, R.; Afridi, S.; Forde, C.; Rutherford, S.A.; Hammerbeck-Ward, C.; Lloyd, S.K.; Freeman, S.M.; Pathmanaban, O.N.; et al. Radiation treatment of benign tumors in NF2-related-schwannomatosis: A national study of 266 irradiated patients showing a significant increase in malignancy/malignant progression. *Neuro-Oncol. Adv.* **2023**, *5*, vdad025. [CrossRef]
10. Plotkin, S.R.; Stemmer-Rachamimov, A.O.; Barker, F.G.; Halpin, C.; Padera, T.P.; Tyrrell, A.; Sorensen, A.G.; Jain, R.K.; di Tomaso, E. Hearing Improvement after Bevacizumab in Patients with Neurofibromatosis Type 2. *N. Engl. J. Med.* **2009**, *361*, 358–367. [CrossRef]
11. Blakeley, J.O.; Ye, X.; Duda, D.G.; Halpin, C.F.; Bergner, A.L.; Muzikansky, A.; Merker, V.L.; Gerstner, E.R.; Fayad, L.M.; Ahlawat, S.; et al. Efficacy and Biomarker Study of Bevacizumab for Hearing Loss Resulting From Neurofibromatosis Type 2–Associated Vestibular Schwannomas. *J. Clin. Oncol.* **2016**, *34*, 1669–1675. [CrossRef]
12. Sponghini, A.P.; Platini, F.; Rondonotti, D.; Soffietti, R. Bevacizumab Treatment for Vestibular Schwannoma in a Patient with Neurofibromatosis Type 2: Hearing Improvement and Tumor Shrinkage. *Tumori J.* **2015**, *101*, e167–e170. [CrossRef] [PubMed]
13. Hochart, A.; Gaillard, V.; Baroncini, M.; André, N.; Vannier, J.-P.; Vinchon, M.; Dubrulle, F.; Lejeune, J.-P.; Vincent, C.; Nève, V.; et al. Bevacizumab decreases vestibular schwannomas growth rate in children and teenagers with neurofibromatosis type 2. *J. Neurooncol.* **2015**, *124*, 229–236. [CrossRef] [PubMed]
14. Alanin, M.C.; Klausen, C.; Caye-Thomasen, P.; Thomsen, C.; Fugleholm, K.; Poulsgaard, L.; Lassen, U.; Mau-Sorensen, M.; Hofland, K.F. The effect of bevacizumab on vestibular schwannoma tumour size and hearing in patients with neurofibromatosis type 2. *Eur. Arch. Otorhinolaryngol.* **2015**, *272*, 3627–3633. [CrossRef]
15. Morris, K.A.; Golding, J.F.; Axon, P.R.; Afridi, S.; Blesing, C.; Ferner, R.E.; Halliday, D.; Jena, R.; Pretorius, P.M.; UK NF2 Research Group; et al. Bevacizumab in neurofibromatosis type 2 (NF2) related vestibular schwannomas: A nationally coordinated approach to delivery and prospective evaluation. *Neuro-Oncol. Pract.* **2016**, *3*, 281–289. [CrossRef] [PubMed]
16. Huang, V.; Bergner, A.L.; Halpin, C.; Merker, V.L.; Sheridan, M.R.; Widemann, B.C.; Blakeley, J.O.; Plotkin, S.R. Improvement in Patient-reported Hearing After Treatment With Bevacizumab in People With Neurofibromatosis Type 2. *Otol. Neurotol.* **2018**, *39*, 632–638. [CrossRef]
17. Sverak, P.; Adams, M.E.; Haines, S.J.; Levine, S.C.; Nascene, D.; Sommer, K.; Dusenbery, K.; Huang, T.C.; Moertel, C. Bevacizumab for Hearing Preservation in Neurofibromatosis Type 2: Emphasis on Patient-Reported Outcomes and Toxicities. *Otolaryngol.—Head Neck Surg.* **2019**, *160*, 526–532. [CrossRef]
18. Chiranth, S.; Langer, S.W.; Poulsen, H.S.; Urup, T. A systematic review of targeted therapy for vestibular schwannoma in patients with NF2-related schwannomatosis. *Neurooncol Adv.* **2023**, *5*, vdad099. [CrossRef]
19. Morris, K.A.; Golding, J.F.; Blesing, C.; Evans, D.G.; Ferner, R.E.; Foweraker, K.; Halliday, D.; Jena, R.; McBain, C.; McCabe, M.G.; et al. Toxicity profile of bevacizumab in the UK Neurofibromatosis type 2 cohort. *J. Neurooncol.* **2017**, *131*, 117–124. [CrossRef]
20. Plotkin, S.R.; Messiaen, L.; Legius, E.; Pancza, P.; Avery, R.A.; Blakeley, J.O.; Babovic-Vuksanovic, D.; Ferner, R.; Fisher, M.J.; Friedman, J.M.; et al. Updated diagnostic criteria and nomenclature for neurofibromatosis type 2 and schwannomatosis: An international consensus recommendation. *Genet. Med.* **2022**, *24*, 1967–1977. [CrossRef]
21. US Department of Health and Human Services. *Common Terminology Criteria for Adverse Events (CTCAE)*; US Department of Health and Human Services: Washington, DC, USA, 2017.
22. Gardner, G.; Robertson, J.H. Hearing Preservation in Unilateral Acoustic Neuroma Surgery. *Ann. Otol. Rhinol. Laryngol.* **1988**, *97*, 55–66. [CrossRef]
23. Committee on Hearing and Equilibrium Guidelines for the Evaluation of Hearing Preservation in Acoustic Neuroma (Vestibular Schwannoma): Committee on Hearing and Equilibrium. *Otolaryngol. Head Neck Surg.* **1995**, *113*, 179–180. [CrossRef] [PubMed]
24. House, J.W.; Brackmann, D.E. Facial Nerve Grading System. *Otolaryngol. Head Neck Surg.* **1985**, *93*, 146–147. [CrossRef] [PubMed]
25. Dombi, E.; Ardern-Holmes, S.L.; Babovic-Vuksanovic, D.; Barker, F.G.; Connor, S.; Evans, D.G.; Fisher, M.J.; Goutagny, S.; Harris, G.J.; Jaramillo, D.; et al. Recommendations for imaging tumor response in neurofibromatosis clinical trials. *Neurology* **2013**, *81*, S33–S40. [CrossRef]
26. Carlson, M.L.; Link, M.J. Vestibular Schwannomas. *N. Engl. J. Med.* **2021**, *384*, 1335–1348. [CrossRef]
27. Plotkin, S.R.; Halpin, C.; Blakeley, J.O.; Slattery, W.H.; Welling, D.B.; Chang, S.M.; Loeffler, J.S.; Harris, G.J.; Sorensen, A.G.; McKenna, M.J.; et al. Suggested response criteria for phase II antitumor drug studies for neurofibromatosis type 2 related vestibular schwannoma. *J. Neurooncol.* **2009**, *93*, 61–77. [CrossRef] [PubMed]
28. Dunn, I.F.; Bi, W.L.; Mukundan, S.; Delman, B.N.; Parish, J.; Atkins, T.; Asher, A.L.; Olson, J.J. Congress of Neurological Surgeons Systematic Review and Evidence-Based Guidelines on the Role of Imaging in the Diagnosis and Management of Patients With Vestibular Schwannomas. *Neurosurgery* **2018**, *82*, E32–E34. [CrossRef] [PubMed]

29. Kanzaki, J.; Tos, M.; Sanna, M.; Moffat, D.A. New and Modified Reporting Systems from the Consensus Meeting on Systems for Reporting Results in Vestibular Schwannoma. *Otol. Neurotol.* **2003**, *24*, 642–649. [CrossRef]
30. Charabi, S.; Thomsen, J.; Mantoni, M.; Charabi, B.; Bjarne, J.R.; Sven Erik, B.R.; Gyldensted, C.; Tos, M. Acoustic Neuroma (Vestibular Schwannoma): Growth and Surgical and Nonsurgical Consequences of the Wait-And-See Policy. *Otolaryngol.—Head Neck Surg.* **1995**, *113*, 5–14. [CrossRef]
31. Plotkin, S.R.; Duda, D.G.; Muzikansky, A.; Allen, J.; Blakeley, J.; Rosser, T.; Campian, J.L.; Clapp, D.W.; Fisher, M.J.; Tonsgard, J.; et al. Multicenter, Prospective, Phase II and Biomarker Study of High-Dose Bevacizumab as Induction Therapy in Patients With Neurofibromatosis Type 2 and Progressive Vestibular Schwannoma. *J. Clin. Oncol.* **2019**, *37*, 3446–3454. [CrossRef]
32. Slusarz, K.M.; Merker, V.L.; Muzikansky, A.; Francis, S.A.; Plotkin, S.R. Long-term toxicity of bevacizumab therapy in neurofibromatosis 2 patients. *Cancer Chemother. Pharmacol.* **2014**, *73*, 1197–1204. [CrossRef]
33. Plotkin, S.R.; Merker, V.L.; Halpin, C.; Jennings, D.; McKenna, M.J.; Harris, G.J.; Barker, F.G.I. Bevacizumab for Progressive Vestibular Schwannoma in Neurofibromatosis Type 2: A Retrospective Review of 31 Patients. *Otol. Neurotol.* **2012**, *33*, 1046–1052. [CrossRef] [PubMed]
34. Farschtschi, S.; Kollmann, P.; Dalchow, C.; Stein, A.; Mautner, V.-F. Reduced dosage of bevacizumab in treatment of vestibular schwannomas in patients with neurofibromatosis type 2. *Eur. Arch. Otorhinolaryngol.* **2015**, *272*, 3857–3860. [CrossRef] [PubMed]
35. Killeen, D.E.; Klesse, L.; Tolisano, A.M.; Hunter, J.B.; Kutz, J.W., Jr. Long-Term Effects of Bevacizumab on Vestibular Schwannoma Volume in Neurofibromatosis Type 2 Patients. *J. Neurol. Surg B Skull Base* **2019**, *80*, 540–546. [CrossRef] [PubMed]

MDPI AG
Grosspeteranlage 5
4052 Basel
Switzerland
Tel.: +41 61 683 77 34

Cancers Editorial Office
E-mail: cancers@mdpi.com
www.mdpi.com/journal/cancers

www.ingramcontent.com/pod-product-compliance
Lightning Source LLC
Chambersburg PA
CBHW061624210926
51850CB00009B/2423
* 9 7 8 3 7 2 5 8 7 1 9 8 8 *